PRACTICAL PATHOLOGY INFORMATICS

Demystifying informatics for the practicing anatomic pathologist

John H. Sinard, MD, PhD

Director, Pathology Informatics Program
Department of Pathology
Yale University School of Medicine
New Haven, CT

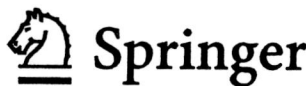 Springer

John H. Sinard, MD, PhD
Director, Pathology Informatics Program
Department of Pathology
Yale University School of Medicine
New Haven, CT
USA

Library of Congress Cataloging-in-Publication Data

Sinard, John H.
  Practical pathology informatics : demystifying informatics for the practicing anatomic
pathologist / John H. Sinard.
      p. ; cm.
  Includes bibliographical references and index.
  ISBN-13: 978-0-387-28057-8 (alk. paper)
  ISBN-10: 0-387-28057-X (alk. paper)
    1. Pathology. 2. Medical informatics. 3. Anatomy, Pathological. I. Title.
    [DNLM: 1. Medical Informatics—methods. 2. Pathology—methods. QZ 26.5 S615p 2005]
    RB25.S52 2005
    65.5'04261—dc22   2005050011

ISBN -10 0-387-28057-X   e-ISBN 0-387-28058-8
ISBN -13 978-0-387-28057-8   e-ISBN 978-0-387-28058-5
Printed on acid-free paper.

Printed in the United States of America.

9 8 7 6 5 4 3 2 1   SPIN 11013969

springeronline.com

PRACTICAL PATHOLOGY INFORMATICS

This book is dedicated to my nieces and nephews:

Thomas, Rebecca, Claire, and Andrew

Contributing Author

(Chapter 11):

Michael Krauthammer, MD, PhD
Department of Pathology
Yale University School of Medicine
New Haven, CT

Preface

Almost all areas of intellectual pursuit in which there is an element of subjectivity share an interesting internal paradox. At first exposure, the field is a complete mystery. Then, as one acquires some of the domain knowledge and learns about the rules, the field starts to make sense, and before long may even seem trivial. However, as one delves deeper and acquires experience, complexities and subtleties begin to re-emerge, as well as realization of the validity of some of the exceptions to the rules, and the field is suddenly less obvious and clear than it was before. This is the value of experience; this is where true insight starts to emerge. Informatics shares this internal paradox. When I peruse the books available on informatics, it is this insight which I am seeking. The details of the data I can look up on the internet, but the insight is harder to find, and only comes from having developed and implemented (or at least tried to implement) various solutions. It would be absurd to suggest that any one solution, no matter how successful in a particular environment, will work well in every other environment, and I personally question the insight of any author who claims that a particular solution to an information management problem is the <u>one</u> right solution. Of course, insight can only be presented in the context of information. This book is a mixture of information, interpretation, perspective, and, I would like to think, a little insight.

When I lecture or give a conference to pathology residents about gross, autopsy, or ophthalmic pathology, I have a pretty good idea going in what level of knowledge I can expect from my audience, from the first year residents up through the fellows. Lecturing on informatics topics, however, is more difficult, not because the material is any more esoteric, but rather because the range of knowledge of my audience can be enormous: some have already designed and deployed complete computer-based solutions to some problem, while others still approach the keyboard and mouse with some degree of apprehension. The target audience for this book is equally broad. Designed around the curriculum I developed for teaching informatics to pathology residents, the goal of this book is to introduce and demystify a variety of topics in the broad discipline of pathology informatics. In no way have I attempted to cover the entire scope of this discipline, but rather have focused on issues of particular relevance to the practicing anatomic pathologist. It is not my intention to turn anyone into an informatician (?informaticist?). Rather, I hope to provide the reader with enough information about the pros and cons of various elements of the field, and to share some insight into their complexity, so that the reader will be able to evaluate the topic in an educated fashion. It is up to the reader to weigh the competing factors presented and then, tempered with an understanding of their own unique environment, to make an individualized assessment as to the best approach from the perspective of their needs.

Toward that end, what follows are multiple relatively short chapters, each introducing and discussing some aspect of pathology informatics. The scope, in my opinion, represents the fund of knowledge with which a typical practicing pathologist should be familiar. In fact, the early chapters contain basic information about computers and databases which is applicable to any discipline, with the later chapters containing more anatomic pathology specific topics. The scope of this text would also be an appropriate core for residency training in pathology informatics. In an attempt to appeal to a broader audience, I have included both basic as well as some less basic information. Since I have always felt that it is better to understand something than to simply memorize it, the detail provided is sufficient for the reader to obtain an understanding of the topic being presented. I have also included, where appropriate, my views of the pros and cons behind the more controversial aspects of each topic. For the most part, I present information and analysis (although I must confess that the first and last chapters are really more like editorials). The chapters can be read in any order. Each chapter is divided into several short sections. If at any point a section drifts into the "too obscure", simply go on to the next section. Throughout the discussions, I will not recommend specific vendors or products, but rather focus on general principles and processes which will remain applicable as the vendors and products come and go. If each reader takes away at least a different perspective on the breath of pathology informatics, its role as a tool in the daily practice of pathology, and an appreciation for how informatics will be key in shaping the way we practice medicine in the future, I will consider my efforts in writing this book worth while.

Acknowledgments

First, I would like to thank my informal consultants, the members of the operational informatics unit of Yale Pathology, for helping to create an environment which allowed me to pursue my interests in this area, as well as for working hard enough to give me the time to write this book. These include Agatha Daley, Peter Gershkovich, Katie Henderson, János Löbb, Brian Paquin, Sophia Gyory, Emma Walz-Vaitkus, and Mark Mattie. Secondly, I want to thank the residents of the Anatomic Pathology Residency Training Program at Yale-New Haven Hospital for giving me a forum to "try out" some of my material, and for consistently reminding me of the importance of informatics training for our future pathologists. In particular, thanks to Yuri Fedoriw, my first "informatics rotation" resident, for input and suggestions which helped me get through some of the more difficult parts of this book. Similarly, thanks to Wally Henricks for helpful comments on a portion of this book, and Jon Morrow for many discussions on the future of pathology informatics. Finally, I want to thank the anonymous person who, on their evaluation of the first presentation of my informatics short course at the United States and Canadian Academy of Pathology annual meeting, wrote simply "when are you going to write your book?"

Copyrights and Trademarks

This book contains some specific examples, and as such must refer to products either copyrighted or trademarked (registered or otherwise) by various manufacturers. Reference to these products is for educational purposes only, and is in no way intended to represent advertisement, endorsement, or any claim of intellectual property on my part. The owners of these trademarks are acknowledged here rather than throughout the text.

Netscape Communications Corporation: Netscape
The Open Group: UNIX
Oracle Corporation: Oracle
Radio Corporation of America: RCA
Robotic Vision Systems, Inc: DataMatrix (placed in public domain)
Scan Disk Corporation: CompactFlash
Sony, Inc.: iLink
Sun Microsystems, Inc.: Java, JavaScript
Sybase, Inc.: Sybase, Adaptive Server, PowerBuilder
Syquest Technology, Inc.: Syquest
Twentieth Century Fox and Matt Groening: the Simpsons
Linus Torvalds: Linux
Unicode, Inc.: Unicode
University of Illinois: Eudora (licensed to Qualcomm Inc.)
University of Manchester, UK: GALEN
Walt Disney Corporation: Donald Duck, Mickey Mouse
Warner Brothers and J.K. Rowling: Harry Potter, Dudley Dursley
Western Digital, Inc.: EIDE, IDE
Wi-Fi Alliance (formerly Wireless Ethernet Compatibility Alliance, Inc.): WiFi
World Wide Web Consortium, Massachusetts Institute of Technology: HTML, XML

Contents

Contributing Author..vii

Preface...ix

Acknowledgments..xi

Copyrights and Trademarks..xiii

1. The Scope of Pathology Informatics 1

Pathology Informatics: What is it?... 1

"Why do I need to know about Pathology Informatics?"..................... 5

The Spectra of Pathology Informatics 6

    Is informatics science or engineering?..8

    Is informatics an "academic" activity? 9

Pathology Informatics as a Subspecialty 13

    Implications for pathology training programs...............................15

Selected References 16

2. Desktop Computers: Hardware.. 19

What's in the box?... 19

    Integrated vs Modular Design 20

    Data Storage in a Computer...21

    Computer Memory Chips 23

Basic Components of a Desktop Computer....................................... 26

    Processor..26

    Main Computer Memory 30

    Video Display Controller..31

    Input/Output Devices 34

    Network Connection 45

Computer Specifications.. 49

3. Desktop Computers: Software.. 51

Executable Software.. 51

    Operating Systems 52

    Operating System Add-ons...53

Application Software 55
Non-Executable Software 65
    Digital Data Representation..66
    Non-Executable (Data) File Formats 76

4. Networking and the Internet... 83
    Network Topologies...84
        Star Network...84
        Ring Network 85
        Bus Network 86
    Communication on a Network...87
        Network Protocols..88
        Bandwidth...89
        Network Communication Logic 91
        Network Interconnectivity Devices.....................................98
    The Internet...102
        A Brief History of the Internet 103
        TCP/IP..105
        The World Wide Web 111
        Electronic Mail 115

5. Databases 121
    Database Terminology 122
    Database Architecture 124
        Single Table Databases...124
        Multi-table Databases 127
        Relational Databases...131
        Entity-Attribute-Value Data Models...................................139
    Database Management Systems 140
        Application Access to Databases 141
        Database Abstraction 144
        Capabilities of a "Full-Featured" DBMS 145
    SQL – A Database "Language"...161
        The SELECT Statement...163
        Processing SQL Statements...165
        SQL Access to Database from Computer Programs.............166

6. Pathology LIS: Relationship to Institutional Systems...........173
    Medical Intranets..173
    Distributing Application Functionality to Desktops 176
        Mainframe Systems...176
        Client-Server Systems (Distributed Processing) 179
        Thin-Client Technology...181

Philosophical Spectra of Information System Management 183
    Enterprise vs Specialty Solution 185
    Off-the-Shelf Software vs Custom-Built Software.................... 187
    Institutional vs Departmental Management................................ 188
Electronic Medical Record Systems 189
    A Resurgence of Interest... 190
    Some Issues of Data Centralization Unique to Health Care.... 192
    Models for "Centralized" Data Storage and Access 195
    Obstacles to the Adoption of an Electronic Medical Record System...... 199
    Anatomic Pathology Outreach Services: A unique EMR Problem 205

7. Evaluating Anatomic Pathology Information Systems 207
General Principles 207
    Workflow... 207
    Traps and Pitfalls.. 209
Evaluating Informatics Activities in Anatomic Pathology................ 211
    Categories of Information Technology Impact 211
    Traditional Features of Anatomic Pathology Information Systems........212
    Newer "High Technology" Features... 215
    Informatics Activities Not Integrated into LISs....................... 227
Data Recovery from Legacy Information Systems............................ 228
    Custom Conversion Programming... 229
    An Alternative Approach.. 231

8. Digital Imaging in Anatomic Pathology 233
Digital Imaging vs. Traditional Photography 234
Basic Digital Imaging Concepts and Terminology........................... 236
    Digital Image Specifications 236
    Storing Images in Files 242
Elements of a Digital Imaging System 245
    Image Acquisition 246
    Image Storage.. 246
    Image Utilization... 247
Practical Aspects of Clinical Imaging for Pathology......................... 248
    Image Utilization... 248
    Image Acquisition 254
    Image Storage.. 257
Complete Clinical Imaging Solutions... 258
    Integrated Imaging 258
    Modular Imaging: "Yale Pathology Solution".......................... 261

9. Video Microscopy and Telemicroscopy...................................265
Video Microscopy Technology 266

Video Cameras 266
Video Signals..268
Video Cables and Connectors 269
Digital Video 271
Video Microscopy for Pathology Conference Rooms............................273
Telemicroscopy Systems 276
Telemicroscopy Technology 276
Uses for Telemicroscopy 279
Wide-field digital microscopy and the future of pathology 281

10. Electronic Interfaces and Data Exchange 287
Architecture of an Interface..287
Communication Handler...288
Interface (Translation) Processor 289
Interface "Languages" 289
Common Interfaces for Pathology Information Systems 293
Admission/Discharge/Transfer (ADT) Interface 293
Billing Batch Interface...296
Results Interface...297

11. Case Identification by Diagnosis...............................303
Evolution of Coding and Information Retrieval 304
The Terminology for Terminologies...305
Coding Systems used in Anatomic Pathology.......................................310
Current Procedural Terminology (CPT)..310
International Classification of Diseases (ICD)..311
Systematized Nomenclature of Medicine (SNOMED)..........................314
Unified Medical Language System (UMLS) 316
Information Retrieval and Natural Language Processing..................316
Keyword-based information retrieval...317
Natural Language Processing..319
NLP-assisted information retrieval 323

12. External Regulations Pertinent to LIS Management...........325
Health Insurance Portability and Accountability Act 325
Background: Privacy, Confidentiality, and Security 327
History, Elements, and Implementation of HIPAA 328
General Provisions 330
Electronic Transactions and Code Sets..331
Privacy Regulations 332
Security Regulations 337
National Identifiers...340
College of American Pathologists' Checklists....................................342

American College of Surgeons...346
Clinical Laboratory Improvement Amendments of 1988..................348
Clinical and Laboratory Standards Institute 350

13. Pathology Informatics and the Future of Medicine 355
A Look Ahead Into the Future...355
Forces Reshaping Medicine..356
Two Views of the Future 358
Building a Path – Making a Future 361
Whole-slide Imaging...362
Create Pathology Informatics Programs...362
Pathology and Computerized Patient Records 364
New Information Systems Structured for Outcomes Research...............368
Pathology Informatics and Biomedical Research 372
"Basic" Informatics Research...374
Summary and Conclusions 379
Index...381

Chapter 1

THE SCOPE OF PATHOLOGY INFORMATICS

Pathology Informatics: What is it?

Pathology informatics is a term which has been in use for several years, and one might think that the author of a book entitled "Practical Pathology Informatics" must know what informatics is if he is writing a book about it. Unfortunately, defining this term is not as uncontroversial as one might think. We'll get back to this in a moment. For the time being, lets simply define it as the application of informatics to the pathology domain. That's pretty safe. What, then, is informatics?

For many, "informatics" means simply anything that has to do with computers. Unfortunately, this emphasizes the tools of the discipline rather than what those tools are used for. Molecular biologists use gels and bacteria as tools to explore the structure and function of DNA, yet no one would define molecular biology as "anything to do with bacteria." Informatics, in its purest sense, is the study of how data is acquired, stored, processed, retrieved, analyzed, and presented, in such a way as to turn data into information. Notice that I have not used the word "computer" in the definition. The field could just have easily existed a hundred years ago, before computers in the conventional sense were in use anywhere. What has changed since then, however, is not so much the invention of the computer, but rather the explosion of data available at all levels, and the drive to maximize the use of that data. The sheer volume of data has forced us to rethink and formalize how we attempt to deal with that volume, and this has led to the development of new processes and new tools for information management. Non-electronic manipulation or storage of that information is impractical, and thus the computer becomes an indispensable tool for the discipline of informatics. The data itself is fundamental to the practice of informatics. In contrast to computer science where the emphasis is, in fact, on developing better generic tools, independent of the content, in informatics, the content is crucial.

The practice of informatics is a process (Figure 1-1), which includes reducing and redefining complex problems, formulating models to solve those problems, developing information systems based on those models, deploying those solutions, and ultimately assessing the impact and redesigning the model and systems accordingly. In many ways, informaticians serve as brokers between biomedical professionals, computer

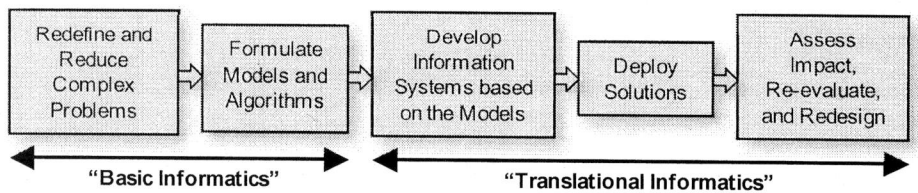

Figure 1-1: The informatics process. Informatics is a tool/process by which complex problems are analyzed and reduced to algorithms, and then information system-based solutions are developed and deployed. The first steps constitute "basic informatics" while the latter steps make up "translational" or applied informatics.

scientists, and end users. Informatics requires a thorough understanding of the "domain" and assimilation of many disparate skill sets, including considerable familiarity with computers, creative problem solving skills, and engineering capabilities. The design of user interfaces even involves elements of sociology. But in addition to drawing from many disciplines, the informatics process is also deeply integrated into them.

Is informatics, then, a field unto itself (my spell-checker keeps suggesting that it is not a real word), or is it simply a process? Can it exist without well defined boundaries? It has been said that "medical informaticians obviously enjoy discussing the existence of their field and reflecting upon it" (Haux, R.; Methods Inf Med 2002; 41:31-5), and there is certainly plenty of literature to support this claim. The value of the informatics process is certainly not in question. Where the controversy arises is in defining the core principles that underlie all of the sub-fields of informatics, and in delineating the scope and boundaries, if any, of the discipline.

Let's address the issue of scope. What is included when one uses the term "informatics", or one of its major subdivisions such as "medical informatics", "bioinformatics", or "clinical informatics"? The term "medical informatics" is not consistently used. For some, it is a larger grouping, which includes bioinformatics. For others, it is a separate discipline, disjoint in scope from bioinformatics. To distinguish between these uses, the term "biomedical informatics" has sprung up, clearly intending to join bioinformatics and medical informatics into one coherent group. Likewise, "clinical informatics" is often used to contrast itself from bioinformatics.

Bioinformatics is perhaps the best defined sub-division of informatics. Bioinformatics is the study of how information is stored in biological systems, from the molecular to the macromolecular level. A large part of the focus has been on DNA, RNA, and protein sequences. The advent of microarray technology and advances in modeling molecular structures had resulted in a tremendous explosion in the popularity of bioinformatics. Processing such large data sets requires, in addition to consideration of the data/information contained within them, significant mathematical and computational power, and therefore the term computational biology has become almost inseparably linked to bioinformatics. Bioinformatics and computational biology is a flourishing field in academic institutions, and significant funding is being funneled to support research in this discipline.

Clinical informatics is less well defined, largely because the associated domain, medicine, is so vast, and so unlike other fields of science. The information structure of medicine is incredibly complex, with layers upon layers of data, building upon itself and spanning from the molecular level to whole organisms. The methodologies in medicine are different from the cleaner "basic" sciences, in that experiments can't be easily designed, and many of the variables are not even known, let alone controllable. Most observations in medicine are the result of an intricate interaction between many different causes, and modification of even a single element has repercussions across multiple systems. As such, clinical data tends to be

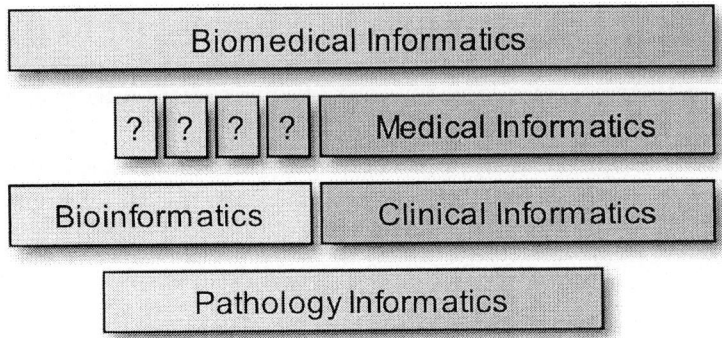

Figure 1-2: Overlapping spectra of informatics disciplines. Pathology informatics combines elements of both "clinical informatics" and the more basic science oriented "bioinformatics".

more inconsistent and subjective. In a sense, bioinformatics is "simpler" than clinical informatics because the data is more objective and the rules are better understood, making more rigorous computational approaches possible. However, the separation between clinical informatics and bioinformatics is beginning to become less distinct. As diseases become understood at a molecular level, underlying genotypic differences are influencing diagnostic and treatment decisions. While molecular diagnosis and pharmacogenomics are bridging the gap between basic science and clinical medicine, gene expression arrays on patient samples, proteomics, and mining of treatment outcomes data is reuniting bioinformatics and clinical informatics into the broader discipline of biomedical informatics.

So where is pathology informatics in all of this? All large pathology departments are already quite familiar with dichotomies, and at academic institutions the "peaceful" coexistence of research and clinical missions within a pathology department is commonplace. Not surprisingly, therefore, the scope of pathology informatics similarly runs the gamut from basic bioinformatics (e.g. microarray analysis) to clinical systems development and support (e.g. synoptic reporting). In addition to these two dimensions, however, the subfield of pathology informatics takes on yet another dimension, and that is knowledge of and familiarity with the instruments and equipment used to collect, communicate, and distribute the information which we manage. In this dimension, the dividing line between "pathology informatics" and "technical support" blurs, but the reality is that designing, developing, evaluating, and using instruments which collect data requires understanding what that data means, and therefore falls well within the scope of pathology informatics. In laboratory medicine (technically "clinical pathology", which is an unfortunate term since anatomic pathology is also quite clinical), numerous instruments are used on a daily basis. Most are automated, and certainly a detailed understanding of the design, robotics, and mechanics can be separated from informatics. The data stream emanating from these machines, however, cannot, since these feed into information systems, often via some sort of intermediate interface, and those information systems have to understand the data: not only its format, but other issues such as accuracy, precision, and reliability. Fewer instruments exist in anatomic pathology, but anatomic pathology is a heavily image-based discipline, and thus the growing need to acquire, analyze, and transmit images has folded an understanding of image acquisition devices, both analog and digital, into the scope of pathology informatics. In addition, although it has always been a good idea for a practicing anatomic pathologist to have a basic understanding of the theory behind microscopy, the ability to image an entire glass slide (virtual microscopy) has even pushed elements of optics into the scope of pathology informatics. Thus, the field of pathology informatics is quite large, and the rapid development of molecular pathology promises to expand the scope of pathology informatics even more.

"Why do I need to know about Pathology Informatics?"

Pathologists like to do pathology – that's why we're pathologists. In general, we would rather not worry too much about non-pathology matters – billing, specimen tracking, coding. These are things we recognize as important (at some level), but would often just prefer that someone or something else take care of them. To the extent to which computer systems can help us do the things we don't want to do, we happily embrace them (in contrast, pathologists are more reluctant to adopt computer systems which try to do what we like to do, namely make diagnoses). The original pathology information systems were generally written by pathologists – after all, we are the ones who know what we want them to do and how we want them to do it. When it works, we are all too happy to let the computers handle the details of the day-to-day activities like specimen tracking and workflow management. The more the computer does well, the more we ask it to do. Freed from these non-medical details, we can devote more time to making diagnoses, and take on larger workloads. Before long, we become dependent upon the computers to do their part, because we no longer have the time to do what they do. Then the computer needs to be upgraded. We don't have the time to adapt the computer programs to a new operating system, so we hire programmers and other IT (information technology) people to do that. They do a good job, but they are not pathologists, and their implementation of a solution might achieve the same end result, but in a slightly different way. Rather than hassle with trying to understand why it is different, we just change, perhaps ever so slightly, how <u>we</u> do things, to fit better with how the computer does them. The more complex the computer tasks get, the more we are willing to let other people solve those problems. Over time, and after many small changes, we come to realize that now the computer is telling us how to do what we do. But there is now such a separation between the people who know the pathology and the people who know the pathology information systems that it often seems as if they don't even speak the same language anymore.

There is no *a priori* reason why pathologists have to abdicate all responsibility for their information systems; it's just easier. There is a lot of ground between knowing everything about information systems and knowing nothing. A basic knowledge of fundamental concepts will allow pathologists to not only better employ the tools which we use on a daily basis, but also to make more informed decisions about how these tools are deployed and used in their practices. Pathology informatics is not a passing trend, because the amount of data pathologists are expected to assimilate is only going to continue to increase. It is the need to collect and manage that data that has driven the growth of pathology informatics as a discipline in its own right. This is not a prediction – it has already happened. In a very real sense, pathologists need to get on board, or they will be left behind.

The Spectra of Pathology Informatics

Regardless of what the dictionaries, journal articles, or textbooks might say, words are really defined by how they are used, and the term "informatics" is no exception. How the term is best defined for any given person at any given institution is likely to vary based on the interests of that person and the needs of that institution. Therefore, no two pathology informatics programs are likely to be exactly the same. I don't believe in the concept that some programs are doing "real" informatics while others are not. It's all informatics. In much the same way that chocolate ice cream and strawberry ice cream are both ice cream, there are a number of flavors of pathology informatics programs, and no one is fundamentally better than any other, assuming they each meet the needs of their institution, department and program faculty.

Members of pathology departments are already quite familiar with spectra, and exploring the vast grey areas which exist between the two extremes of an apparent dichotomy is part of our daily lives. Pathology informatics is no different. At one end of the dichotomy are general core principles such as ontology definitions, systems modeling, problem solving methodologies, and artificial intelligence. These can be termed "basic informatics." I would like to propose using the term "translational informatics" to refer to the rest of the spectrum. At the far end are more practical service related issues such as clinical information systems management, desktop computer support, and digital camera selection. In between are issues such as decision support, workflow management, organizational learning, and knowledge management tools. Where in the spectrum between underlying core concepts and technical support services is the "right" place for pathology informatics to be?

Many informaticians argue that the technical support services, what are often referred to as "Information Technology Services" or ITS, should be segregated from informatics proper. Is this really practical? Is this equivalent to trying to separate a surgeon's technical skills in the operating room from his/her patient management skills, which clearly can't be done, or is it more like separating histotechnology skills from the practice of anatomic pathology, which is routinely done? For many informatics groups, the service component is their main reason for existence. However, if the role of the informatics program is simply one of maintenance, support, even deployment, this undermines the status of informatics in academic medical centers.

I would argue that the operational services and the developmental ends of the spectrum have to coexist to define the field of informatics. As I presented above, informatics is a process, which starts with problem analysis and ends with the development, deployment, and support of information systems formulated to address those problems. Informatics is fundamentally an applied discipline, and if the basic underlying concepts never make their way into real-life solutions, the value of the discipline is limited. Every step along the way is important. Granted, not every informatician works at the same point in this process, and the informatics process is therefore most commonly accomplished via a team approach. However, those individuals who purport that the particular point along the spectrum on which they have

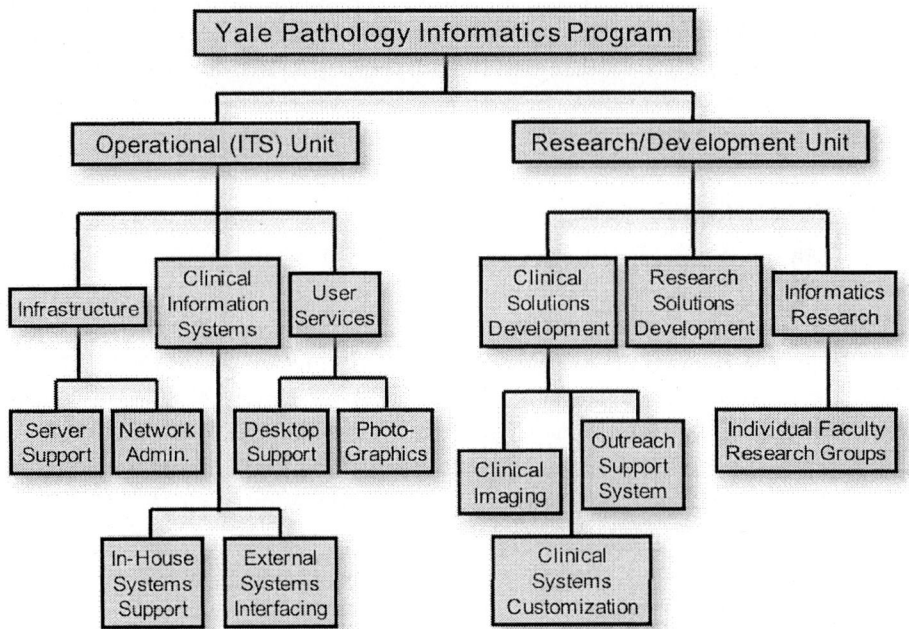

Figure 1-3: The Yale Pathology Informatics Program. The informatics program in the pathology department at Yale Medical School is an example of a hybrid program, combining both an operational unit with responsibilities for the day-to-day maintenance of desktop computers and production information systems, with a more "academic" research/development unit involved both in development of departmental systems as well as externally funded research in medical informatics.

chosen to focus is in fact the true core of informatics, in my opinion, hurt the discipline as a whole.

In the Pathology Department at the Yale University School of Medicine, our Pathology Informatics program (Figure 1-3) has two arms: an "operational" oriented arm, the ITS unit, and a "research" oriented arm, the developmental informatics unit. The faculty are more closely associated with the latter, some working predominantly on externally funded research projects, others focusing more on developing computer-based solutions to meet the department's clinical, research, and teaching missions. The ITS unit, consisting predominantly of non-faculty professionals, provide desktop support services, network and server management, and clinical information systems management for the department as a whole, as well as supporting the activities of the developmental informatics unit. The two arms of the informatics program work closely together. The ITS unit provides server and systems support for the developmental informatics faculty, while solutions developed by the faculty are deployed within the department by the ITS unit, who then assume the responsibility for support and maintenance of those solutions. The entire program is relatively small, with each individual serving multiple roles in the organizational structure shown. However, the structure appears to be working well, although it is still too early to tell if this program will survive the financial and academic advancement constraints of an academic medical center.

Is informatics science or engineering?

An issue that has often been debated amongst informaticians is whether the discipline of informatics is best classified as a science or as engineering. I must confess that I have always considered engineering to be a science, and even Webster's revised unabridged dictionary defines engineering as "the art and science by which the mechanical properties of matter are made useful to man in structures and machines." Science, on the other hand, has several definitions, all centered around the word "knowledge", the most pertinent of which is "accumulated and established knowledge, which has been systematized and formulated with reference to the discovery of general truths or the operation of general laws." The debate between the labels "science" vs "engineering" translates to attempting to locate where informatics should reside on the spectrum between seeking new knowledge and building new solutions, between discovery and creation, between an experimental approach and an organizational one. Is informatics a science in its own right, or a tool for the medical and biological sciences? Informatics is not a natural science, in that it does not seek to discover new knowledge about the physical universe, but beyond that disclaimer I would argue that informatics has elements of both science and engineering, with different parts of the informatics process containing different relative amounts of these two approaches. In the early steps, informatics uses hypothesis-driven analyses to define a problem, test possible approaches, and design a solution. This process requires not only knowledge of the details of the technology tools which might be used to ultimately deploy the solution, but also extensive domain knowledge about the data which is being manipulated and managed. As the informatics process progresses, engineering skills play a more important role to craft, build, and deploy the solution designed. At the end, scientific methods are again used to evaluate the tools developed and assess how well they address the underlying problem. For data mining problems, use of the informatics tools may lead to discovery of new relationships and suggest new hypotheses for further investigation, either via additional informatics tools or more traditional experimental approaches. For clinical management problems, the tools may lead to new models and new opportunities for patient care delivery.

It is important not to confuse the informatics process with the discipline in which the problem being addressed resides. For example, bioinformatics tends to be more readily recognized as a "science" because the problems relate to questions in the arena of basic science, whereas clinical informatics is less readily accepted as scientific because the problems addressed are more applied with implications for patient management. However, in both cases, the underlying informatics process is essentially the same.

Is informatics an "academic" activity?

Non-medical environments, which accept mathematics, computer science, statistics, and probability as academic, have been willing to accept informatics as an academic discipline. In contrast, this acceptance, in general, has not been as forthcoming within medical schools.

Medical schools as academic institutions have wrestled for years with the dichotomy between basic study of disease and the treatment of patients. What is becoming increasingly clear is that these are not two separate things, but rather two ends of a spectrum – the middle ground encompassing what is often now called translational research. Whether or not one end of the spectrum is "better" or "more important" than the other is a matter about which many have strong opinions, but, when it comes to academic advancement, it is certainly true that academic centers are more comfortable with the basic research end, because it is what most clearly separates them from the "private practitioners". I am not going to try to debate this issue here, but rather want to point out that this dichotomy extends into informatics. Clinical informatics is associated with the practice side of the spectrum, and bioinformatics with the research side. This perhaps explains why academic medical centers have been much more willing to accept bioinformatics as an academic discipline than clinical informatics. Pathology departments are but a microcosm of the entire medical school, and every large pathology department is well familiar with the struggle between the research and patient care missions of the department. In the pathology informatics arena, those faculty engaged in bioinformatics are readily accepted as doing scholarly work. Those working on more clinically related projects, however, are not as readily received.

Many academic medical centers have not yet figured out what to do with medical informatics. A number of factors are likely to be contributing to this situation. One is simply history. Computers initially made their appearance in medicine to assist with the predominantly non-professional activities of billing and scheduling. Although information systems in medicine have grown far beyond these initial activities, and now incorporate workflow management and decision support, the origin of these systems, as well as, often, the management by administration, have caused individuals closely associated with these systems, including faculty, to be viewed as predominantly technical and therefore not scholarly.

A second factor harming the academic status of faculty working on developing medical information systems relates to the life cycle of the informatics process. As discussed above, this process begins with problem definition and reduction, proceeds through solution design and development, and ends with deployment and re-evaluation. There are many who would argue that only these early steps, what I term "basic informatics" constitute scholarly activity, and that the later "translational informatics" steps do not. Consider, as an analogy, the process of developing a new diagnostic test. New information about a particular enzyme suggests that alteration of that enzyme function may be involved in the development of a hereditary disease. A partial gene sequence is obtained, and linkage studies are performed in two pedigrees confirming tight linkage to the disease. The gene for the enzyme is cloned and sequenced, identifying a significant difference in the sequence between affected and unaffected individuals. The same variation is found in both pedigrees. This difference is used to develop a PCR based test for the presence of the mutation. Additional patients and pedigrees are sought and identified, further validating the test. Soon two or three specimens a week begin arriving from all over the world for evaluation, and this becomes a routine activity within the research lab. A pharmaceutical company hears about the test, purchases licensing rights to it, and after conducting a series of clinical trials ultimately obtains FDA approval for a now commercially available test which detects the mutation. This test becomes available in reference labs across the country. Few would argue that this process clearly started out as an academic endeavor. Similarly, few would argue that at the end of the process, ordering this test on a patient or performing the test in a reference lab does not constitute an academic activity. At what point in the process did this become no longer academic? Was it when the test began being performed on individual patients not known to have the disease? Was it when the licensing rights were purchased by a pharmaceutical company, or during the clinical trials, or when the commercial test became available, or when it became available at multiple testing sites? It is likely that academicians would not all be in agreement about when this process changed from being a scholarly activity to being a technical one. In an analogous way, medical school faculties have different opinions about which steps in an informatics process constitute an academic activity and which do not. This analysis is further compromised by the fact that whereas the development of a new drug generally takes years, the life cycle of an informatics solution is much shorter, often only weeks.

Academic medical institutions seem to define themselves not so much by what they are but rather by what they are not: in particular, they are not industry, they are not private practice, and ideally they are not providers of routine clinical care. To the extent that informatics projects produce successfully deployed solutions which assist in patient care, they become less academic. It is unfortunate that the potential for commercialization and the overall usefulness of an informatics solution in the day-to-day care of patients both appear to contaminate the perception of that solution as being academic. Early commercial information systems focused only on financial and administrative concerns. It was academic institutions which embellished these by adding data management, workflow management, and decision support. Development of these new "state of the art" patient management systems spurred the establishment and even the acceptance of academic groups in medical informatics. However, as these elements have transitioned into commercially available systems, their view as an academic contribution has faded. This is not a new problem, nor one restricted to informatics. In his analysis of the evolution of medical centers in the United States entitled "A Time to Heal", Kenneth Ludmerer comments that "In general, only the scholarship of discovery, and not the scholarship of teaching, integration, and application, was considered the appropriate standard for faculty advancement"[1]. Although he was referring to academic medical centers of the 1980s, the situation has changed only slightly today.

---

[1] Ludmerer KM. <u>Time to Heal: American Medical Education from the Turn of the Century to the Era of Managed Care</u>. New York: Oxford Univ. Press; 1999. p309.

Once deployed into routine use, or integrated into a commercially available product, the perception of informatics solutions by academic centers is clearly altered. However, as previously mentioned, ultimate deployment is arguably an essential component of any informatics solution, and routine use is generally the goal. This creates almost a no-win situation for medical informaticists, except for those who restrict their activities only to the very early stages of the overall informatics process.

A final factor which has compromised the perception of informatics as an academic discipline has, ironically, been the success of the solutions developed. This has been alluded to above. As the use of computer systems has become more common in medicine, and those systems have become more user-friendly, the contributions made and being made by informatics are less appreciated. The underlying "academic" contributions become abstracted and subsequently viewed as technical. In addition, the more successful and usable a solution it is, the more likely it is to become a target for commercialization. Perhaps the ultimate irony is that homegrown systems, once the pride of academic medical informatics, are being turned off and replaced by commercial systems. Why? Because the day-to-day operations of most health care organizations have simply become too dependent upon these systems. Administrations, uncomfortable with being reliant on the one or two individuals with the skills and knowledge needed to maintain these systems, prefer the backing and support of larger, external, presumably more stable commercial organizations. The success of medical informatics in building valuable solutions has contributed to its own downfall.

What should be the standard by which institutions determine whether or not an activity is academic? Rather than trying to set specific criteria, most institutions have essentially outsourced this decision, relying upon the peer-review process or determining what is publishable and what is externally fundable. In general, these categories have not included solution deployment, but that environment is now changing. With the recognition that sound, deployed informatics solutions represent not only a good idea but rather an essential infrastructure enabling the future advancement of medical care and research, a number of journals are beginning to accept for publication manuscripts describing the details of some of these deployments. In addition, the federal government is beginning to fund the actual development and deployment of software. Elements of the relatively recent caBIG (cancer Biomedical Informatics Grid) project (see cabig.nci.nih.gov) include specific funding for the development of open source modular software for use by the medical community. This is a clear change from prior practices, and may therefore represent a sign that the scope of informatics activities which have traditionally been viewed as academic might also be poised for a change.

Pathology Informatics as a Subspecialty

Many practitioners of the discipline of pathology informatics have lobbied for the designation of pathology informatics as a subspecialty area within pathology, complete with fellowship training programs and specialty board certification. There are many excellent justifications for this. Much like the other subspecialty areas in pathology, there is no question that pathology informatics comprises a unique skill set. Requiring a specialized knowledge base and a unique approach to problems within the discipline, the practice of pathology informatics draws on specialized training beyond what is generally in the scope of "basic" pathology training programs. Organizations with well trained pathology informaticians rapidly set themselves apart from peer organizations as a "center of excellence" in this area. Additionally, pathology informatics goes beyond simply knowing about computers, and the yields obtained from having a pathologist with a special interest in informatics directing an informatics program generally exceed those obtained when the "computer related" activities are relegated to administrative computer support staff. A subspecialty designation would also benefit the discipline greatly, increasing its recognition and validating interest in this area as a scholarly activity.

Another reason for promoting the designation of pathology informatics as a formal subspecialty in pathology relates to the overall future of the discipline. As discussed more fully in the last chapter of this book, the future practice of medicine will involve some discipline taking a more prominent role in integrating data from multiple sources. I strongly feel that the pathologist should fill this role. Informatics tools will be needed to aid in this process. Establishing pathology informatics as a recognized subspecialty, making pathology the first major field in medicine to designate an informatics subspecialty, will help to secure this role for the pathologist.

Despite these justifications and benefits, however, I am going to take the somewhat controversial position of suggesting that such a subspecialty designation might not be in the best long-term interests of the field of pathology. I say "controversial" because I am clearly a strong supporter of the value of informatics to the field, and most of my colleagues would expect me to advocate for such a subspecialty designation. In defense of my position, I would like to contrast the current "attitude" of general practicing pathologists to hematopathology and to immunohistochemistry. Hemato-pathology has been accepted as a subspecialty area in pathology. Cases which fall into the domain of this subspecialty are segregated from the rest of the cases and handled not only in a unique way but also by a subset of pathologists. In contrast, immunohistochemistry is considered a "tool" for the pathologist, whose applicability and use crosses all of the accepted subspecialties. This is in spite of the fact that selecting, performing, and interpreting immunohistochemical stains requires specialized knowledge and skills. As a pathologist who openly acknowledges a lack of "specialty" training in hematopathology, I find that when I am evaluating an active surgical pathology case, once I make the determination that I am likely to be dealing with a hematopoietic malignancy, I can almost feel my brain backing off from engagement with the case, because I know that it will be referred for ultimate diagnosis to a colleague who either has specialty training or at least a special interest in hematopathology. This is not because I feel that either this case in particular or hematopathology in general is beyond my abilities, but rather because hematopathology has been accepted as a subspecialty area in pathology, and my clinical responsibilities do not include "doing" hematopathology. However, if I receive a case consisting of a proliferation of poorly differentiated cells, my brain seamlessly begins building a list of immunohistochemical stains which I plan to order as part of the evaluation of that case, and I would never consider claiming that this case falls outside of my practice domain and refer it to an immuno-histochemistry specialist. Use of immunohistochemistry as a tool to evaluate cases has been integrated into not only mine but every pathologist's practice, and it is difficult to imagine how the diagnostic power of the field of pathology could have advanced to where it is if the use of immunohistochemistry had been relegated to a subset of pathologists. In a similar way, I feel that use of informatics tools must be integrated, across subspecialty disciplines, into the daily life of practicing pathologists. This does not mean that every pathologist needs to understand how to write computer programs, any more than every pathologist is expected to know how horseradish peroxidase converts diaminobenzidine into a deposit which is visible through the light microscope, or how the combination of lens elements made of glass with different dispersion properties is used to chromatically correct achromatic objectives. However, as will be discussed more thoroughly in the last chapter, the future of the practice of pathology lies in adopting a central role in integrating data from multiple sources, not just the histologic section, and that data assimilation role will require informatics tools. To some degree or another, every pathologist will have to learn to use these tools. Designation of pathology informatics as a subspecialty within pathology may result in those not in that subspecialty feeling they are exempt from any need to learn these skills. Granted, pathology informatics is certainly more complex than immunohistochemistry, and undoubtedly individuals will have varying proficiencies with informatics tools, but some core skills will have to be learned by all pathologists.

The astute reader will be quick to point out that molecular pathology has been relatively recently designated as a subspecialty field of pathology, and part of the justification for that designation was the need for specialized knowledge and familiarity with special techniques. I feel this designation was a mistake, and rather than promoting the advancement of molecular pathology may in fact hinder its adoption. Fortunately, molecular pathology tests are being interpreted, for the most part, in a consultative role, and most pathologists are still integrating the results of these interpretations into their overall evaluation of the cases involved.

A forum does exist for pathologists, and others working with pathologists, who have a particular interest in informatics to interact with other similarly inclined individuals. The Association for Pathology Informatics (API) (www.pathologyinformatics.org) supports advances in the field of pathology informatics through research, education, scientific meetings, electronic and printed communications. Other goals include developing standards for data reporting and storage, as well as building relationships with other societies and industry partners which share similar interests. The API sponsors or co-sponsors several educational sessions at a number of national meetings each year, and is establishing itself as a resource for informatics expertise within the discipline of pathology.

Implications for pathology training programs

Independent of my personal opinions on the subject, one of the obstacles faced by advocates of designating pathology informatics as a recognized subspecialty area of pathology is the overall lack of a clear definition as to what precisely pathology informatics is. Without drawing some boundaries to determine what is part of pathology informatics and what is not, it is difficult to define learning objectives, core competencies, and credentialing requirements. How can you train someone for subspecialty certification when the trainers can't agree on what to train? This represents a real problem, not only for possible fellowship training, but also for incorporation of basic informatics training into pathology residency programs. As a result many programs are in a quandary as to how to define and address this need.

A number of "models" for pathology informatics training are beginning to emerge at training programs across the country, and opinions differ as to what should be included in a core training program. This is certainly an area where it is easy to go too far in setting goals and expectations, especially in light of the rapid evolution of hardware and, to a lesser degree, software, but some underlying core concepts are definable. Topics such as basic elements common to desktop computers, features of clinical information systems, database concepts and terminology, information security, inter-system communication, and digital imaging are so fundamental to the pathology informatics process that they represent good launching points for informatics training. Toward that end, it is my hope that this book will address the needs of some programs and pathologists looking to expand their familiarity with this discipline in a very practical way.

It is important to remember, however, that regardless of the level of complexity of a formal training program in pathology informatics, pathology residents today are being already exposed, knowingly or not, to a number of important informatics tools and solutions. In contrast to residents completing their training only a few years ago, it is unusual for a trainee today not to have routinely used a clinical information system, or to have taken digital photographs, or prepared digital case presentations. MEDLINE searches, interacting with other hospital information systems, and using electronic mail are nearly daily activities in the lives of pathology residents. The desire to use these tools and to access the information which these tools unlock is clearly present, and it is the responsibility of training programs to make these tools available to their residents and guide them in their use.

Selected References

Balis UJ, Aller RD, Ashwood ER. Informatics training in U.S. pathology residency programs. Results of a survey. Am J Clin Pathol. Oct 1993;100(4 Suppl 1):S44-47.

Becich MJ, Gross W, Schubert E, Blank G. Building an informatics training program for pathology. Semin Diagn Pathol. Nov 1994;11(4):237-244.

Becich MJ. Information management: moving from test results to clinical information. *Clin Leadersh Manag Rev.* Nov-Dec 2000;14(6):296-300.

Becich MJ. The role of the pathologist as tissue refiner and data miner: the impact of functional genomics on the modern pathology laboratory and the critical roles of pathology informatics and bioinformatics. *Mol Diagn.* Dec 2000;5(4):287-299.

Buffone GJ, Beck JR. Informatics. A subspecialty in pathology. *Am J Clin Pathol.* Jul 1993;100(1):75-81.

Friedman BA. Informatics as a separate section within a department of pathology. *Am J Clin Pathol.* Oct 1990;94(4 Suppl 1):S2-6.

Goldberg-Kahn B, Healy JC. Medical informatics training in pathology residency programs. *Am J Clin Pathol.* Jan 1997;107(1):122-127.

Harrison JH, Jr., Stewart J, 3rd. Training in pathology informatics: implementation at the University of Pittsburgh. *Arch Pathol Lab Med.* Aug 2003;127(8):1019-1025.

Harrison JH, Jr. Pathology informatics questions and answers from the University of Pittsburgh pathology residency informatics rotation. *Arch Pathol Lab Med.* Jan 2004;128(1):71-83.

Haux R. Health care in the information society: what should be the role of medical informatics? *Methods Inf Med.* 2002;41(1):31-35.

Henricks WH, Healy JC. Informatics training in pathology residency programs. *Am J Clin Pathol.* Aug 2002;118(2):172-178.

Henricks WH, Boyer PJ, Harrison JH, Tuthill JM, Healy JC. Informatics training in pathology residency programs: proposed learning objectives and skill sets for the new millennium. *Arch Pathol Lab Med.* Aug 2003;127(8):1009-1018.

Jones R, O'Connor J. Information management and informatics: need for a modern pathology service. *Ann Clin Biochem.* May 2004;41(Pt 3):183-191.

Kulikowski CA. The micro-macro spectrum of medical informatics challenges: from molecular medicine to transforming health care in a globalizing society. *Methods Inf Med.* 2002;41(1):20-24.

Lun KC. Challenges in medical informatics: perspectives of an international medical informatics organization. *Methods Inf Med.* 2002;41(1):60-63.

Maojo V, Martin F, Crespo J, Billhardt H. Theory, abstraction and design in medical informatics. *Methods Inf Med.* 2002;41(1):44-50.

Marchevsky AM, Wick MR. Evidence-based medicine, medical decision analysis, and pathology. *Hum Pathol.* Oct 2004;35(10):1179-1188.

Musen MA. Medical informatics: searching for underlying components. *Methods Inf Med.* 2002;41(1):12-19.

Sarachan BD, Simmons MK, Subramanian P, Temkin JM. Combining medical informatics and bioinformatics toward tools for personalized medicine. *Methods Inf Med.* 2003;42(2):111-115.

Shahar Y. Medical informatics: between science and engineering, between academia and industry. *Methods Inf Med.* 2002;41(1):8-11.

Sinard JH, Morrow JS. Informatics and anatomic pathology: meeting challenges and charting the future. *Hum Pathol.* Feb 2001;32(2):143-148.

Sprogar M, Lenic M, Alayon S. Evolution in medical decision making. *J Med Syst.* Oct 2002;26(5):479-489.

Stefanelli M. Knowledge management to support performance-based medicine. *Methods Inf Med.* 2002;41(1):36-43.

Talmon JL, Hasman A. Medical informatics as a discipline at the beginning of the 21st century. *Methods Inf Med.* 2002;41(1):4-7.

van der Lei J. Closing the loop between clinical practice, research, and education: the potential of electronic patient records. *Methods Inf Med.* 2002;41(1):51-54.

Chapter 2

DESKTOP COMPUTERS: HARDWARE

The paradigm for the interaction of people with computers has completely inverted itself over the past three decades. In the 1970's, the model was of large main-frame computers serving the needs of many, often hundreds of users. The 1980's brought us the era of the personal computer, and suddenly the model was one person – one computer. Finally, the expansion of networking and explosion of the world-wide-web in the 1990's created an environment where multiple computers, sometimes hundreds, were needed to serve the needs of one person. Yet, even under this new paradigm, the desktop computer remains the predominant interface between the user and the electronic world. This chapter will discuss the basic architecture of a desktop computer, specifically the major hardware components. The next will deal with how the various types of software interact to make this such an indispensable tool.

What's in the box?

Probably the single question I am most frequently asked is "I need to get a new computer... which one should I get?" This question stems from a lack of understanding of what the various elements of a computer's "specifications" mean, and what the significance of each is. This will be the topic of this section.

The main internal components of all desktop computers, in addition to a power supply and fan, are the processor, main memory, video interface, and input/output controllers. Each of these components will be discussed separately below. First, however, brief consideration should be given to a few fundamental concepts: how are these components connected to each other, how is data stored in the computer, and what are the differences between different types of memory chips?

Integrated vs Modular Design

Manufacturers use two basic configuration approaches to fit all of the core components of the computer into the "box": integrated and modular. The approach chosen is largely responsible for the variation in the size and shape of desktop computers. The difference is much like the difference between a component sound system, in which one buys the receiver and the amplifier and the tape deck and the CD player as separate devices and hooks them together, versus an integrated system, in which one unit contains all of these functionalities.

In the integrated configuration for assembling the core internal components, sometimes called "monolithic", all of the electronic circuitry is contained on essentially a single circuit board, perhaps with a small number of more customized slots for insertion and removal of components which frequently vary, such as memory chips. The integrated configuration is generally less expensive to produce and takes up less space, so integrated configuration computers often cost less and are smaller than the equivalent modular configuration. However, because most of the electronics are built into the circuit board, the user has fewer choices at the time of purchase, and subsequent upgrading of any of the integrated components is not an option.

In contrast, in the modular configuration, each of the components of the computer are manufactured separately, sometimes by different manufacturers, and then connected to each other inside the desktop computer. This allows individual components to be replaced, upgraded, or added, without having to buy a whole new computer. It also allows the user to select, at the time of purchase, what level of each component he or she wants. Traditionally, one large circuit board, called the "mother board", contains the circuitry for the components to communicate with each other via a number of standardized multi-pin slots into which smaller circuit boards comprising the component circuitry are inserted. Traditionally, the processor was placed on the mother board, although it is now more common for even this component to be placed on a removable board. The smaller, removable boards include memory cards, video display cards, input/output controllers, and a modem, for example. An internal "bus" connects all the expansion slots, usually in a way which makes each slot functionally equivalent. Thus, pin 1 of slot 1 would connect to pin 1 of slot 2 and pin 1 of slot 3, etc. Likewise, pin 2 of each slot would all be connected to each other. The "bus architecture" determines what each of the pins are used for, and therefore dictates what expansion cards can be plugged into these expansion slots – only cards designed for a particular bus architecture can be used in that bus.

A number of different bus architectures have been used in desktop computers, but fortunately this is becoming less complicated as most manufacturers have standardized on a single choice. This is the "Peripheral Component Interconnect" standard, or PCI (*pee-see-eye*) bus. There are actually two different PCI standards, a 32 bit one and a 64 bit one (see the next section for a definition of a "bit").

The circuit boards themselves are complex, multi-layered, and can contain dozens or even hundreds of components. (Ironically, they are sufficiently complex that other computers are used to design them.) For all intents and purposes, a completed circuit board becomes a single entity. If a component of a circuit board fails, it is usually too difficult to figure out which component failed, and even if one could, is it unlikely that it will be possible to replace it without destroying the board. Therefore, diagnosing problems with computer hardware means figuring out which circuit board has the problem, and then replacing that board. If one has an integrated configuration computer in which all of the circuitry is on one board, and some component on that board fails, it is time to get a new computer.

Data Storage in a Computer

The fundamental unit of digital storage in all computer systems is the "bit", short for "binary digit." Electronically, this is represented by a single microscopic device which can exist in one of two states: "on" or "off". In an abstract state, these two electronic states are represented by a "1" or a "0", respectively. This device, initially a transistor, responds differently based on which state it is in, and thus other electronic circuitry can determine whether a 1 or a 0 is currently being stored. Of course, not much information can be stored in a single bit, so collections of bits are generally used together to form a more useful unit of

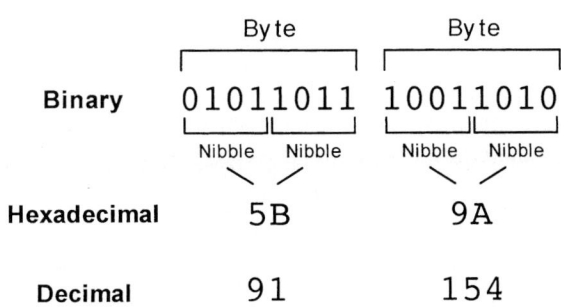

Figure 2-1: Binary representation of digital data. A byte consists of 8 bits, or two nibbles, each composed of four bits. Each nibble can be expressed as a single hexadecimal digit. Therefore, two hexadecimal digits represents one byte.

storage. The most common of these, by far, is the "byte" (*rhymes with kite*), a collection of eight bits (Figure 2-1), each of which can have a value of 0 or 1. Therefore, the byte can have 2^8 or 256 possible states. The value of a byte can be represented in one of three ways: as a binary number between 00000000 and 11111111, as a decimal number between 0 and 255, inclusive, or as a sequence of two hexadecimal (base 16) digits, each corresponding to a four bit block, otherwise known as a "nibble" (because it is half of a byte). Thus, in hexadecimal representation, a single byte can have a value between 00 and FF, inclusive.

The next larger unit of digital data storage is known as a "word". This term, however, is more loosely defined, and whereas a byte is a byte on any computer system from any manufacturer, the use of the term "word" varies from system to system. In general, it is used to describe the size of the standard instruction set for the particular computer system. In the not too distant past, computers used 2-byte (16-bit) instructions, and thus a word was a two byte block. More recently, 32-bit (4-byte) instructions have become more common, so the "word" size has doubled to 4-bytes. Some of the newest processors are beginning to use 64-bit (8-byte) words.

Now for something really obscure. When two or more bytes are combined together to form a single "word", there are two ways to do this. Take the two bytes shown in the example above, with values of 91 and 154 decimal, in that order. If one were to combine these two bytes into a single word, the first byte (at the lower address location) could represent the lower order bits, in which case the entire word would have a value of 91 + (154 * 256) = 39,515. Alternatively, the first byte could represent the higher order bits, in which case the entire word would have a value of (91 * 256) + 154 = 23,450. Clearly, it is important to know which representation one is using. The term "little-endian" (*end-eee-enn*) is used for the first case because the lower order bits come first, whereas the term "big-endian" is used for the second case where the more significant bits come first. The little-endian convention is used by Intel processors, whereas Motorola and other RISC processors tend to use the big-endian convention. The terminology derives from Gulliver's Travels by Jonathan Swift, in which the Lilliputians were at war with the inhabitants of the nearby island of Blefuscu over whether soft-boiled-eggs should be opened from the little-end or the big-end. In computers, the distinction between these two choices, based on technical merits, carries about the same significance.

Of course, memory usage in computers involves literally millions of bytes, so additional terminology is needed to refer to large collections of bytes. Since all data storage in computers is binary, and since the most common small blocks of data usage are also binary, memory chips are manufactured with binary quantities of bytes. Unfortunately, large powers

Table 2-1: Terms used to describe large quantities of bytes.

Abbrev	Name	Approx power of 10	Actual power of 2	Actual # of bytes	Approximation
KB	kilobyte	10^3	2^{10}	1,024	thousand
MB	megabyte	10^6	2^{20}	1,048,576	million
GB	gigabyte	10^9	2^{30}	1,073,741,824	billion*
TB	terabyte	10^{12}	2^{40}	1,099,511,627,776	trillion*
PB	petabyte	10^{15}	2^{50}	1.126×10^{15}	quadrillion*
EB	exabyte	10^{18}	2^{60}	1.153×10^{18}	quintillion*

Although standard metric terminology is used, these are merely approximations to actual powers of two. (*Note: The American usage of the terms "billion", "trillion", etc. is different from how they are used in most European countries.)

of 2 are not easy to represent in terms of abbreviations, so a certain amount of rounding error occurs when referring to large blocks of memory by more commonly used "power of ten" abbreviations. For example, 1 KB or kilobyte of memory, which one might expect would be 10^3 or 1000 bytes, is actually 2^{10} or 1024 bytes. Similarly, 1 MB or megabyte of data is not 10^6 or 1,000,000 bytes of data but rather 1024 "kilobytes", or 2^{20} bytes, which is actually 1,048,576 bytes (about a million bytes). Larger memory blocks are described in Table 2-1.

Computer Memory Chips

There are basically three different types of memory chips, all containing many bytes of data storage. Understanding the differences between these types is important in understanding their role in the computer.

The first major type of memory chip is Random Access Memory, otherwise known simply as RAM (*pronounced like the male sheep*). RAM is called "random access" because any of the memory locations can be accessed directly, either to put something into it ("write") or to find out what has already been stored there ("read"). Random is in contrast to "serial", where one can only start reading at specific points, and then has to read the next byte, and the next byte, etc., until the desired memory location is reached. One thing that all RAM has in common is that when the power supplied to the chip is removed (usually because the computer is turned off), all of the information stored in the memory is lost.

RAM comes in two different types, static and dynamic. Static RAM, also known as SRAM (*ess-ram*) will remember whatever is written to it as long as power is applied to the chip. SRAM is very fast (data can be written to and read from memory very rapidly), but is also relatively expensive to manufacture and thus to buy. Dynamic RAM, or DRAM (*dee-ram*), only remembers what is written to it for a brief period of time, usually less than one one-hundredth of a second (0.01 sec). This would seem to make it rather useless. However, with the addition of a small amount of circuitry, the contents of the memory locations can be repeatedly refreshed, so that it acts more like SRAM. DRAM is slower than SRAM, but it is a lot cheaper to make and therefore much less expensive to buy. Just to make this a little more confusing, a special type of DRAM exists, known as SDRAM (*ess-dee-ram*), which stands for synchronous DRAM. SDRAM is faster than standard asynchronous DRAM in that it can synchronize its operation with the same clock cycle that the central processor is using. Once synchronized, the processor can be assured that memory reads and writes occur within a certain time period, and therefore does not have to check to see if the operation has been completed before using the data retrieved. Since SDRAM must synchronize itself with the processor's clock cycle, one needs to match the speed of the SDRAM to the speed of the processor when putting these components together.

The second major type of memory chip is Read Only Memory, or ROM (*rhymes with bomb*). ROM is designed to remember it's contents, even if the power to the chip is completely removed. In the initial ROM chips, the contents of the memory locations had to be hard-wired into the chip at the time of manufacturing, which required close cooperation between the individuals designing the chips and those deciding what information needed to be stored on the chips. This type of ROM chip is much less commonly used today, but when it is used it is referred to as "masked" ROM, to distinguish it from the newer types of ROM. The next generation of ROM chips were Programmable Read Only Memory, or PROM (*pronounced like the high school dance*). PROM chips are manufactured blank (they have no pre-defined contents). A special circuit can then be used to write contents into the memory chip, a process known as "programming" or "burning", but this can only be done once. Once written, PROM chips retain their contents even in the absence of power, but cannot be erased or reused. However, this allows the chip manufacturers to make the chips without having to know in advance what to store in them, significantly decreasing the cost of the chips.

The next major advance in ROM technology was the Erasable and Programmable Read Only Memory chip, or EPROM (*eee-prom*). Like other PROMs, the EPROM is manufactured blank and then programmed using a PROM burner. However, the chip is also manufactured with a quartz window on the top of the ceramic chip case. Removing the chip from the circuit board and bombarding it with strong ultraviolet radiation through the window will erase the contents of the chip, allowing it to be reprogrammed. In general, this can be done approximately 100-1000 times before the chip wears out and becomes unreliable.

The final major type of memory chip attempts to combine features of both RAM and ROM, in particularl the re-writability of RAM and the non-volatility of ROM. Sometimes referred to as "hybrid" chips, these account for the majority of the ongoing development of chip technology. I will simply discuss three major types here. The first is known as Electrically Erasable and Programmable Read Only Memory, or EEPROM (*double-eee-prom*). Like EPROM, these are manufactured blank, can be written to, and can be erased. However, EEPROMs can be erased electrically, and therefore do not need a quartz window or even to be removed from the circuit in order to be erased. EEPROM chips have to be erased and re-written one byte at a time, so write times are very slow (compared to RAM), and the chips are much more expensive than RAM chips, especially for large storage capacities. Depending upon the manufacturer, EEPROMs can support anywhere between 10,000 and 1,000,000 erase-write cycles before they become unreliable.

To address the very slow write times of EEPROMs, Flash ROM was developed. Flash ROM, or Flash Memory, is nonvolatile like EEPROM, but is lower cost and faster both for reads and writes. This is accomplished by changing the way erases are handled. Rather than being able to be erased and re-written one byte at a time, Flash memory must be erased in blocks of bytes, known as sectors. The size of the sector is determined by the manufacturer, but generally is between 512 bytes and 16 KB, depending upon the total memory capacity. In this way, Flash memory is much like a hard disk. Once a sector is erased, writes and reads can be done one byte at a time. Since Flash memory is usually used to store blocks of data, the requirement for erasing whole sectors at a time is not really a problem, and allows much faster access than having to erase each byte individually. Like EEPROM, Flash memory has a limited number of erase-write cycles, usually about 10,000-100,000, after which the chip becomes unreliable.

The last type of hybrid memory chip is called non-volatile RAM, or NVRAM (*en-vee-ram*). This is simply SRAM with a battery to maintain power to the chip even after the power to the computer is removed. NVRAM is very fast, has an unlimited number of erase cycles, does not "wear out" until the battery dies, but is very expensive and therefore not generally used.

Two other terms which I may as well throw into this discussion are SIMM (*sim*) and DIMM (*dim*). SIMM stands for Single Inline Memory

Module, and is a small circuit board with multiple memory chips attached to it. It allows blocks of memory to be added or upgraded. These small memory boards insert into special slots on the mother-board of the computer. Dual Inline Memory Modules (DIMMs) are essentially the same thing, except that the pins on opposite sides of the board are different from each other, thereby doubling the number of connections for the same physical slot size and allowing more information to be exchanged simultaneously.

Basic Components of a Desktop Computer

As previously mentioned, the main components of a desktop computer are the processor, the main computer memory, the video display controller, the input/output controllers, and the network interface card (Figure 2-2). Each will be discussed separately.

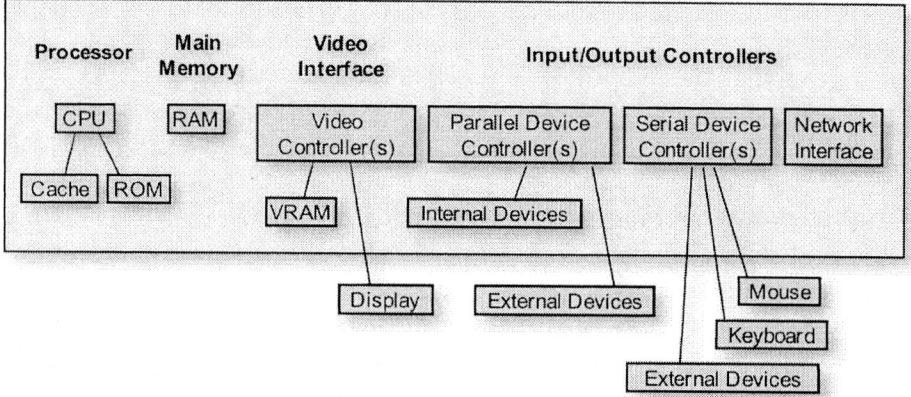

Figure 2-2: Major components of a desktop computer. This diagram displays the major elements of a standard desktop computer. Those inside the large rectangle are usually found inside the "box" which is the "computer". The others are usually attached as peripherals.

Processor

The "brain" of any computer is the processor. Everything the computer does is done by the processor, and, in general, the "type of computer" which you have is determined large by the type of processor in the computer. Manufacturers usually name their processors. The "Power PC" (developed by IBM and Motorola) has been the processor for the Apple Macintosh computers, and there have been a number of generations of this chip, the most recent at the time of this writing being the G5. "Windows" machines run on Intel's processors, the most recent of which is the Pentium series. Traditionally, the Power PC chip has only been available in Apple built computers, whereas, in contrast, Intel sells its processor chips to a number of computer manufacturers, such as Hewlett-Packard and Dell. Recently, Apple announced it would be switching to Intel processors in future versions of the Macintosh.

The main component of the processor assembly is the Central Processing Unit or CPU (*see-pee-you*). In addition to having a name, the CPU is also designated with a "speed". This refers to how quickly the processor can perform individual steps of a task. Each step may involve moving data around or adding two numbers, etc. This is done electronically and takes time. If the processor tries to move on to the next step before the first is completed, the system will stop operating (a system "crash"). The speed with which a CPU can perform these steps is determined by a large number of factors built into the design of the chip. In order for the CPU to know how long to wait before starting another task, each step of the operation of the CPU is driven by an external "clock", a chip which puts out a signal at regularly spaced intervals, currently about every billionth of a second. This clock drives and synchronizes all of the tasks which the computer performs. If a slow clock is used in the computer, it will still do all of the same tasks – they will simply take longer. Therefore, one wants to use the fastest clock which the CPU can keep up with. The maximum clock speed at which a CPU can run is referred to as the processor speed. This is currently measured in gigahertz.

When comparing two processors of the same type but with different speeds, the ratio of the speeds will give a pretty good indicator of the relative speeds of the two machines (note that this only applies to calculations, since often the rate limiting step for any real task is access to a disk or other long-term storage device). However, one cannot directly compare the speed of a processor of one type with the speed of a processor of a different type. This is not intuitively obvious, and warrants a bit of explanation. The "speed" of a CPU indicates the number of processor cycles which occur each second. Unfortunately, what one really wants to know is how long it will take the processor to perform a certain task, and the number of processor cycles which occur each second is only a part of the equation. Every task that a processor performs must first be broken down into a combination of many discrete steps, referred to as machine instructions. The range of possible machine instructions available for a given processor comprises the instruction set for that processor. The amount of time it takes for the CPU to perform the task is determined by the number of machine instructions necessary to perform that task, multiplied by the number of processor cycles

$$\frac{time}{task} = \frac{machine\ instructions}{task} \times \frac{processor\ cycles}{machine\ instruction} \times \frac{time}{processor\ cycle}$$

Figure 2-3: Computer processing speed. Although most people refer to the number of processor cycles per unit time as the "speed" of the processor, there are a number of other elements which factor into determining how long it will take a given processor to perform a given task.

it takes for each machine instruction, multiplied by the amount of time for each processor cycle (Figure 2-3). The last of these three terms is the inverse of the processor speed. The first two are determined by the architecture of the processor.

The term "processor architecture" refers to the details of the functional design of the CPU. As just mentioned, this is intimately linked to the instruction set for the processor. Two basic architectures exist: Complex Instruction Set Computing, or CISC (*sisk*) and Reduced Instruction Set Computing, or RISC (*risk*). Intel processors use a CISC architecture, whereas the PowerPC uses a RISC architecture. In the former case, the instruction set is large, and each instruction can perform complex operations. As such, fewer machine instructions are needed to perform a given task, but it takes many processor cycles for each machine instruction to be completed. In contrast, in RISC processors, the instruction set is relatively smaller. More machine instructions are needed to perform the same task, but each instruction can execute in a small number of processor cycles, often only one. Therefore, for a particular task, a 1.5 GHz RISC processor might complete the task faster than a 2.0 GHz CISC processor. However, for a different task involving a different set of machine instructions, the balance may tip in the other direction. Therefore, there is no "conversion factor" which will allow comparing the speed of processors of different architectures across all tasks.

Parallel computing is a term used to refer to the situation in which two or more processors are doing different things simultaneously. In the not too distant past, only large server-level computers had multiple processors. This has begun to filter down into desktop computers, and now most high end desktop computers come with at least the option of getting them with two or more processors. However, having two processors does not mean that everything will happen twice as fast, just as putting two engines in a car will not necessarily make the car go twice as fast. In the car analogy, there are still only four wheels, and they all have to turn at the same rate. Similarly, computers with two or more processors still have only one set of main memory, one mother board, and have to access the same peripheral devices, and the constraints placed by these factors limit the increase in efficiency. More importantly, however, is that most software has traditionally been written to do one thing at a time, finish it, and then move on to the next thing. If one runs such software on a dual processor computer, one processor does all the work and the other just sits there. To take advantage of multiple processors, programs have to be redesigned to do multiple things at once. This is referred to as "multi-threaded". Then, each thread can be handed off to a different processor, yielding the increased speed. Although many operating systems have been redesigned to take advantage of multiple processors, application software is only beginning to catch up.

Other elements of the processor design, beyond the scope of this discussion, also influence the overall performance of the processor. This includes such things as the number of stages in the processor pipeline and the logic behind its speculative operation (processors attempt to increase their efficiency by "guessing" what they will need to do next).

Two other core components are present in essentially every computer system and are so intimately tied to the CPU that it makes sense to think of them as part of the whole processor. These are the ROM and the cache. The ROM is usually made up of PROM chips, described above. These are pre-programmed by the manufacturer and store elements of the operating system. The ROM is generally only accessible by the processor and cannot be directly accessed by a programmer. Since ROM cannot be rewritten once burned in at the factory, one could potentially be faced with an inability to upgrade the operating system without replacing the ROM chips. To get around this limitation, most operating systems have the ability to override the information stored in ROM by dedicating a section of RAM for storage of any updated routines.

The cache (*kash*) is a small block of fast memory used to store recently accessed data or routines so that subsequent access to the same information can occur more quickly. When data is read from main memory, a copy of that information is stored in the cache. The cache monitors all requests for data from memory. If the cache happens to be storing a copy of the requested data, the cache intercepts the request and provides the processor with the requested information directly, much quicker than it would take to retrieve the information from main memory. If the requested data is not in the cache, it is fetched from main memory, and a copy is stored in the cache. Of course, everything can't be stored in cache, so how the cache is designed and managed can significantly effect the performance of the processor. The size of the cache is also an important determining factor. The goal for management is to try to maximize the percentage of memory requests which can be satisfied from the cache.

Most processors have some cache built directly into the CPU chip casing. Because cache has to be fast, it is generally made of static RAM (SRAM). Many processor also support additional cache external to the CPU chip. This additional cache is variably called "secondary cache", "level 2 cache", or "backside cache". It may be made up of SRAM or DRAM.

Main Computer Memory

Main computer memory makes up the active "work-space" for the computer. All of this memory is dynamic and volatile – once you turn off the computer, anything stored in the main memory is lost. Main computer memory is almost always made up of DRAM chips, as described above. Therefore, this is what one is referring to when you are asked "How much RAM do you have in your computer?" The chips may insert individually into the mother board, or more commonly are inserted as small circuit boards known as inline memory modules (SIMMs or DIMMs – see discussion above under Computer Memory Chips).

Essentially any and everything has to be transferred into main computer memory in order to be used. This includes any programs you may want to run, any data files you may want to open, or even any files you simply want to copy from one long term storage location to another. As such, the amount of main memory in a computer is an important factor in determining what that computer will be able to do. Most desktop computers currently come with between 512 megabytes (MB) and 2 gigabytes (GB) of RAM. The maximum amount of memory you can have is limited by how much money you want to spend and by the type of "memory addressing" used by the processor in the computer.

Data is generally stored in memory in consecutive memory locations (bytes). Since it can be stored anywhere in memory, the processor needs to be able to know where to find it and how to retrieve it. This is done by giving each memory location an "address", simply a sequential number uniquely identifying each memory location in the computer. The processor keeps track of where things are in memory by remembering the address at which the storage of each thing in memory begins. Of course, this memory address needs to be stored in memory, and the number of bytes used by the processor to store the memory address determines how much memory can actually be addressed. Early computers used 16-bit (2-byte) memory addressing, and therefore could only address up to $2^{16} = 65,536$ memory locations, or 64 KB. This is why early computers had a 64 K memory limit – one could put more memory in the box, but the processor couldn't address it. In an attempt to break through this barrier, some computers added what was called "extended memory". This was memory above the 64 K addressable limit, so a variety of electronic contortions were necessary to get access to this memory, including swapping its contents with memory addresses below the 64 K limit. Eventually, modern computers moved to 32-bit (4-byte) memory addressing. This allowed for up to 2^{32} = 4 GB of memory addresses. However, even this limit is proving too restrictive for some applications, and some of the newest computers are beginning to use 64-bit (8-byte) memory addressing, allowing up to sixteen million terabytes of data to be accessed dynamically.

Video Display Controller

In order for the user to be able to interact with the computer, desktop computers need some sort of video display. Originally, these were all based on cathode ray tubes (CRTs), but now a variety of liquid crystal and plasma displays are available. Some of the integrated computers, including laptop computers, have the display built directly into the computer casing, whereas the display is a separate device in the modular computer design. A multi-pin connector and multi-wire cable are used to connect the display and the computer.

Circuitry is needed to control the display. This circuitry may be built into the mother board of the computer, but is more commonly found on its own circuit board, the video display controller. The video card has a multi-pin connector on one end to plug into the internal bus of the computer, and one or more additional multi-pin connectors to which the monitor(s) is connected. A variety of video cards are available from a variety of manufacturers, and although some are proprietary, most commonly available video cards can be used with most monitors. Remember that the standard "tube-based" monitors are inherently analog devices, and take an analog signal. Much of the circuitry on the video card involves taking the digital display built in memory and converting it to an analog signal. Newer monitors are digital, and can take a direct digital input. Some of the newer video cards support both analog and digital video outputs.

One of the most important features differentiating monitors from each other is the screen resolution: the screen is divided, in each dimension, into a large number of discrete points of light, or pixels (*piks-ells*), which can be individually manipulated by the computer to display different colors and form patterns which we recognize as text or pictures. The more pixels which can be displayed in each dimension, the higher the resolution of the monitor. Originally, standard monitors supported 640 pixels wide by 480 pixels high, since that was a direct extrapolation of the most common video signal technology used by CRTs (see Chapter 9 on Video Microscopy). However, it is uncommon to find monitors with such a low resolution currently, and resolutions of at least 800 x 600 pixels, or more commonly 1024 x 768 are now standard. To support the increasing use of computers to display video, including DVDs, wide-screen format monitors are becoming more common. These deviate from the standard aspect ratio of 4:3 (the ratio of the number of pixels in the horizontal dimension to the number in the vertical dimension). Many modern monitors have the ability to switch between multiple different resolutions, displaying more or fewer pixels in the same amount of physical screen space (multi-synch monitors).

Of course, there is a "terminology" for video resolutions in the digital display environment. Although the acronyms "VGA", "XGA", etc. actually define a specific analog video standard, they are most commonly used to refer to the maximum resolution (in pixels) which that standard accommodates. VGA, XGA, and SXGA are the most common, corresponding to screen resolutions of 640 x 480, 800 x 600, and 1024 x 768, respectively. Table 2-2 provides a "key" to this terminology.

There are also "Wide" versions of most of the above formats with the same number of pixels vertically but more pixels horizontally, changing the aspect ratio from 4:3 to approximately 16:9. For example, WXGA (Wide-

Table 2-2: Standard digital display resolutions.

Acronym	Name	Width x Height	Total Pixels
CGA	Computer Graphics Adapter	320 x 200	64,000
QVGA	Quarter Video Graphics Array	320 x 240	76,800
EGA	Enhanced Graphics Adapter	640 x 350	224,000
VGA	Video Graphics Array	640 x 480	307,200
SVGA	Super Video Graphics Array	800 x 600	480,000
XGA	Extended Graphics Array	1024 x 768	786,432
SXGA	Super Extended Graphics Array	1280 x 1024	1,310,720
SXGA+	Super Extended Graphics Array Plus	1400 x 1050	1,470,000
UXGA	Ultra Extended Graphics Array	1600 x 1200	1,920,000
QXGA	Quad Extended Graphics Array	2048 x 1536	3,145,728
QSXGA	Quad Super Extended Graphics Array	2560 x 2048	5,242,880
QUXGA	Quad Ultra Extended Graphics Array	3200 x 2400	7,680,000
HSXGA	Hex Super Extended Graphics Array	5120 x 4096	20,971,520
HUXGA	Hex Ultra Extended Graphics Array	6400 x 4800	30,720,000

These acronyms refer to the most common video standards for monitors and video projectors. Other pixel resolutions are also possible.

Extended Graphics Array) supports a resolution of 1366 x 768 for a total of 1,049,088 pixels.

Video display controllers keep track of what is supposed to be displayed at each pixel location, and constantly refresh the display. This information is stored in memory chips on the controller card, referred to as video-RAM or VRAM (*vee-ram*). VRAM is usually made up of DRAM chips. This memory is not included in the total amount of main computer memory for the computer, but rather is generally quoted separately. The amount of VRAM present determines the maximum display resolution which the memory card can support, but one also has to take into account color when determining how much VRAM is needed.

For each pixel location on the display, any of a number of different colors can be displayed. The details of color encoding are described later in the chapter on digital imaging. For now, suffice it to say that the number of colors available depends on how much memory is dedicated to each pixel location. "Full color" usually requires 3 bytes of memory per pixel. Thus, for an XGA display at full color, one would need 1024 x 768 x 3 = 2,359,296 bytes, or 2.25 MB of VRAM.

Most video display controllers have a simple "processor" on board to handle the constant refreshing of the display. However, some come with a more sophisticated processor which can perform complex image manipulation tasks. These can significantly improve the performance of image editing software, since the CPU of the computer can off-load some of the processing tasks to the processor on the video controller.

If a computer has multiple video controllers, then it can support multiple simultaneous displays. For users who like to have multiple documents open at the same time, adding an additional display can increase the screen "real-estate" available. The resolutions of the two monitors can be different. An operating system program is used to define how each of the display areas relate to each other in forming a large virtual desktop, such that, for example, an object dragged off the right edge of one screen appears on the left edge of the second screen.

Rather than using the second monitor to increase the size of the virtual desktop, the two monitors can be set to display the same information, an arrangement known as mirroring. Although at first this might seem pointless, it makes a lot of sense when the second display is a video projector. In this way, the computer screen displays the same thing which is being projected. Keep in mind that when two different display devices are set up to mirror each other, the maximum resolution usable is limited by the smaller of the resolutions of the two devices being mirrored.

One last thing to keep in mind is the type of connector needed to attach a monitor to the video display controller. This connector port is usually marked on the back of computer with the international icon for a monitor (Figure 2-4). Standard connectors are available for both analog and digital displays, but they are different from each other. Converters can be used to convert one standard to the other. The analog standard contains three rows of 5 pins each as is referred to as a VGA connector. Despite the same name as a low resolution video standard,

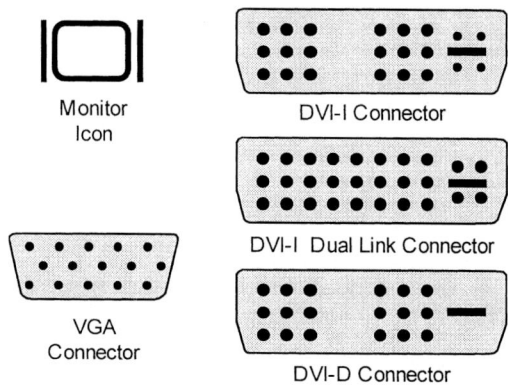

Monitor Icon

DVI-I Connector

DVI-I Dual Link Connector

VGA Connector

DVI-D Connector

Figure 2-4: Icon and connector diagrams for video display connections.

VGA connectors can support a wide variety of resolutions. The standard digital connector is the DVI or Digital Video/Visual Interface connector. There are two types of DVI connectors: DVI-D contains only the digital signals, whereas DVI-I contains both analog and digital signals. The DVI-I is the most common. This consists of 2 3x3 arrays of pins, and a small plate-shaped connector flanked by two pairs of pins (these flanking pairs of pins are absent from DVI-D connectors). Another variation known as "dual link" DVI connectors have 6 additional pins between the two sets of 9 pins.

Input/Output Devices

The processor, main computer memory, and video interface represent the core of the computer system. All other devices are considered "outside" of this core, and therefore are often referred to as "peripherals". The designation as peripheral is based on how these devices communicate with the core system, which is via one of several Input/Output or I/O (*eye-oh*) interfaces (input/output indicating bidirectional communication, although in some instances the communication is predominantly input, such as a keyboard, and in others it is predominantly output, such as a printer). Peripheral devices include such items as the keyboard, mouse, floppy disk drives, hard disk drives, compact disc (CD) drives, printers, bar-code scanners, digital cameras, etc. This includes some devices which may be physically located inside the computer box, such as the main hard drive, and hence the terms "internal peripheral devices" and "external peripheral devices" are used. Internal devices often cost less than a corresponding external device because they do not require an outer casing and can generally draw power from the computer's power supply, eliminating the need for their own power supply. A subset of peripheral devices, mainly a hard disk, keyboard, and mouse, are essentially "required", since they are all present on the vast majority of desktop computers. A special type of I/O device is the network interface card. This is special because although the method of communication is in many ways similar to other I/O devices, there is often no actual device connected. Network cards will be considered separately.

A variety of different types of I/O connections are possible for any different computer. These are often compared to each other by the rate at which information can be exchanged between the device and the computer. Data communication rates are generally expressed in bits-per-second, or bps (*bee-pee-ess*). As will be seen below, bits-per-second makes more sense as a standard for comparison than bytes-per-second because some of the communication methods transmit one bit at a time rather than one byte at a time. Nonetheless, manufacturers tend to use bytes-per-second for disk drives, so be careful about this distinction. In this book I will use a lower case "b" in "bps" to indicate bits-per-second and an upper case "B" in "Bps" to indicate bytes-per-second (usually with an "M" in front of it for Megabits or Megabytes), but not everyone follows this convention.

Many common peripheral devices can connect to the core computer by different methods, based on how they are designed. Therefore, discussions of the devices can get intermixed with discussion of the communication methods. I will first discuss the communication methods, and then briefly mention a few of the specific devices. The communication methods divide into two broad categories: parallel and serial, and devices connected by these methods are subsequently referred to as parallel or serial devices, respectively.

Input/Output Controllers – Parallel Devices

Parallel communication refers to a data exchange method in which multiple bits of information are transmitted simultaneously on different wires. Depending upon the configuration, this can be 8, 16, or 32 bits at a time. Simultaneous communication requires multiple wires, so the connectors are more complex and the cables are thicker. This makes for bulky and expensive cables, and as a result these cables often tend to be shorter in length than serial cables.

One of the earliest parallel connections on a personal computer was the "printer port", very common on earlier Intel-processor-based personal computers. This connector supported eight lines for data transfer to a printer, but could also be used to connect other devices such as scanners. With the increasing popularity and speed of new serial communication protocols, this printer port is less frequently used, and is beginning to disappear from the newer desktop computers.

The most common parallel devices are long-term storage devices such as magnetic disk drives and compact disc drives. Although these are usually built into the computer box, and in the case of the main hard disk drive may not even be visible to the user, they are still technically "peripheral" devices. The two most commonly used communication methods are IDE (ATA) and SCSI. Both of these communication standards currently incorporate DMA or Direct Memory Access, which means the device controller is allowed to directly access the main memory of the computer and does not have to involve the processor when reading or writing large blocks of data. This results in much greater efficiency of data transfer.

The Integrated Drive Electronics or IDE (*eye-dee-eee*) standard also goes by the names ATA (Advanced Technology Attachment) and ATAPI (Advanced Technology Attachment Packet Interface). The "Packet Interface" was introduced at ATA version 4 and added support for CD-ROM drives. The ATA standard supports the connection of two devices, a master and a slave, to the computer through a single controller. Because only two devices can be connected to an IDE controller, these are "always" internal devices, and there is no cabling standard for an external IDE device (therefore, there should not be an IDE connector on the back of the computer). An alternate version of this standard, known as EIDE for Extended IDE, supports both a primary and a secondary path, each with a master and slave device, and therefore can accommodate four devices. The circuitry for IDE communication is relatively simple (compared to SCSI), and therefore it is less expensive and for single isolated accesses can be very fast. Maximum data transfer rates for the most recent versions can be as high as 44.4 – 66.7 MBps (ATA-5) or even 100 MBps (ATA-6).

SCSI (*skuz-eee*) stands for Small Computer Systems Interface. It is a more sophisticated standard with more complex electronics, and supports a higher bandwidth, command queuing, and optimized seek patterns. The SCSI standard supports both internal and external devices. Computers with a SCSI controller usually have a cable connection site on the back. A number of "standards" exist for SCSI cables (Figure 2-5). The DB-25 connector is unique to the early Macintoshes. This connector, although physically the same as that used for the parallel port on early Intel-based personal computers, uses a completely different pin-connection standard. More commonly, the Centronics 50 cable is used for external SCSI connections. Recently, smaller, "high density" connectors have become more popular. The external devices are connected to each other in a fashion known as "daisy-chaining", which means the first device connects to the connector on the back of the computer, the second device connects to a second connector

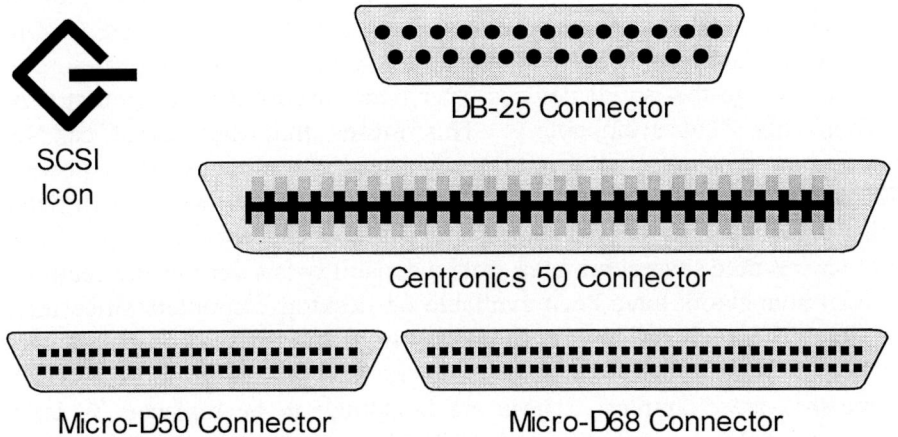

Figure 2-5: Small Computer System Interface (SCSI) icon and connectors. The DB-25 connector was used on early Macintosh computers, but because it was often confused with the identical appearing parallel port on Intel-based computers, its use was discontinued. The micro-connectors are the ones most commonly in use today.

on the first device, the third to the second device, etc. The last device in the chain must be "terminated": a special blank connector is placed in the unused connector. This prevents signals from echoing along the cable.

The SCSI-1 standard supported up to 8 devices in a chain (the processor counted as one of those devices) and had maximum communication rates of 5 MB/sec. SCSI-2 supported 8, 16, or 32 devices, depending upon whether "wide" cables were used, with 16 or 32 data lines. Maximum communication rates of 10-40 MBps were attainable. SCSI-3 supports up to 32 devices and has a maximum communication rate of 160 MBps.

Purely by looking at the transfer rate specifications, IDE (ATA) and SCSI seem to be comparable in speed, and when a single device is connected to the computer, that is in fact the case. However, when multiple devices are connected, the increased sophistication of the SCSI interface becomes apparent, and SCSI significantly out-performs the IDE (ATA) devices.

Input/Output Controllers – Serial Devices

Serial communication refers to a data exchange method in which each bit of data is sent individually and successively as a stream of bits along a single communication medium, usually a single wire. Because fewer wires are needed than for parallel communication, the connectors tend to be smaller, and wire runs can often be longer. Serial communication has traditionally been slower than parallel, because data is sent one bit at a time rather than one or more bytes at a time, although new serial communication protocols are overtaking parallel communication methods (in fact, both the IDE (ATA) and SCSI standards are being redeveloped for serial communication).

An advantage that serial devices offer over parallel devices is that they are frequently "hot swappable." This means that the device can be connected or disconnected from the computer without having to power-down either the computer or the device. Since shutting down the computer so that a device can be connected or removed and then re-booting the computer can take several minutes, hot-swappability is a very useful feature.

Serial connectors have been available on desktop computers since their inception. The keyboard and mouse ports on the Intel-based computers, and the "Apple Desktop Bus" for connecting the keyboard and mouse to early Macintoshes are examples. These are beginning to be replaced by USB devices (see below). In addition, the "COM" ports on the early Intel-based computers and the "Printer" and "Modem" ports on the early Macintoshes were also examples of serial ports. These seem to have completely disappeared. These early serial connections could support data transfer rates in the range of 1.0 – 1.5 MBps.

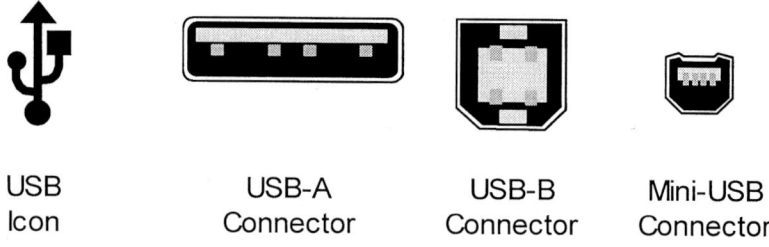

USB	USB-A	USB-B	Mini-USB
Icon	Connector	Connector	Connector

Figure 2-6: Universal Serial Bus (USB) icon and connectors. USB has rapidly become the most popular serial communication protocol for desktop computers.

The most common serial communication method used by desktop computers today is the Universal Serial Bus, or USB (*you-ess-bee*). It can support up to 127 devices, is hot-swappable, and can even provide limited power levels to some external devices (like the keyboard, mouse, some disk drives, bar-code scanners, etc.). A few different styles of connectors are used for USB connections (Figure 2-6). The most common, the USB-A, is a flat, rectangular connector with an internal spacer on one side to maintain proper polarity. A somewhat smaller USB-B connector is also occasionally seen. A mini-version, the Mini-USB connector, is most commonly used on digital cameras and other small devices with limited space for large connectors. Version 1.1 of the USB communication protocol supports data transfer rates of 12 Mbps (1.5 MBps), but the more modern version 2.0 supports a remarkable 480 Mbps (60 MBps) !

The other big player in current serial communication standards is IEEE (*eye-triple-eee*) 1394. IEEE stands for the Institute of Electrical and Electronic Engineers. This organization develops and certifies communication standards, and 1394 is the standard number for this protocol. Unfortunately, IEEE 1394 is not a very catchy name, and since Apple was one of the first to implement this standard on their desktop computers, they coined the name "Firewire" to refer to it. Sony referred to their implementation of the same standard in their digital cameras as "iLink", but that name has not caught on like Firewire. Technically, the name Firewire should only be used to refer to Apple's implementation, but it is used unofficially to refer to any implementation of this standard. Like USB, Firewire devices are hot-swappable, and like SCSI, the devices can be connected to each other in a daisy-chain configuration, although no terminator is needed. Up to 63 devices can be connected. The more common connector is also a flat, approximately rectangular connector, slightly smaller than the USB-A connector, but the female end of the connector has its internal spacer centrally placed, and one of the narrow ends of the connector is slightly tapered (Figure 2-7). This six-pin connector can provide limited power to the attached device. A smaller, four-pin version of the connector also exists which cannot provide any power to the attached device. The first version of this standard supported communication rates of 400 Mbps (50 MBps). The updated version (IEEE 1394b) doubles this to 800 Mbps (100 MBps) and uses a nine-pin connector. New versions with rates up to 3200 Mbps (400 MBps) will soon be available.

With the increasingly mobile world we live in, some mention should be given here to wireless communications. Three are worthy of brief note. The

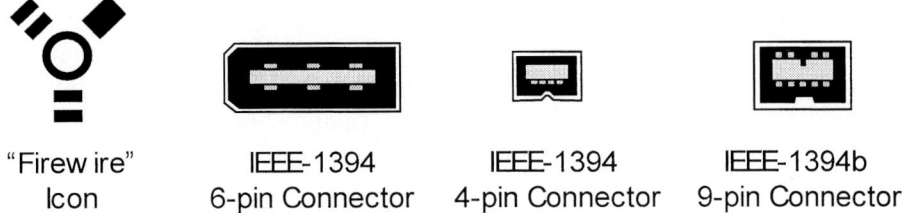

"Firew ire"   IEEE-1394   IEEE-1394   IEEE-1394b
Icon   6-pin Connector   4-pin Connector   9-pin Connector

Figure 2-7: IEEE-1394 (Firewire) icon and connectors. The different versions of the connector each have a different number of contacts. The four-contact connector cannot supply power to the peripheral device. The "Firewire" protocol supports data transfer rates that rival those of parallel communication standards.

first is IrDA (Infrared Data Association), which uses low energy light waves to send information. This is used by television and stereo remote controls, and for transmitting data between personal digital assistants (PDAs). It can be and has been used by desktop computers, but is limited by the fact that it accommodates only line-of-sight transmission, and therefore has not caught on. A second, much more robust wireless communication protocol is IEEE 802.11a-g, sometimes referred to as "Wi-Fi" (*why-figh*) for Wireless Fidelity. This is used for networking, and is discussed in greater detail later.

A wireless communication protocol which is becoming more commonly used to connect desktop computers to peripheral devices like printers and headphones is known as "Bluetooth", developed by a group of electronics manufacturers known as the "Bluetooth Special Interest Group". The code-name "Bluetooth" was taken from a 10th century Danish King. Bluetooth uses the 2.45 GHz frequency band used by some cordless telephones, baby monitors, and garage door openers, and can transmit voice or simulate a serial connection between two devices. The technology is inexpensive (the chip costs less than $5), and is beginning to be incorporated into a large number of devices. The transmission range is relatively short, about 10 meters (30 feet), but this limits interference with other devices. Bluetooth technology is "plug-and-play", in that it requires no intervention by the user. When two devices with Bluetooth chips enter each other's transmission range, they automatically identify themselves and connect to each other. Because Bluetooth is wireless, there probably won't be any connectors on the back of the computer. If a connector is present with the Bluetooth icon by it (Figure 2-8), this is most likely a connection for an external antennae. When simulating a serial connection between a computer and, for example, a printer, communication rates of approximately 1 Mbps (125 KBps) can be attained. This would be painfully slow for transferring data to a mass storage medium, but is actually quite adequate for connecting many peripheral devices (for example, few people can type at speeds of 125 thousand characters per second).

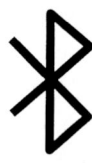

Figure 2-8: Bluetooth icon. Since Bluetooth is a wireless protocol, if a port is labeled with the Bluetooth icon, that connection is for an external antenna.

Input/Output Controllers: Summary

Table 2-3 summarizes the maximum data transfer rate for the various types of communication standards discussed. Keep in mind, however, that these are only the maximum rates attainable with the interface. One must

Table 2-3: Summary of maximum data transfer rates for different input/output communication methods.

	Communication Method	Maximum Data Transfer Rate
Parallel	IDE (ATA-5)	44.4 – 66.7 MBps
	IDE (ATA-6)	100 MBps
	SCSI-2	10-40 MBps
	SCSI-3	160 MBps
Serial	USB 1.1	1.5 MBps
	USB 2.0	60 MBps
	IEEE 1394 (Firewire)	40 MBps
	IEEE 1394b (Firewire 2)	80 MBps
	Bluetooth	0.125 MBps

also keep in mind the data transfer rate of the device connected. For example, if one connects a 1x CD drive (explained below) which has a maximum data transfer rate of 150 KBps, it doesn't matter whether one uses an IDE, SCSI, USB, or Firewire interface, since the maximum transfer rate attainable is limited by the device itself rather than the communication method.

Keep in mind that the transfer rates quoted here can be misleading. The value quoted for the data transfer rate of a given device or connection method refers to the rate for continuous transmission of contiguous chunks of data, and does NOT take into account the time needed to collect that data or to process that data once received, and these can often limit the data exchange rate to well below the quoted maximum data transfer rate.

Peripheral Data Storage Devices

Having discussed the various methods by which peripherals can be connected to a computer, it is worth briefly summarizing the major mass storage devices which exist, since every computer must have one or more of these devices.

The most common of these are magnetic storage devices or disks. Magnetic disks are broadly divided into "floppy" and "hard", based on whether the medium is flexible or not. The contents of these disks are read and written by "heads" which travel radially over the disk. To obtain access to the entire disk, the disk spins beneath the heads. Hard disks can be spun much faster than floppy disks, and therefore have much higher access speeds.

Magnetic disks have to be formatted before data can be written to them. Most come pre-formatted. Unfortunately, the formatting standard used by Intel-based personal computers and Macintosh personal computers is different, so a disk formatted for one of these processors cannot necessarily be read by the other (traditionally, Macintoshes have been able to read floppy disks formatted either for the Macintosh or for an Intel-based PC, whereas Intel-based PC's generally cannot read disks formatted for the Macintosh.)

Floppy disks are rapidly becoming of historical interest only. The first floppy disks were 5.25 inches in diameter and could store 360 KBytes of data. High density 5.25 inch floppies could store 1.2 MBytes. Then came 3.5 inch floppy disks, which were smaller, easier to carry, and less subject to damage, since they were in a hard case. Regular and high density 3.5 inch floppy disks have capacities of 720 KBytes and 1.44 MBytes, respectively. Early floppy disk drives had "custom" connections to the motherboard, but USB floppy drives are now available. The main advantage floppy disks offered over hard disks was that they were removable, in theory allowing for "unlimited" storage capacity on the computer by swapping out disks containing files not currently being used.

The most common magnetic storage medium is the hard disk. Hard disks may consist of one or more "platters", but they are accessed as if they are one logical device, so the specifics of the internal configuration is not of great relevance. As little as 20 years ago, a 10 MByte hard disk was considered large. Now, even laptop computers routinely come with built-in 60 GByte hard disks. Hard disks can be internal or external, and can be connected by essentially any of the communication methods described above. The disk drives themselves are usually sufficiently fast that the maximum data transfer rates attainable are limited only by the communication method being used to connect them to the computer.

Data is stored on disks as blocks of bytes, and has to be read and written in full block increments. The size of the "block" is determined at the time the disk is formatted, and is usually a multiple of 512 bytes. Higher capacity disks tend to have larger blocks. One can see this phenomenon by saving a very small text file on disk, say one containing only a single character, and seeing how much disk space the file takes up. For example, on my 60 GByte hard disk, the minimum file size is 4 KBytes.

The next most common method of mass storage is optical. By far, the most common of these is the compact disc, or CD. There are three basic types of CDs: CD-ROM, CD-R, and CR-RW. Each is analogous to one of three types of ROM: masked ROM, PROM, and Flash ROM, respectively. CD-ROMs (read only) are manufactured with the contents pressed into them. They cannot be written to. CD-R (recordable) discs are manufactured blank and can be written to once, a process known as "burning". Once written, they cannot be erased and rewritten, but they can be read indefinitely. Sometimes, the acronym "WORM" which stands for "Write-Once, Read Many" is used to refer to this type of device. CD-RW (rewritable) discs can be read, erased, and re-written. The erasing and rewriting has to be done in blocks (like Flash ROM), but that is the way magnetic disks work as well. CD-RWs can be used like a hard disk, but they are much slower. CD-RWs started to gain some popularity because of their capacity as a removable medium, but they have been largely replaced by alternate technology. All three types of CDs have a storage capacity of 650 - 700 MBytes, sometimes expressed in minutes (74 minutes − 80 minutes). These times reflect the original use of this medium to store audio: a 650 MByte CD can hold 74 minutes of audio, and a 700 MByte CD can hold 80 minutes of audio.

All CD drives have the ability to read CD-ROMs and already written CD-Rs. The speed of data access for CD drives is often given as "1x", "2x", "8x", "24x", etc. This refers to the data transfer rate relative to the original audio standard. Thus, an "8x" CD drive can read an 80 minute CD in 10 minutes. Those CD drives which can both read CDs and write (burn) CD-Rs often list two speeds in their specifications, such as "8x/16x". In this case, the first speed is the write speed, and the last is the read speed. Finally, CD drives which can read and write both CD-R and CD-RW discs usually list three speeds, traditionally in the order of write/rewrite/read speeds such as "8x/4x/16x". Of course, these speeds refer to maximum speeds, and the actual performance will be somewhat slower. In terms of actual data transfer speeds, a "1x" drive corresponds to approximately 150 KBps (0.15 MBps), so "1x" CD drives are very slow compared to hard disks.

Another optical storage medium is the Digital Video/Versatile Disc, or DVD. DVD writing is more complicated than CD writing, with even more formats, some incompatible with each other. These include DVD-ROM, DVD-R, DVD-RW, DVD-RAM, DVD+R, and DVD+RW. DVD-R and DVD-RAM are the two formats most commonly used for data storage. Like CD-R and CD-RW, DVD-R and DVD-RAM are write-once-read-many and rewritable formats, respectively. The discs are also the same size as CDs. The advantage that DVDs offer over CDs is much higher data storage capacity. The capacity depends upon whether one is using single or double sided discs, and whether one is using single or double layered discs. Single-sided single-layered (SS-SL) discs hold 4.7 GBytes of data. Double-sided single-layered (DS-SL) discs hold twice this amount, 9.4 GBytes. Single-sided double layered (SS-DL) discs hold 8.5 GBytes, because the second layer cannot hold as much data as the first layer. Finally, DS-DL discs have a capacity of 17 GBytes of data, which is more than 24 times the capacity of a CD. As with CD drives, DVD drives can be read only, read-write, and read-write-rewrite. Speeds are also expressed as multiples of the base video standard, which is 1.4 MBps. Thus, a 1x DVD drive is approximately 10 times as fast as a 1x CD drive.

In general, drives which can read DVDs can also read CDs. Writing is another matter, however. Some drives can read or write CDs, but can only read DVDs. Some can read and write both CDs and DVDs, but not re-writable CDs or DVDs. Pay attention to the drives capabilities when selecting one. Both CD and DVD drives come in IDE (ATA), SCSI, USB, and IEEE 1394 varieties.

An issue which has relatively recently become of concern is the life expectancy of CDs and DVDs. Initially, it was thought that these might represent "permanent" storage. Official estimates remain at 100-200 years for both CD-R and DVD-R, with the RW variants lasting only about 25 years. In reality, the lifespan depends upon temperature and humidity. Leaving a disc on the dashboard of a car will significantly shorten its lifespan. With proper care, however, 10-50 years is probably a reasonable expectation for CD-R and DVD-R discs.

One of the most recent peripheral mass storage devices is the "Flash memory drive", also known as a memory-stick. Made of Flash memory (Flash ROM) as described above under "Computer Memory Chips" and usually using a USB communication method, Flash drives are fast, hot-swappable, and come in a variety of capacities, from 128 MBytes up to 1 GByte. They are also "cross-platform", meaning they can be used with either a Macintosh or an Intel-based personal computer. However, because of the technology used, they do wear out after repeated rewriting.

Removable long term storage media

In addition to the peripheral data storage devices discussed above, a number of other devices using removable "cartridge" type disks exist. The first of these were the floppy drives already discussed, but others include Syquest and Zip drives. Removable media devices offer three key advantages over fixed media devices: 1) Increased dynamic storage for day-to-day use (can swap in a removable device corresponding to whatever project is currently being worked on); 2) Archival storage (data which does not need to be constantly available, but isn't ready to be thrown out); and 3) Transporting data from one computer to another

However, each of these functions can also be served, often more successfully, by alternate storage devices. Internal hard drives have become so large, and external hard drives are so cheap that there is less need for increased dynamic storage, and any such need can be met by adding an external Firewire drive, which is routinely faster than removable media drives. CD-R and DVD-R discs are more suited for archival storage of data than rewritable media, and have a large capacity. Finally, data transfer between computers is more rapidly and easily accomplished with Flash drives.

Network Connection

The last component(s) common to essentially all desktop computers is some method to connect to either a local network or to the internet, usually both. Networking allows two or more computers to share information and resources. Depending upon the size and configuration of the network, the "other computer" with which you are communicating could be across the room or across the world. There so many ways to connect to the internet with so many possible configurations, and the number of options is increasing so frequently that they cannot all be discussed here. However, I will mention some of the most common.

First, lets address local networking, which is generally accomplished via additional hardware in the desktop computer known as a Network Interface Card or NIC (*nick*). This card provides an additional port on the back of the computer into which a network cable can be plugged. By far, the most common network communication method currently used by desktop computers is Ethernet. The details of this communication method will be discussed in Chapter 4 on networking, as will other issues related to network design and use. For now, suffice it to say that Ethernet provides for rapid data exchange, originally at 10 Mbps, then 100 Mbps, and now 1 Gbps Ethernet is becoming available. (Note that when discussing data transfer rates over a network connection, it is more conventional to quote rates in bits-per-second rather than Bytes-per-second.) The connector for the Ethernet cable, called an "RJ-45 connector", is similar to a modular telephone jack, only wider (Figure 2-9). The simplest method of connecting to the network is to plug an Ethernet cable into this jack, and the other end into a wall-plate which has been previously wired into an

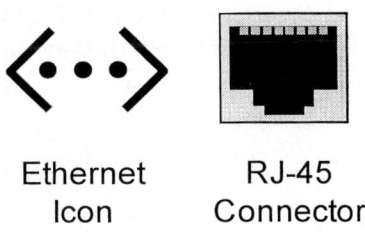

Ethernet   RJ-45
Icon   Connector

Figure 2-9: Ethernet icon and connector. The Ethernet port is used for high speed network connections, including cable modems.

institutional network. This connects your computer to the "Local Area Network" or LAN (*rhymes with can*). That LAN then provides connection to other devices on the network such as other desktop computers, file servers, and networked printers. Also, via this local network, it can be possible to connect to the internet.

In addition to this approach, desktop computers can use a "modem" to connect via other commercial lines such as phone lines or a cable line directly to a company which provides access to the internet. This bypasses any local network, and therefore a modem connection does not provide access to other local devices such as printers.

The most common type of modem is a dial-up modem which uses standard phone lines. A dial-up modem can be either internal to the computer box or external. When internal, an "RJ-11" (standard modular telephone) connection jack will be present on the back of the computer (Figure 2-10). If external, the modem is usually connected to the computer through a serial port. Dial-up modems use your standard telephone line to place a call to a receiving modem at an Internet Service Provider or ISP (*eye-ess-pee*), a company which sells temporary connections to the internet (Figure 2-11). Dial-up modems convert the data to be transmitted into sound and sends that sound along the phone line, similar to a fax machine. To humans, it sounds like static or screeching, but modems can convert this sound back into digital data. One

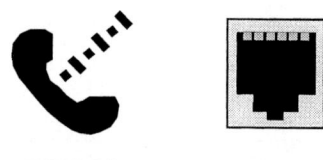

Dial-Up   RJ-11
Modem Icon   Connector

Figure 2-10: Dial-up modem icon and connector. The RJ-11 connector is a standard modular telephone jack.

of two methods is most commonly used to communicate along the phone line. Serial Line Internet Protocol or SLIP (*like one might do on ice*) is an older protocol which did not allow for authentication, and therefore is being replaced by Point-to-Point Protocol or PPP (*pee-pee-pee*). The rate at which data can be transmitted over phone lines is limited by the fact that phone lines can contain a lot of noise. For normal voice transmissions, our brains can filter out that noise and piece together the words being spoken. For digital transmissions, however, every bit of data counts. Therefore, transmission rates cannot be faster than the frequency of the noise. Modern dial-up modems communicate at 28.8 Kbps or even 56.6 Kbps, but those are only maximum transmission rates – the actual rate of data transfer is generally slower.

Other types of modems are available which provide faster transmission rates (Figure 2-11). These include ISDN, cable, and DSL modems. These

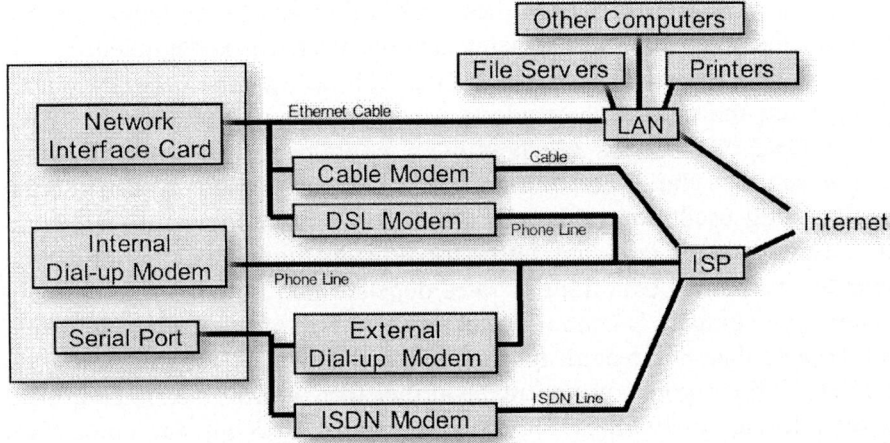

Figure 2-11: Options for connecting a desktop computer to the "internet". A variety of solutions are available. Direct local area network connections allow access to local devices like networked printers. However, a number of different types of modems can be used to obtain an internet connection through an internet service provider. Modems can be internal or external, and connect through a variety of different ports.

modems are rarely built into the computer, since they are either less common or dependent upon standards used by local companies. Integrated Services Digital Network (ISDN) lines are separate lines run by the phone company which can support transmission rates of 128 Kbps. Since these lines are designed specifically for digital transmission, one can usually achieve the advertised 128 Kbps. Special modems are needed when using these lines. They usually connect to a serial port on the computer.

Cable modems use the same cable line which carries television signals. Since this is a direct-wired line, and usually a shielded coaxial cable (unlike phone lines), it can carry data with a greater fidelity and therefore at a faster rate. The speed attainable depends upon the service in your area, but speeds around 1 Mbps are common. Often, the data transfer rates are asymmetric; that is, the rate at which data can be transferred to your computer is different than the rate at which data can be sent from your computer to the internet. The sending or upload rate is generally much slower than the download rate. The fast download speed or "bandwidth" represents the rate between the cable and the cable modem. To attain that speed in the computer, the modem has to connect via a communication method which will support a high data transfer rate. For this reason, most cable modems connect into the Ethernet port of the computer's network interface card or to a USB port. A disadvantage of cable modems is that you and your neighbors share the bandwidth in your area. Therefore, as more and more of your neighbors use cable modems, the overall performance any one user sees is degraded.

Another high-speed option is a Digital Subscriber Line (DSL) modem. DSL lines use the same type of wiring used by regular phone service. Two types of DSL connections are possible. Asymmetric DSL (ADSL) can communicate over the same wire used for telephone service, even while the phone is being used, and is the most common service found in residential areas. Data transfer rates are faster for downloading than for uploading. Maximum theoretical data transfer rates depend upon how far you are from the telephone company's central switch box, with the fastest rates attainable if you are less than 800 feet away, and the slowest rates at 18,000 feet (about 3.5 miles). DSL signals do not travel further than 18,000 feet. Theoretical transfer rates up to 9 Mbps for download and 640 Kbps for upload are attainable. This requires a device installed in your house called a splitter. Another alternative ADSL protocol referred to as "Splitterless DSL" or "G.lite" does not require a splitter at the house, and therefore is easier to install, but has slower data transfer rates (1.5 Mbps for download, 128 Kbps for upload). Symmetrical DSL uses dedicated lines, performs uploads and downloads at the same rate, and can support rates up to 2 Mbps in both directions. This service is usually only available to businesses. Both types of DSL modems traditionally connect into the Ethernet port or USB port on the computer. Since phone lines are not shared with others in your neighborhood, there is no sharing of the bandwidth as occurs with a cable modem.

One final category of networking options which is becoming more popular is wireless connection. Two types of connections are common. In the first, a cellular telephone is used in place of a standard land-line telephone. This phone plugs into either an internal or an external modem. Connection speeds are no better than attainable with a standard dial-up modem, and may in fact be slower owing to the less predictable quality of the cellular connection.

The most common wireless networking standard is known as Wireless Fidelity, or "WiFi" (*why-figh*). The actual name for the communication standard is IEEE 802.11. A WiFi card in the computer transmits to a WiFi base station. WiFi uses the 2.4 GHz frequency range for transmission, the same range used by many cordless telephones. This signal can pass through walls and ceilings/floors, and has a maximum range of about 200 feet. However, cordless phones can interfere with the signal. Since the communication from the computer

Figure 2-12:
Since this is a wireless communication standard, a port marked with this icon is for connecting an external antenna.

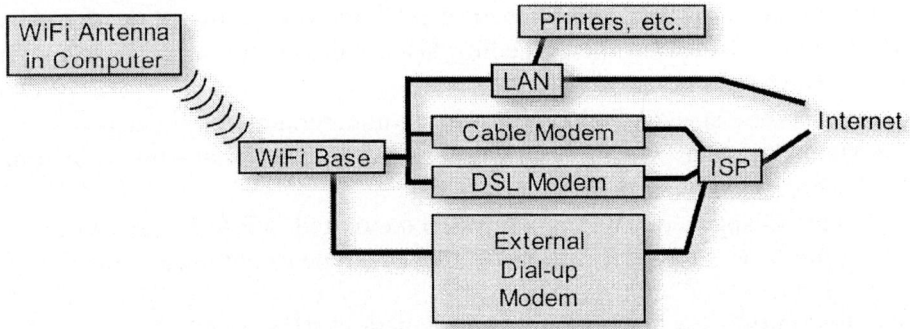

Figure 2-13: Using wireless networking. The best way to think of wireless networking is as a way to place your computer's network card outside of the computer. Anything you might plug into the network card is plugged into the WiFi base station.

is wireless, there is traditionally no port on the computer for this communication method. If a port is present marked with the Wi-Fi icon (Figure 2-12), it is for an external antenna, which can improve the range. Perhaps the best way to think of this wireless communication method is to approach it as a way of placing your computer's network interface card outside of your computer in the WiFi base station. Then, anything which you might plug into your interface card's Ethernet port, such as a connection to a local area network or a cable modem or a DSL modem, can be plugged into the base station, and it acts as if it is plugged directly into your computer (Figure 2-13).

There are a number of WiFi communication standards designated IEEE 802.11b-g. Data transmission rates range from 11 to 54 Mbps for 802.11b to 802.11g, respectively. Keep in mind, however, that the communication rate seen is often limited by what is downstream of the base station. If the base station is connected to a DSL modem, for example, that will limit the communication rate. In addition, most WiFi base stations act as hubs. That is, each station can maintain communication with a number of computers simultaneously. When this is occurring, the connected computers share the downstream bandwidth, potentially further compromising the observed data transfer rate.

Computer Specifications

When evaluating a computer's specifications, there are a relatively small number of core elements which determine the capabilities of the computer. These details constitute the computer "specifications". Most computer manufacturers allow the consumer to select from a range of options for each specification. Based on the preceding discussions, things which one might want to consider would include:

- Processor: "speed", type (architecture), number, amount of cache
- Main Computer Memory: how much RAM?, additional slots for adding more, maximum
- Video Display: maximum resolution supported (VRAM), presence of a processor, support for multiple displays, type of connectors (analog or digital)
- Hard Disk: capacity, communication method (IDE vs SCSI)
- CD/DVD: read only or read/write or read/write/rewrite
- I/O Connection port options: number and type (SCSI, USB, Firewire)
- Network Interface Card: speed, protocol
- Built in modem (if needed)
- Built in Wireless networking
- Expansion slots (ability to add more electronics, like a Bluetooth card)

Chapter 3

DESKTOP COMPUTERS: SOFTWARE

In computer terms, software includes any part of the computer system which is not in and of itself tangible (so "soft" is a bit of an over statement). Note that the ability to touch media used to store software, such as CDs, removable magnetic disks, or even paper, does not make it tangible.

All software must be loaded into memory before it can be executed, used, or accessed. Therefore, CDs and disks are simply storage locations for the software. Software is not used directly from its storage medium. However, it is generally not necessary to load the entire software file into memory at one time – only the portion or portions which are being used need to be in memory. This allows computers to run very large application programs which are too large to fit into memory all at once.

Software can be divided into two large groups: executable and non-executable. Some restrict the use of the word "software" to executable files, referring to the non-executable files as simply data. However, a file which is executable on one system may not be executable on another, and then would become data. Also, command files and other scripts are not executable per se, but when processed by the operating system do result in the execution of commands. For this reason, I prefer to consider all files to be software.

Executable Software

Executable software is composed of a series of machine-language commands, specific for a particular processor, which can be fed directly into the processor and are responsible for everything the computer "does". Executable software can be roughly divided into system software and application software. System software represents the core elements which the computer needs to run. They create the environment and access to resources which application software then uses to accomplish specific tasks.

An application is an executable computer program which creates and/or manipulates data files. By convention, the term is used to distinguish programs which run within an operating system (applications) from programs which are part of the operating system.

Operating Systems

The main component of the system software is the operating system itself. This is what gives the computer its look-and-feel. Examples of operating systems include DOS, Windows 98, Windows NT, Windows 2000, Windows XP, Mac OS 9, Mac OS X, Unix, Linux, etc. Operating systems are invariably complex, and can even be layered. For example, Windows 98 runs within a DOS shell, whereas Windows XP does not, and Mac OS X runs within a Unix shell, whereas Mac OS 9 does not. It is through the operating system interface that users interact with the computer, request files from the attached storage locations, and run the computer programs which have been installed. All of the software is built upon the operating system, which is perhaps why the operating system is often referred to as the "platform" (as in "this program was written for the Mac OS X platform").

The details of what makes one operating system different from another are beyond the scope of this text. However, I should comment briefly on the ongoing search for the "best operating system". A lot of quite bright individuals have spent a surprisingly large amount of time arguing over which operating system is better than another. In many respects, I consider this argument akin to arguing over which is the best religion: at some level, they all address the same issues, albeit in somewhat different ways, and probably the factor most influencing your choice is which one you were brought up with. Also, not unlike religions, there are some zealots and some individuals which can easily transition from one operating system to another without much notice or concern. Granted, some operating systems have traditionally been known for "expertise" in certain areas. For example, the Macintosh initially was far ahead of Windows operating systems with respect to integrated graphics capabilities, but that "lead" has largely dissipated. From a practical point of view, however, your choice of operating system will be largely determined by your environment and by what applications you need to run. For a work computer, your department or institution may have pre-determined rules about which operating systems they will and will not support. Although you still have freedom to choose whatever operating system you want for your home computer, most people try to match whatever they have at work, to facilitate transferring information back and forth, and to eliminate the need to learn how to do everything two different ways. As for applications, although most basic types of applications like word processing software and presentation software are available for many operating systems (platforms), custom applications such as pathology information systems are traditionally built for a specific platform, and if you want to use a specific information system, you will have to use the platform for which it was written.

Operating systems are written to be run on specific processors. The bytes which make up the code for the operating system contain instructions which must be compatible with the instruction set of the processor. As new versions of a processor become available, the instruction set for that processor evolves. New versions of the operating system are developed to take advantage of those new instructions. Therefore, when a new processor becomes available, if the instruction set for that processor is different than its predecessor, a new version of the operating system will most likely be required.

Operating System Add-ons

It is never possible, when writing an operating system, to consider in advance all of the things which that operating system might be asked to do. In addition, one would rather not have to release a new version of the operating system every time a new disk drive or monitor becomes available on the market. Therefore, most operating systems are designed with the flexibility to add-in support for future needs. The two main types of add-on supporting software are device drivers and services.

Device Drivers

Device drivers address the need created by the fact that computer components are manufactured by many different companies, and they do not always operate in the same fashion. In much the same way as processors have their own unique instruction sets, devices created by different manufacturers have to receive commands in different ways to perform tasks. For example, the way in which data files are stored on a brand X's disk drive may be very different than they way files are stored on brand Y's CD-ROM drive. The operating system has a generic request: "get me the file named ABC and put it in memory at location D". For brand X's disk drive, this might mean looking up the file in the directory located at one part of the disk, finding out what physical location the file starts at, going to that location, reading that disk block, finding out from it where the next part of the file is stored, etc. For brand Y's CD-ROM drive, the same request might mean spinning up the CD if it is not already spinning, looking up the file in its directory located at a specific sector, finding the location and size of the file which is known to consist of consecutive sectors, and then reading those sectors. Device drivers are generally small programs (relatively speaking) which translate generic system requests into hardware specific requests. They are specific both for the operating system in which they will run and the device which they are expected to control. When a manufacturer creates a new device, it also writes a driver for that device. When you connect that device to your system, you have to install the driver for that device into your operating system so that the operating system will know how to access that device. All communication between the operating system and the device passes through the device driver.

The modularity of device drivers not only allows users to add support for devices which did not exist at the time the operating system was written, but

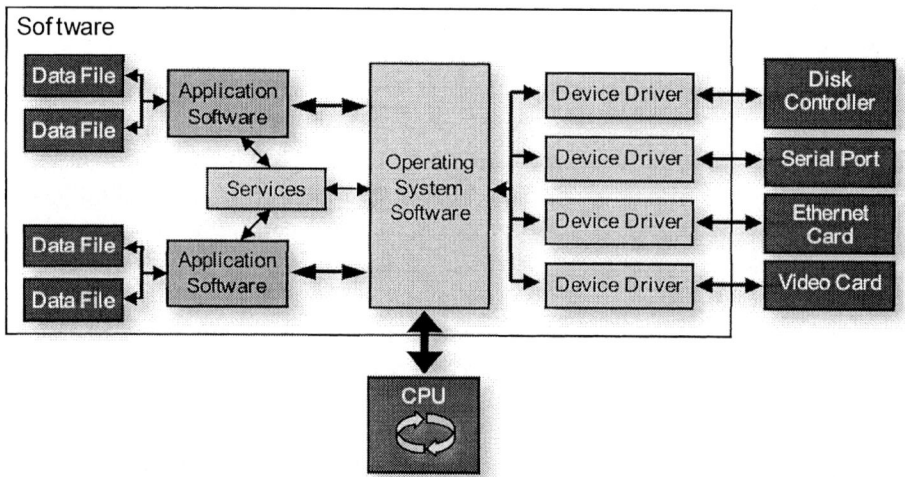

Figure 3-1: Simplified diagram showing the inter-relationship of the various types of executable software. All access to the central processing unit (CPU) goes through the operating system. Application software stores information in data files. Applications can communicate with each other through operating system services, and communicate with devices via device-specific drivers.

also allows operating systems to be smaller. Rather than building into the operating system compatibility with all known devices, drivers for those devices can be provided separately, and the user installs only those drivers which correspond to the devices which they have connected to the computer.

All of the standard input/output connection ports built into the computer such as the USB port and the Firewire port described in Chapter 2 on "Hardware" have associated with them generic drivers. These drivers support a series of the most common commands used by devices, and provide those commands using a standardized method. Many manufacturers of external devices design their devices to accept these standardized commands. When this is the case, no special driver needs to be installed to operate the device, since the already present generic driver will suffice. In this instance, the device is often referred to a "plug-and-play", because the user simply has to connect it and can start using it without any set up or configuration required.

Services

A second type of operating system add-on is known as a "service". This is a less well defined concept than the device driver. Whereas device drivers allow the operating system to communicate with specific hardware devices, services allow one piece of software, either an application or the operating system itself, to communicate with another. Examples of services might include things like web serving, file sharing, or task scheduling. Many of these appear, in practice, to be so fundamental to the operation of the computer that they are viewed as being part of the operating system itself, but they actually represent add-on functionalities which generally can be configured or even turned off.

Application Software

Application software is essentially a computer program written to perform a certain task, usually involving the creation and manipulation of some sort of data file. Applications may consist of a single file or a collection of multiple files, some storing data needed to run the application. Because of this, the term "application" is preferred over "computer program", since when one thinks of a "program" one thinks of a single file, whereas "application" refers to the entire collection of files needed to do what the program was designed to do. However, "application" specifically excludes the files which store the user's data. For example, a word processing program, including any associated dictionaries or settings files, constitute an application, but the files created containing the user's letters or documents are not part of the application.

Just as operating systems are designed to run with specific versions of a processor, application software is written to run with particular versions of an operating system. Applications interact with the operating system, and the operating system must therefore support those interactions. However, whereas a change in the processor instruction set almost always requires a new version of the operating system, a new version of the operating system may not require a new version of the application software. This is because the operating system can protect the application from changes in the processor by translating processor changes internally so that the applications themselves do not have to change. In general, the evolution of operating systems involves the addition of new features rather that removing older features. Therefore, operating system vendors try to preserve what is known as "backward compatibility"; that is, the operating system is compatible with previous versions of itself. This means that applications written to run in an older version of an operating system are likely to run in a new version of the operating system. However, applications written for the new version of an operating system will not necessarily be able to run under older versions of the operating system. This makes sense, since the application may use new features of an operating system or processor which were not present in older versions. Sometimes, the changes in the processor or the design of the operating system are so fundamental that backward compatibility cannot be preserved. When that happens, you will have to purchase new versions of the application software which are compatible with the new operating system. However, be cautious about buying a new version of either the operating system or the application software just because it is available; as described below, this may introduce incompatibilities with previous documents. If you are not forced to upgrade by external factors (you are a member of a group, and everyone else has upgraded) or by hardware changes (you need to use new hardware which does not run with the previous software version), critically evaluate what the new software offers, and whether or not you really need that feature, since upgrading can take a lot of time and introduce more problems than it is worth.

Computer Programming

Rest assured, this section will not try to teach you how to write computer programs; that is well beyond the scope of this book. However, understanding the process can be helpful not only in understanding the terminology used but also in determining why some programs can be run under multiple operating systems whereas others cannot.

Computer programs, just like any other executable software, must be converted into machine language compatible with the instruction set of the particular processor on which they will be run in order to be executed. There are no exceptions to this. However, the programming environment used and the computer language chosen determine whether that conversion happens in advance, or at the last minute (more accurately, at the last microsecond, or nanosecond).

Computer programs are generally written using simple text editors, and the programs themselves are simply text files. The programming "language" chosen (discussed more below) determines how that text file needs to be formatted, what command words can be used, and what structure those commands need to conform to. Collectively, these rules are known as the "syntax" for the language. The resulting file or files produced, written in the syntax of the language chosen, constitute the **source code** for the computer program. Source code is considered "human readable" because it is composed of letters, numbers, and symbols which will make sense to anyone familiar with the computer language in which the program was written. Of course, the central processing unit of the computer cannot execute the program in this form. Each line of the source code must first be converted into the machine instructions needed to perform the task represented by that command. The machine instructions which result from this conversion constitute the **object code** for that program. This conversion is most commonly done by a special computer program known as a "compiler".

Compilers are specific both for the computer language used in the source code and for the machine language needed in the object code (which is determined by the CPU which will be asked to run the program). The compiler goes through each line of the source code, verifies and interprets the syntax, and then produces the corresponding object code. Depending upon the computer language chosen, each line of the source code may produce five or six machine instructions, or hundreds to thousands of machine instructions. The object code itself is not editable: even if someone were to go through the object code byte by byte and cross reference a translation of the machine instructions used by a particular CPU, the slightest modification is likely to disrupt the relative locations of various parts of the object code to itself and result in nonsensical instructions for the processor. If/when one asks the processor to execute a machine instructions which is not properly constructed, the processor stops processing, resulting in a system crash. Therefore, if one wants to modify a computer program, one makes the modification in the source code, and then recompiles the source code to generate new object code. This separation of the modifiable source code from executable object code is what has allowed programmers to preserve their intellectual property. When the user buys a computer program, they are generally provided only with the object code, and therefore they cannot make any modifications to it without collaborating with the author/owner of the source code. De-compiling object code, sometimes referred to as reverse engineering, in order to try to produce a modifiable source is essentially impossible, and is specifically prohibited by the license agreements used by most software vendors.

If the computer program is simple enough, the same source code might be compilable by different CPU specific compilers to produce multiple CPU specific object codes (Figure 3-2). In this way, the "same program" could run on multiple platforms (operating systems). However, in this case, it is not really the same program which is being run on the different platforms,

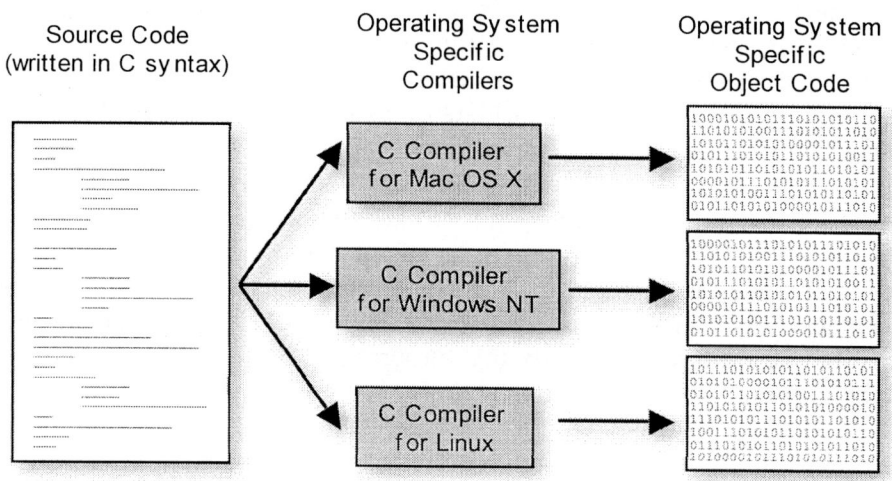

Figure 3-2: Relationship between source code and object code. Source code is text, written in a language-specific syntax. Source code is therefore essentially operating system independent. Operating system specific compilers convert source code into operating system specific object code, which is directly executable, but only on the operating system for which it was compiled.

but rather different object codes produced from the same source code. This can be done in one of two ways. Initially, source code files were simply flat text files (this term is described in greater detail below, but simply means the files consist only of text without any formatting or other coded information). Flat text files can be moved from one platform to another. If a programmer writes a computer program in C (a computer language) as a flat text file, he/she can compile that on a Macintosh using a C compiler to produce object code which will run on the Macintosh. He/she can then copy the source code file to a Windows machine, use a Windows specific C compiler, and produce object code which will run under Windows. Since most of the popular computer languages are available for most platforms, this is a relatively simple process.

However, many computer programs are not written as simple flat text files, but rather as more complicated files produced from within a more complex program known as an Integrated Development Environment, or IDE (*eye-dee-eee*). IDEs have the source code text editing capabilities, the compiler, and often multiple debugging tools all built into one program. The source code files produced by these IDEs generally cannot be simply moved from one platform to another. However, the IDEs often have multiple compilers, some of which can produce object code for different operating systems, often referred to as "cross-compilers". Thus, one can use one operating system to develop and maintain the source code (the development operating system), yet produce object code which can only be run on a different operating system (the target operating system). A single source code can then be used to produce multiple object codes targeted to different operating systems.

Although this one-source to many-objects model would be ideal for software developers, since they would only have to maintain one source code but could still sell object code to users of multiple different computer platforms, this model usually breaks down. Most complex software draws upon operating-system specific libraries, as is usually needed for the graphical user interface, and appropriate libraries with identical capabilities may not be available for all desired target operating systems. When this happens, developers are forced to maintain different platform-specific versions of the source code, which is why the "same" application may have slightly different capabilities when run from one platform rather than another.

The process of converting source to executable object code can actually be a little more complex than described, and in fact three approaches are commonly used (Figure 3-3). The one already described is a one-step pre-compiling: the entire source code is converted to processor specific object code and stored in an executable file. At run time, this pre-compiled object code is simply executed by the CPU. Alternatively, no preprocessing of the source code is done. Rather, at execution time, each line of the source code is translated, one line at a time, into processor specific machine code by an **interpreter**. That machine code is then executed, and the interpreter moves on to the next line. This process is slower than pre-compiling the whole source code, especially for loops where the same line of source code is translated over and over again for each iteration of the loop. However, it can be advantageous during the development stage. Compiling a large program can be time consuming, taking minutes. When developing or debugging a portion of the code, it is frequently necessary to make small changes and then re-run the code. Using an interpreter does not require completely re-compiling the entire source code, and portions of the program which are not being executed do not have to be translated. It is not uncommon to use an interpreter during development and then a compiler when the program is complete.

A third approach which is becoming more popular is a combination of the above two, and adds the feature of processor independence. In this approach, the source code is pre-compiled to an intermediate, processor independent point referred to as bytecode. This is based on the concept that although each operating system has its own look-and-feel, the elements of the user interface are very similar, and include such things as windows,

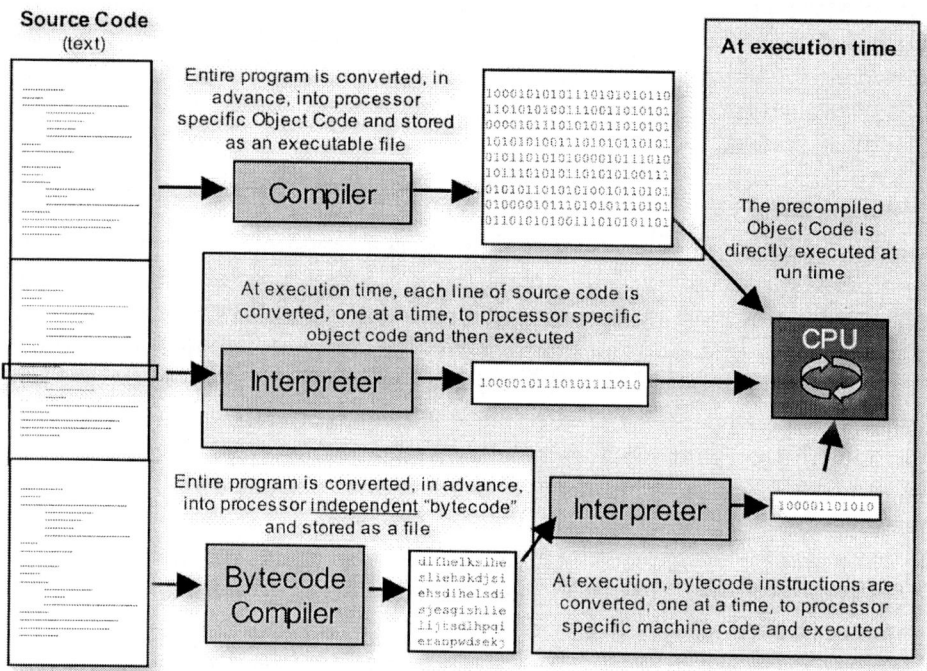

Figure 3-3: Execution of computer programs. Computer programs, written as source code in text, can be executed in one of three ways. A compiler can pre-convert the entire program into executable object code, which at run time can be directly executed by the processor. Alternatively, at run time, each line of the source code can be individually translated into object code by an interpreter and then executed. Finally, the source code can be pre-converted to a processor independent "bytecode", which is then converted to processor specific object code at execution time.

icons, buttons, and scroll bars. These concepts can be represented in the bytecode in a processor independent fashion. At execution time, this bytecode is then linked to a processor specific library which does the final translation step into processor specific machine code which can then be executed.

Perhaps the best example of a language using a bytecode compiler is Java. With the appropriate versions of the Java Runtime libraries, the same bytecode file can be executed on different operating systems. This is what allows Java "applets" (mini-applications) to run in web browsers on multiple different platforms. The speed of execution is intermediate between that of fully compiled object code and interpreted source code.

Computer Languages

Computer programs are written in any of a number of different computer languages. For the most part, computer languages are pretty similar, in that they do essentially the same sort of things. (In much the same way that different human languages are simply different ways of expressing concepts which are common to all societies.) For example, all computer languages have variables which can store data, procedures for assigning values to these variables and manipulating those values, conditional expressions (do X only if Y is true), loops (do X, and continue to do X until Y is true), and some mechanism for interacting with the user. The details of how these are accomplished, and the level of control the programmer has over these interactions is what makes one language different from another. Specific computer languages are designed to offer different levels of control, and are optimized for different tasks (Figure 3-4). "Low level languages" use

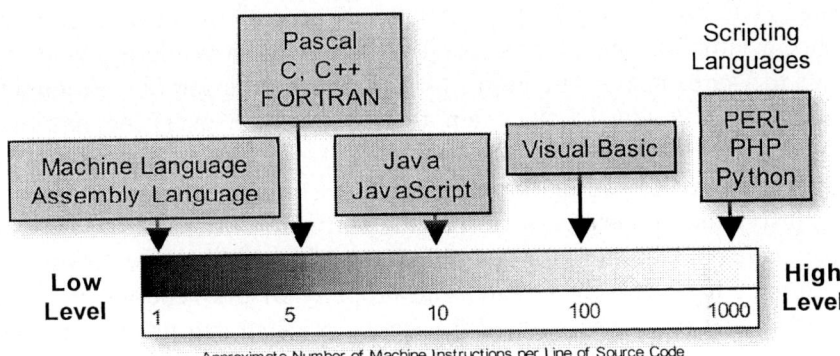

Figure 3-4: Spectrum of computer languages. Computer languages are often divided, rather arbitrarily, into "low" or "high" level, based on how much "work" can be accomplished with each line of source code. In reality, this is actually a spectrum, and many languages are designed to accomplish some tasks, like computation, more easily than others.

instructions which are relatively close to machine language instructions. These programs take a long time to develop. The source code is very long, because many lines of source program are required to do relatively simple tasks. In addition, the programs usually have to handle their own memory management and device management needs. The advantage is that, when properly written, the programs compile into very efficient object code, and will generally perform tasks at rates of 10 to 100 times that of comparable programs written in a high level language. Therefore, low level languages are the preferred choice for programs which do extensive computations. In contrast, "high level languages" allow the source code to contain single instructions which represents large blocks of machine language instructions. As such, a lot can be accomplished with relatively few lines of source code, so the source code tends to be smaller, and the development time for an application can be much shorter. However, the corresponding object code tends to be large and inefficient. Execution can be slower and require more memory. This used to be a major drawback when processors were slow and memory was expensive, but the modern processors and cheaper memory have allowed many developers to take advantage of the more rapid development cycles allowed by the higher level languages.

Software Licensing

All commercial software is sold with a license agreement. This is the small type printed all over the sealed envelope containing the installation CD, and the screen-full of small type displayed when the user installs the software. The user is required to click on "I accept" in order to continue with the installation, and this is usually done without reading any of the terms of the agreement. Therefore, in part as a public service, I thought I would touch on a few of the main things to which everyone has been agreeing.

Most software license agreements contain a phrase similar to "grant a non-exclusive individual license to use the software". Despite the fact that you may have paid a lot of money, you have not actually acquired ownership of anything. The software remains the property of the vendor. For your investment, you have been granted the rights to install and use the software on one computer. Sometimes, even the media upon which the software is sold remains the property of the vendor. Usually, you are restricted from reselling, renting, or sublicensing the software to anyone else. Some agreements allow you to transfer ownership to another, providing you remove all copies of the software from your own computer. All software license agreements restrict you from attempting to decompile, reverse engineer, or otherwise convert the software to a "human-perceivable" form, that is, to attempt to covert the provided object code back into source code.

One way in which software license agreements can differ is in the number of copies they allow you to install and use. Some specifically state you can install the software on only one computer. Others allow installation on two computers, both of which are primarily used by the purchaser, with the understanding that two people will not use the program at the same time on two different computers. Examples of this would be installing the software on both a home and office computer (presumably a person can only be in one of the two places at a time), or a desktop and a portable computer.

Some license agreements are designed for multi-user environments, and may specify the number of computers or number of simultaneous users rather than the number of individual users.

The internet has become a very common way of distributing software. Users can go to a developers web site, enter a credit card number, and download a copy of the software specific for their operating system. There is a good deal of instant gratification associated with this practice. If you are not sure whether or not you want to buy the software, many vendors offer a demonstration or trial version of their software which can be downloaded for free. This version will have several of the key features of the package turned off, like the ability to save files or to print, but give the user an opportunity to determine whether or not the software will meet their needs. If it looks promising, paying the purchase price will get you either a fully functioning version, or a key-code to convert your demonstration copy into a fully functioning version. Vendor web sites are also a good place to look for free upgrades or bug-fixes for your already purchased and licensed software.

Other models for software distribution exist. "Shareware" is software developed usually by a single individual, often as a hobby rather than a profession. It is generally distributed via the internet or in software bundles which are given out by the larger software vendors packaged along with their own products. Shareware is software distributed on the honor system. You can generally download a fully functional version of the product to try out. If you find you like it and plan to continue using it, there is usually an address to which you are asked to send a small fee, usually on the order of $20 - $50 dollars, to support the developer's efforts. In my opinion, this is a great way to encourage the development of useful software solutions which may not have sufficiently large markets to attract the major vendors, and I encourage individuals who take advantage of shareware to actually pay the requested fee.

"Freeware", like shareware, is distributed as fully functional software, but the developer has no expectation of receiving any fee. Although there are a few real gems to be found here, in most cases you get what you have paid for.

"Open Source" software has been around for many years, and recently is beginning to become more popular. Open source software is free, and as its name implies you can download not only the object code but also the source code. The bulk of the initial development is usually done by an individual or a small group of individuals, but then others continue and add to the development process. Since any user can download the source, any user (with the appropriate level of knowledge) can modify and enhance/improve the software, or customize it for a particular purpose. The individuals involved in creating and enhancing open source software, needless to say, comprise a relatively small cross section of society, but the multi-user development can result in rapid testing, debugging, and advancement of the product. Examples of the great success of the open source approach include the Linux operating system, Apache web server, PHP (a server-side web programming language), Perl, Python, and MySQL.

Open source development embraces a philosophy very different from that of commercial software vendors. In addition to the obvious difference in price, commercial software is driven by two incentives: lock in a user base, and constantly add new features to attract new purchases. Locking in a user base is a natural result of storing information in a proprietary format. If you have hundreds of documents created with brand X word processor, and those documents can only be opened from brand X word processor, you are going to be somewhat reluctant to switch to brand Y word processor. Some vendors use interlocking software packages to promote sales of their other products. Additionally, absence of "forward-compatibility" can be important in driving software purchases. Assume a large number of users share documents created with version n of brand X software. The vendor comes out with version n+1, and a few of the users buy it. The new version of the software can open documents created with the old version, but the old version cannot open documents created with the new version. Once documents created with the new version start circulating among the group, everyone in the group must buy the new version if they want to be able to continue to share documents. How do vendors get users to buy new versions: features. Commercial software development is driven by the incorporation of new features. If people are happy with the software they have, they won't buy new software. Therefore, bigger and better software must continually be developed to not only attract new customers, but also to entice existing customers to upgrade. Unfortunately, the incentive to introduce new features is often at the cost of quality control and user support. In contrast, the driving force behind open source development is quality and elegance. Since this is not a commercial venture, these developers are driven by pride in their work, and distributing their product is a way of showing off their skill. There is less focus on esoteric "bells-and-whistles", since the thought is that individual end users will customize the product locally to meet their specific needs.

One of the major drawbacks with open source software is support. Often, it is not clear who to contact if you have a problem. There may be many unrelated developers, and they are often only minimally interested in trying to determine why a particular user is having trouble figuring out how to make the software work, especially if that user is perceived as a novice. To address this need, a number of user-groups and electronic mail list-serves have sprung up where users can post their questions and more than likely find a sympathetic ear in another user who had a similar problem.

Some controversy exists about the role of open source software in medical environments. Certainly, the low initial cost ($0) is very attractive to members of the healthcare industry, but the concern about long-term support for a mission-critical application is a very real one. Reputable commercial vendors who have been around for a while are likely to continue to be around for a while, and although you may have to pay dearly for it, you can probably be pretty sure that support will be available. In contrast, some open source projects have not caught on, and are eventually abandoned by their developers. For this reason, I would caution against committing a mission-critical solution to new open source ventures. However, if the open source software has been around for a long time, especially if it has developed a strong user base, it is probably safe to assume that even if the initial developers lose interest, someone else will pick up where they left off. I have often heard concern expressed about the fact that since the source code for open source software is freely available, unscrupulous individuals may use that source code to identify security vulnerabilities and compromise the integrity of the data, a risk too great for healthcare information. This has not really been a problem in the open source world, and the protection of the healthcare information depends not on the software itself but rather upon access to the software from outside the institution, something firewalls have been very successful at controlling. Finally, as one who has had to make this choice more than once, I am personally uncomfortable with storing data in a proprietary format which requires the continued cooperation of a vendor for me to maintain access. For example, I am reluctant to advocate for a document archiving system in which the archives can only be interpreted by a particular vendor's software. Even if the vendor has been around for many years, I don't want to get five or ten years of documents locked away in a proprietary format and be subject to a vendor making a business decision that they are no longer going to support access from a particular platform, or that the cost of that access is going to double. Therefore, I much prefer using standardized formats for long term data storage – files which can be opened and read by software from a number of vendors. Some of these file formats are discussed later in this chapter.

Non-Executable Software

Non-executable software includes data files, such as text documents, images, and databases, and "resources" such as fonts, icons, and dialog boxes. It is difficult to discuss data files in general, since there is so much variation in what their contents might represent. However, it is worth considering the general way in which data is stored in a computer, since this discussion will be relevant no matter what operating system or application program you are using.

Digital Data Representation

As introduced in Chapter 2 during the discussion of memory, all information stored in a computer is stored in binary form. The base unit of storage is the byte, and data is stored as either a sequence of bytes or a combination of bytes. Each type of data which can be represented digitally is stored in a slightly different format. For most purposes a user does not have to concern himself or herself with the actual format for the data storage. After all, if one wants to store a value in a variable or in a database, one simply provides the value, and expects to get the same value back when requested. However, understanding a little about the data storage can help in designing the best solution for a problem, and is crucial for many types of data-mining operations.

Storage of Integer Data

Integers are the most straight forward. Integers are stored digitally simply as their binary repre-sentation. When expressed in binary format, this is invariably shown with the most significant bit on the left and the least significant bit on the right, just as one would for a decimal number. If one byte (8 bits) is used to represent an unsigned integer, than any value from 0 to 255 (2^8-1) can be stored (Figure 3-5, top). If two bytes are used to store the integer, values from 0 to 65535 are possible.

	Binary	Decimal
	2^7 2^6 2^5 2^4 2^3 2^2 2^1 2^0	
Unsigned Integer	**01011011** =	91
	11011011 =	219
	S 2^6 2^5 2^4 2^3 2^2 2^1 2^0	
Signed Integer	**01011011** =	+91
	11011011 =	-37

Figure 3-5: Unsigned and signed integers. Unsigned integers are expressed simply in their binary form. For signed integers, the highest order bit represents the sign, but the absolute value of the number is expressed in two's complement.

Four bytes allows values from 0 to 4,294,967,295 (Table 3-1). This number came up before in our discussion of memory addressing. Recall that 32 bit memory addressing (4 bytes) allowed

Table 3-1: Integer storage.

# Bytes used	Range for Unsigned Integer	Range for Signed Integer
1	0 – 255	-127 – +127
2	0 – 65,535	-32,767 – +32,767
4	0 – 4,294,967,295	-2,147,483,647 – +2,147,483,647

The range of possible integers which can be stored is determined both by the number of bytes used and by whether or not the integer is signed.

addressing up to a maximum of 4 gigabytes of memory. (See Chapter 2 under "Main Memory").

Alternatively, to be able to express both positive and negative numbers, one of the bits has be used to indicate the sign. The most significant bit is used to represent the sign of the number, with a zero representing positive and a one representing negative (Figure 3-5, bottom). For a one byte (8 bit) signed integer, this leaves 7 bits to store an actual number, thus allowing values from -127 to +127 to be stored. Two bytes, signed, allow values from –32,767 to +32,767 (the sign bit is only on the most significant byte) (Table 3-1). In many programming languages, 2 byte signed integers are referred to as short integers and 4 byte signed integers are referred to as long integers.

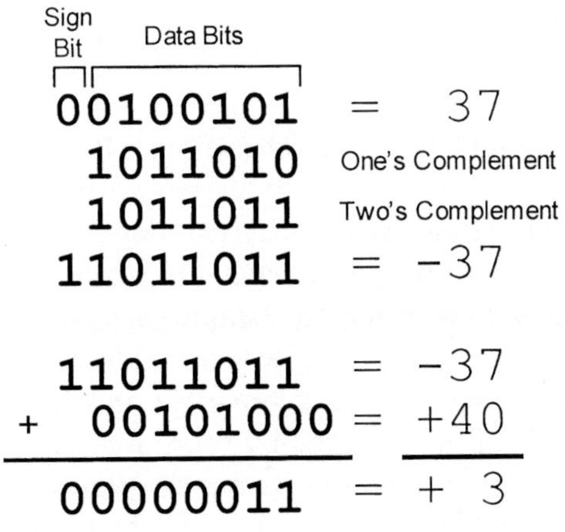

Storing a negative number is not as simple as expressing the number the way one would express the positive version of the number, and then setting the sign bit on. Rather, one expresses the absolute value of the number as its "two's complement". To do this, you start with the binary representation of the absolute value of the number (see Figure 3-6). Then, a "one's complement" is created by flipping each of the data bits to their complementary value (zeros become ones, ones become

```
Sign
Bit     Data Bits
00100101  =   37
 1011010   One's Complement
 1011011   Two's Complement
11011011  = -37

11011011  = -37
+ 00101000 = +40
─────────────
00000011  = + 3
```

Figure 3-6: Negative integers. Negative integers are expressed in two's complement notation. This allows the negative numbers and positive numbers to be added with standard binary arithmetic without the need for special procedures.

zeros). To convert from a one's complement to a two's complement, you simply add one. Then, set the sign bit and you are done. Why would anyone want to store negative numbers in such a complicated way? The reason is because this allows mathematical operations to work the same way for both positive and negative numbers. In the example shown in Figure 3-6, consider adding 40 to the −37 stored in two's complement. Simple addition as one would do for two positive numbers yields the correct result. (Remember, this is binary addition: 1 plus 1 equals 10, which is "zero, carry the one". The left-most carried "1" is "lost" off the end.)

Note that whereas using an unsigned one byte integer permits 256 different values, a signed one byte integer permits only 255 possible values, since there is no difference between negative and positive zero. Whether the stored binary number is interpreted as an unsigned integer or a signed integer is determined by the program storing/using the value; there is nothing specific about the storage which would allow one to determine in which context the byte is being used. Thus, as shown in Figure 3-5, there is no way to tell simply by looking at the data storage of "11011011" whether this is meant to represent 219 or −37.

Essentially all operating system store and interpret integers in the same way, once one knows how many bytes were used to store the integer, and whether it is a signed integer or an unsigned one. The only variation, for multiple byte integers, is the order in which the bytes are stored. Refer to the "little-endian"/"big-endian" discussion from Chapter 2 for determining which is the most significant byte.

Storage of Floating Point Data (Real Numbers)

Real numbers can take on an infinite number of possible values. It is not possible to represent an infinite number of values digitally. Therefore, real numbers are usually stored as approximations with different degrees of "precision". The more bytes used for the value, the greater the precision. Thus, different programming languages may refer to "single precision" (usually 4 bytes) and "double precision" (usually 8 bytes) variables. Of course, real numbers which can be exactly represented in binary form with a small number of digits, such as the result of one divided by four, are stored exactly. However, values whose decimal representation is not simple, such as the result of one divided by three, are stored as approximations. Note that some fractional numbers which can be easily represented in decimal notation, such as 0.2, can only be approximated in binary notation.

The digital storage of floating point numbers is a little obscure. As with signed integers, the reason for this rather complex method of storing floating point numbers is because it facilitates mathematical calculations. Floating point numbers are stored in three parts: a sign bit, an exponent, and a

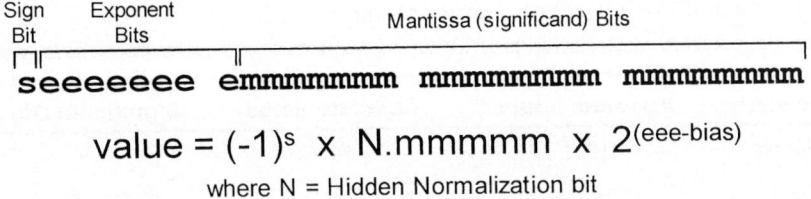

$$\text{value} = (-1)^s \times N.mmmmm \times 2^{(eee-bias)}$$

where N = Hidden Normalization bit

Figure 3-7: A generic single precision floating point number. The binary representation of floating point numbers includes a sign bit, an exponent, and a mantissa. Determining the value requires knowing how many bits are used for each part, as well as knowing the normalization bit and the bias.

"significand", also known as the mantissa or fraction. In a typical 32-bit (4 byte) single precision number, the most significant bit of the first word is the sign bit, followed by 8 bits for the exponent, followed by 23 bits for the mantissa. The sign bit, as for integers, uses zero for positive and one for negative. The 8-bit exponent is stored with a "bias" of 127 resulting in a convention called "excess-127". That means you store, as the exponent, a value which is 127 greater than the exponent you actually want. This is done because, to express fractional values, one may need a negative exponent. To indicate an exponent of "1", one stores "128". Storage of "126" indicates an exponent of "-1". The exponent stored is the power of 2, not of ten (two is referred to as the "radix" of the notation). To obtain the significand or mantissa, one first needs to express the number in binary exponential notation and then "normalize" it so that there is only one "1" to the left of the decimal point. Then, the fractional part of the normalized number is stored as the significand, using as many binary digits as are needed or available, beginning at the most significant bit of the significand. Since the normalized value will always start with "1.", the one is usually assumed and not stored, resulting in a "hidden" normalized bit. This effectively means that whereas for integers, the "values" of the bits from the

seeeeeee emmmmmmmm mmmmmmmmm mmmmmmmmm

00111111 10000000 00000000 00000000 $(-1)^0 \times 1.0000_2 \times 2^{(127-127)} = 1.000 \times 2^0 = 1.00$

11000000 01000000 00000000 00000000 $(-1)^1 \times 1.1000_2 \times 2^{(128-127)} = -1.500 \times 2^1 = -3.00$

01000000 10111000 00000000 00000000 $(-1)^0 \times 1.0111_2 \times 2^{(129-127)} = 1.4375 \times 2^2 = 5.75$

Figure 3-8: Sample floating point numbers. These numbers are stored with a bias of 127 and a hidden normalization bit of 1.

Table 3-2: Real (Floating point) number storage.

# Bytes (Precision)	Smallest Non-zero Absolute Value	Largest Non-Infinite Absolute Value	Approximate # of Significant Digits
2 (Single)	10^{-38}	10^{38}	7
4 (Double)	10^{-308}	10^{308}	16

The range of possible real values depends on the precision of the storage, as well as other specifications which vary from operating system to operating system. Single precision numbers, in general, provide about 7 decimal significant digits, where as double precision numbers allow for about 16.

least-significant to the most significant are 2^0, 2^1, 2^2, 2^3, ..., for the significand, the values of the bits from the most-significant to the least significant are 2^{-1}, 2^{-2}, 2^{-3}, 2^{-4}, ... Figure 3-7 shows how to obtain the value of a floating point number, in its most general form. Figure 3-8 gives some examples for a bias of 127 and a hidden normalization bit of 1.

An 8-bit exponent with a bias of 127 allows single precision real numbers to have absolute values ranging from 10^{-38} to 10^{38} (Table 3-2). Twenty three mantissa bits, plus one hidden bit, allows approximately 7 decimal significant digits. Note that this method of storage does not allow zero to be expressed. To address that, a "special" case is created. When the exponent and significand are both zero, the value is interpreted as a zero. Many operating systems also allow special cases for positive and negative infinity.

Double precision numbers are stored in a similar way, except that 11 bits are usually used for the exponent (stored as "excess-1024") and 52 bits for the mantissa/significand. This increases the range to $10^{\pm308}$, and the precision to approximately 16 decimal significant digits.

There is significant variability between operating systems as to how floating point numbers are stored and interpreted. Variations include the number of bits for the exponent, the exponent bias, whether the data is normalized to the most significant one or zero, whether the normalized bit is included or "hidden", and how many bytes are used for the entire storage. Some operating systems and programming languages do not use a pre-defined number of bytes to store real numbers, either allowing the programmer to specify the number of bytes to use, or even dynamically allocating as many bytes as needed to most accurately represent the value, up to a limit. This results in more accurate values, but slower calculations. The major disadvantage of this variation is that when floating point numbers are stored in a file, such as a database, and that file is moved to a different operating system, the textual data will be interpreted correctly, as will the integer data, but the floating point data probably will not be correctly interpreted without some form of conversion.

Storage of Dates and Times

Dates and times can be expressed in so many different ways. There are American formats (month before day before year) vs European formats (day before month before year) vs interface formats (year before month before day), two digit vs four digit years, military vs standard time, etc. One could simply pick a format and store the data as text (some systems do this), but then one has to be able to break apart the elements if one wants to change the display format. One could also conceive of custom schemes, where 4 bits is used for the month, and 5 for the day, and eleven or twelve for the year, etc.. Of course, if one stores a date/time, then one is going to want to be able to determine when one day is before or after another day. Electronic interfaces usually use the format of YYYYMMDD for dates because if one sorts them numerically (or even alphabetically – see text representation, below), one gets a chronological order. Performing other "mathematical operations" on dates and times, such as determining how much time there is between two different dates, can also be quite complex. Anyone who as tried to write a simple program to determine a person's age given the current date and the date of birth has encountered the complexity of this: it is the difference between the years, but if the current month is before the birth month it is one less, and if the current month is the same as the birth month, then one has to compare the days. Figuring out the number of days between two dates is even worse: let's see, it's "30 days hath September, April, June, and November…", and "a year is a leap year if it is evenly divisible for 4, unless it is divisible by 100, in which case it is not, unless it is divisible by 400, in which case it is…"

To facilitate these "mathematical" operations, most computer systems store dates and times as the number of days, minutes, seconds, or milliseconds after a certain reference date/time. Dates/times after the reference are stored as positive numbers, and those before are stored as negative numbers. This complicates displaying the date in a meaningful way, but greatly facilitates sorting and other mathematical operations. For example, to determine the amount of time between two different dates, one simply subtracts the stored values. Unfortunately, the time increment used, as well as the reference date/time, are different for different operating systems and programming languages. To make things worse, the data is usually stored as a floating point number, whose format is also different across operating systems. Therefore, transferring a file with stored date information from one operating system to another almost invariably requires some form of conversion.

Storage of Textual Data

Digital storage works well for numeric values, but does not readily accommodate text. Therefore, to store text digitally, a coding system is used in which each "character" (meaning any letter, digit, symbol, etc.) is represented by a code number. By far, the most common text encoding system in use by computers today is the American Standard Code for Information Interchange, or ASCII (*as-key*). Despite it's name, this code is even popular outside of the United States. ASCII uses a single byte to store each character of text, stored as a coded value. The codes up to 127 decimal (7F hexadecimal) are standardized across all fonts and are known as the standard ASCII character set.

Table 3-3: Standard ASCII character set.

Char	ASCII Hex	ASCII Dec	Char	ASCII Hex	ASCII Dec	Char	ASCII Hex	ASCII Dec	Char	ASCII Hex	ASCII Dec
NUL	00	0	space	20	32	@	40	64	`	60	96
SOH	01	1	!	21	33	A	41	65	a	61	97
STX	02	2	"	22	34	B	42	66	b	62	98
ETX	03	3	#	23	35	C	43	67	c	63	99
EOT	04	4	$	24	36	D	44	68	d	64	100
ENQ	05	5	%	25	37	E	45	69	e	65	101
ACK	06	6	&	26	38	F	46	70	f	66	102
Bell	07	7	'	27	39	G	47	71	g	67	103
Backsp	08	8	(	28	40	H	48	72	h	68	104
Tab	09	9	)	29	41	I	49	73	i	69	105
LF	0A	10	*	2A	42	J	4A	74	j	6A	106
VT	0B	11	+	2B	43	K	4B	75	k	6B	107
FF	0C	12	,	2C	44	L	4C	76	l	6C	108
CR	0D	13	-	2D	45	M	4D	77	m	6D	109
SO	0E	14	.	2E	46	N	4E	78	n	6E	110
SI	0F	15	/	2F	47	O	4F	79	o	6F	111
DLE	10	16	0	30	48	P	50	80	p	70	112
XON	11	17	1	31	49	Q	51	81	q	71	113
DC2	12	18	2	32	50	R	52	82	r	72	114
XOFF	13	19	3	33	51	S	53	83	s	73	115
DC4	14	20	4	34	52	T	54	84	t	74	116
NAK	15	21	5	35	53	U	55	85	u	75	117
SYN	16	22	6	36	54	V	56	86	v	76	118
ETB	17	23	7	37	55	W	57	87	w	77	119
CAN	18	24	8	38	56	X	58	88	x	78	120
EM	19	25	9	39	57	Y	59	89	y	79	121
SUB	1A	26	:	3A	58	Z	5A	90	z	7A	122
ESC	1B	27	;	3B	59	[	5B	91	{	7B	123
LAr/Hm	1C	28	<	3C	60	\	5C	92	|	7C	124
RAr/End	1D	29	=	3D	61	]	5D	93	}	7D	125
UpAr	1E	30	>	3E	62	^	5E	94	~	7E	126
DnAr	1F	31	?	3F	63	_	5F	95	del	7F	127

The characters with codes less than 32 decimal, and 127 decimal, are known as the non-printing control characters. This is a way to express concepts such as the tab, line feed, carriage return, and delete. Codes above 127 represent the "extended ASCII character set" and can vary from system to system and from font to font within the same system.

With the spread of computer systems across the world, is has become apparent that 127 codes, or even 256 codes, are not sufficient to represent all of the character sets in the world. This is particularly true of many of the Asian character sets. Therefore, another character coding system, called the "Unicode Character Set", has been developed, in which two bytes are used for each character. Currently, its use is pretty much restricted to situations in which the ASCII character set will not suffice, and it is unlikely to replace ASCII in the near future.

When characters are combined together to form multi-character expression, they are referred to as "strings". Within the computer's memory, strings are stored simply as a sequence of their ASCII values. Depending upon the operating system, one or more bytes may be used to store the length of the string, or the string may simply be "terminated" by the first ASCII 0 which is encountered. Some operating systems limit strings to 255 characters. Others allow strings to be any length. When a limit exists on the size of a string, a solution needs to exist for longer sequences of characters. In this instance, a different storage type, usually called "text", is used.

Since each printable character has a numeric value associated with it, it is possible to compare or sort strings. Sorting strings orders them by the ASCII values of the characters. Conveniently, the letters are encoded in ASCII in alphabetical order, so sorting strings alphabetizes them, for the most part. I say for the most part, because the ASCII values for the lower case letters are all greater than the ASCII values for the upper case letters. Therefore, for standard sorting algorithms, "HOUSE" will sort to a lower final position than "ant", because the ASCII code for "H" (72) is less than the ASCII code for "a" (97). Of course, custom sorting algorithms can take this into account. The use of ASCII codes to sort strings "alphabetically" also explains why "327" comes before "CAT", but after "$17".

Storage of Graphical Data

In addition to numeric and textual data, multimedia data such as images, line graphics, movies, and sound also needs to be describable digitally. In this area, there is significant variation in how this problem is solved, and numerous "standards" have been developed, often by individual software developers.

For graphical information, pictures and/or diagrams are stored in one of two ways: bitmapped or raster graphics and vector or object-based graphics.

For bitmapped graphics, usually used for photograph-like pictures, the image is represented as a rectilinear arrangement of "dots" of different colors, known as pixels (*pick-sells*). The range of colors available for each pixel is determined by how much memory (how many bytes, usually one to four) is used to store the color information for that pixel. (This topic is covered in much greater detail in Chapter 8). The overall size of the image in memory is determined by that number, plus the number of pixels in the horizontal and vertical dimension which comprise the image. Each pixel in the image bears no relationship with its neighbors, at least as far as the computer is concerned. "Objects" within a raster image are created simply by putting dots of similar color in some arrangement so as to visually form an image. In contrast, vector images consist of an ordered collection of real objects. The computer stores information about how to draw each object, such as "start 3 cm from the left margin and 2 cm from the top margin, and draw a line which is black, 2 pixels wide, and which ends 5 cm from the left margin and 10 cm from the top margin", or "draw a circle centered at 4 inches from the left margin and 6 inches from the top margin which is 2 inches in diameter; the perimeter of the circle is 3 pixels wide and is red; the circle is filled with solid blue". Text is also easily accommodated in vector images: "starting 4 cm from the left margin and 5 cm from the top margin, draw the text 'Hi there' using Times font, 12 point, bold." The details of how the computer encodes this information varies with the file format. Each time the image is drawn, it is "re-rendered", that is, the computer goes through the objects in order and redraws them given the instructions provided. Computer application programs which allow creation and editing of vector graphics are often referred to as "drawing programs" whereas those which allow creation and manipulation of bitmapped graphics are generally referred to as "painting programs".

The main advantage bitmapped images have over vector images is that there are many things which simply cannot be depicted by a combination of simple objects. "Photographic" quality pictures are the best example of this. One needs the flexibility of being able to control each pixel independently to produce life-like images.

Vector images, however, have a couple of important advantages over bitmapped images. With a vector image, if one draws a black triangle, and then draws a grey square partially overlapping the triangle, the computer still knows that the object behind the square is a triangle (Figure 3-9). If one moves the square, the underlying black triangle is redrawn as it originally existed. If one were to do the same thing with a bitmapped image, the black triangle drawn first is not really a triangle, but rather a collection of black pixels in the shape of a triangle. Drawing the grey square "in front of" the black triangle would replace some of the black pixels with grey pixels. If

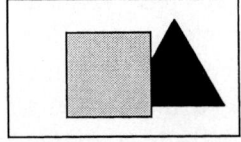

Draw triangle, then square.
Then move the square.

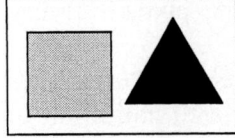
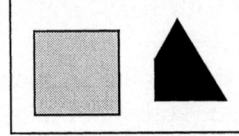

| Result with Vector Image | Result with Bitmapped Image |

Figure 3-9: Vector vs bitmapped images. With vector images, information about how to draw the image is stored. Therefore, if an overlapping object is moved out of the way, the original underlying object can be re-drawn. This is not the case for bitmapped images.

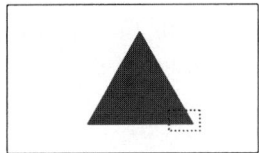

Draw triangle.
Magnify indicated portion.

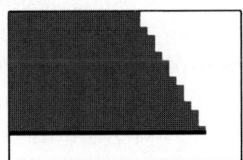

| Result with Vector Image | Result with Bitmapped Image |

Figure 3-10: Vector vs bitmapped images. Digital magnification of bitmapped images results in a phenomenon known as pixelation. This does not occur with vector images, since the information stored about the objects allows them to be redrawn at the new resolution.

one were to then select the gray pixels making up the square and move them, there are no black pixels underneath, so all one sees is what was left of the triangle. More sophisticated bitmap-based image editing programs address this problem by allowing the user to draw in layers, in which an upper layer can obscure pixels in a lower layer without replacing them.

A second advantage is seen with the use of diagonal lines and increasing magnification (Figure 3-10). For vector images, what is stored is the specifications about how to draw each object. Increasing the magnification of the image then becomes simply a mathematical process. Diagonal lines are still re-rendered as diagonal lines, within the resolution of the display device. When one "draws an object" as a bitmapped image, however, that object consists simply of a collection of dots. Those dots are in a rectilinear array. Diagonal lines are approximated by selectively making pixels black or white depending upon how much they overlap this theoretical line. If the pixels are small enough, one perceives the collection of black pixels as a diagonal line. However, when one magnifies the image, the only thing the software can do is "make each pixel bigger", which means that each pixel in the unmagnified image becomes 4 or 9 or 16 pixels in the magnified image. Here, the effect of having defined the initial line as pixels becomes obvious, and the result is not a clean diagonal line. Modern bitmap-based image editing programs mitigate this effect somewhat by blending partially overlapping pixels into the background color, a process known as anti-aliasing. For example, for a black line outlined object on a white background, the original diagonal would have been drawn not simply with black and white pixels but also some grey pixels.

There is a final complication in the distinction between vector images and bitmapped images. Vector images consist of an ordered collection of objects. Although those objects are usually things like lines, squares, and text, bitmapped images can also be objects within a vector image. Application software which allows the user to combine objects such as text, lines, and shapes with bitmapped image objects is sometimes referred to as layout-software or presentation software. Usually, the individual pixels of an embedded bitmapped image are not editable within the object-based software.

Non-Executable (Data) File Formats

Data is stored in "files" on long term data storage devices. The structure of the file system used depends upon the device and the operating system using it. However, the details are generally transparent to the user. The user does, however, need to know how to find his or her data. To accomplish this, each file is given a name. File names have two parts: the actual name part, and the extension. The extension is usually three alphanumeric characters appended to the end of the file name, separated from the main part of the name with a period. (NOTE: The term "alphanumeric character" means any letter or number.) This three character extension identifies the file type, and is usually used by operating systems to identify the computer application used to create and/or interpret the file. If the extension is unique to a particular application, "opening" the file from the operating system will actually run the associated application, which will then open the file. Note that depending upon the operating system and the settings, the file extension may be displayed or may be suppressed, so you may need to use built in tools to display this information.

Older versions of the Macintosh operating system did not use the file extension to determine the file type. Rather, that information was stored in a separate part of the file known as the resource fork. Beginning with OS X, an operating system built on a UNIX core which does not support resource forks, the Macintosh joined the other major types of desktop computers which use a three character extension to determine the file type.

The manner in which the data is stored in the data file depends on what application was used to create that file. For the vast majority of data files, the data is stored in a proprietary format, and as such can be fully interpreted only by the applications which created them. For example, a document file created with one word processing application will store its setting information and formatting information in a manner which is unique to that application, and a different word processing application will, in general, not be able to properly open that file.

The same discussion as above about backward compatibility and versioning of applications applies to files created by application software. An application which is backward compatible will be able to open files created with an older version of itself. This is extremely important for applications, perhaps even more so than for operating systems. If an operating system is not backward compatible, that means that you have to buy a new version of the application program you want to run in order to be compatible with the new operating system. But you can do that. If an application is not backward compatible, and you have dozens or hundreds of files created with an earlier version of that application, you cannot go out a buy new versions of those files, because they contain your personal data. In the absence of some sort of conversion utility, you would have to start over from scratch, and would no longer have access to any of your previous work.

A word about versions. Application version numbers are generally expressed as at least two numbers, separated by a period. Examples would be 2.0, 2.1, 2.1a, 2.1.3. The first number is the "major" version number, and the others are "minor" version numbers. Increments in the minor version number(s) usually represent bug fixes or introduction of new compatibilities. These upgrades are often provided free of charge, and are generally recommended, especially if they fix a bug which you have experienced. Increments in the major version number represent a fundamental change in the application, presumably an improvement. These upgrades are generally not free. This is where potential incompatibilities with previous version of the document files might be introduced. As a general rule, I urge caution when deciding whether or not to upgrade an application. Especially for major revisions, do not upgrade simply because a new version is available; this could be far more trouble than it is worth. Many people feel a need to have whatever the most recent version is. Remember that new major revisions are more likely to have bugs which the vendor has not yet discovered and fixed. Many vendors use users to debug their products. As a rule of thumb, I never upgrade to a new X.0 version of software, preferring to let other users find the bugs, report them to the vendor, and wait until the vendor releases X.1. Also, if you upgrade to a new version and share documents with other computers which may still be running the older version, your documents may not be usable by those computers. Therefore, be sure to critically evaluate what the new version is offering, and determine whether or not that is a feature you really need before simply laying down your money and acquiring it.

There are a number of file formats which are "standard", or at least sufficiently standard so as to be openable by a number of different applications and across operating systems. Some of these will be described here briefly. Note that when using a "standard" file format, you will often have to instruct the computer which application should be used when opening it, but the fact that you have a choice creates, in addition to peace of mind, an opportunity to use different applications with different capabilities in different settings. Also, standardized file formats allow the ability to distribute documents widely, without having to worry about whether or not some of your intended audience has the correct application program on the correct operating system needed to read your document.

Flat-Text Files (.txt)

"Flat-text" files are data files which contain only text data without any formatting information (Table 3-4). This means there is no mechanism to specify the font face, size, or style, and no mechanism to store customized indenting. Flat-text files traditionally have an extension of ".txt", and consist simply of a string of ASCII characters (Table 3-3) specifying the text of the file. Non-printing characters such as carriage returns, line feeds, and tabs can also be included (each tab is often interpreted as either 5 spaces or 0.5 inches). A "nil" character (ASCII 0) usually marks the end of the file.

Table 3-4: "Flat-text" ASCII file.

Sample Flat Text File	Hexadecimal Dump of File								
	54	68	69	73	20	69	73	20	61	20
This is a sample file.	73	61	6D	70	6C	65	20	66	69	6C
This is the second line.	65	2E	0D	54	68	69	73	20	69	73
This is the end.	20	74	68	65	20	73	65	63	6F	6E
	64	20	6C	69	6E	65	2E	0D	54	68
	69	73	20	69	73	20	74	68	65	20
	65	6E	64	2E	00					

Each character in the file is represented by a single byte, expressed here as a two "digit" hexadecimal value. The carriage returns (ASCII = 0D Hex = 13 decimal) and "end of file" characters are highlighted.

Essentially all word processing programs can open flat-text files, and likewise all word processing programs can save text as flat-text files. Be aware, however, that all formatting information will be lost when doing this. Despite the simplicity of this file format, there is still a slight difference between how different operating systems indicate the end of a line. On Macintosh computers, the carriage-return (ASCII 13 decimal, 0D hexadecimal) marks the end of a line. The Unix operating system uses a line-feed (ASCII 10 decimal, 0A hexadecimal), whereas DOS and Windows operating systems use the combination carriage-return plus line-feed. Fortunately, most word processing programs can compensate for this difference and still properly interpret flat text files created by a different operating system.

Portable Document Format (.pdf)

A need existed to be able to produce a formatted textual document which could be transferred from one desktop computer system to another and both look the same on all computer screens and print the same from all computer systems, independent of the operating system used to create it or to view it. Since essentially every word processing application stored its formatting information in a unique, proprietary fashion, this was problematic. Even if the user uses both the Macintosh and Windows versions of the same word processing application, the same document might look different on the two systems, with line breaks and page breaks occurring at different locations. This is often related to the fact that many fonts are not identical across computer systems. The Portable Document Format (PDF, pronounced *pee-dee-eff*) was designed to address this need. Developed by Adobe Systems, Inc, "PDF files" use a standardized approach for storing all of the formatting information, including an ability to embed the fonts within the document. A viewer application (Acrobat Reader) has been developed by Adobe for essentially every operating system, and this application is available free of charge to anyone through Adobe's web site. PDF files look exactly the same on every computer system, and when printed look identical, independent of the system which created them or printed them. Although initially pdf files could only be created using Adobe proprietary software (which was not free), Adobe has licensed this format to numerous software developers, and therefore many word processing applications and even operating systems can produce PDF formatted documents.

For the most part, PDF files cannot be edited. Although viewed as a negative feature by some, this property can actually be very useful, since the producer of the PDF file maintains control of the document, yet can freely and accurately distribute it without concern that altered versions of the document might turn up. This is particularly valuable when one wants to distribute an electronic copy of a medical document, such as a pathology report, and assure that the recipient cannot alter the contents of the document. PDF documents can also be password protected.

Image File Formats

There are literally dozens of "standard" image file formats, so many that one might question why the word "standard" is used. However, these files can be opened and edited by a number of different applications, and therefore the term "standard" is appropriate. There are also a number of proprietary image file formats, specific for particular image editing programs. It is important to keep in mind the fundamental difference between a vector (object-based) image and a raster (bitmapped, pixel-based) image when selecting an image file format or trying to open one. See the discussion above (Storage of Graphical Data) for details on this distinction.

Details about image resolution, color depth, and image compression are discussed later in Chapter 8 on digital imaging. Here I will just briefly catalogue some of the differences between the most common image file formats. Refer to the later discussion for a more thorough explanation of the terms used. However, I need to say something quickly about image compression. Bitmapped digital images can get very large, taking up megabytes of data. These large image files can be cumbersome to move around on a network. As such, a number of approaches, called compression algorithms, have been developed to decrease the size of the image file. Compression algorithms can be "lossy" or "lossless". "Lossy" means that information is lost when the image is compressed, so that the decompressed image does not have the same level of detail as the original image. However, often the differences can be minor and of no great consequence.

Perhaps the most popular and standardized image file format for continuous-tone graphics is JPEG (*jay-peg*), which is an acronym for Joint Photographic Experts Group. The extension ".jpg" is usually used for these files. JPEG files store full-color (i.e., millions of colors) bitmapped (pixel-based) images using a lossy compression algorithm. The JPEG compression algorithm was developed to minimize the perceivable visual distortion of the image while significantly decreasing file size. The amount of compression can be varied at the time the file is saved: high levels of compression result in smaller files, but poorer image quality. Almost every imaging application can interpret JPEG images, and they are the most popular choice for web pages. In addition, most consumer digital cameras store their images in JPEG format.

Graphical Interchange Format or GIF (*giff*) files are another popular choice for web pages, and in fact preceded the use of JPEG files. Developed originally by CompuServe in 1987, GIF images (extension is .gif) are also bitmapped images, and are traditionally compressed. Their main drawback is that they use an indexed color scheme which only allows for a maximum of 256 colors. Therefore, they are not well suited for "photographs" and are more appropriate for icons and diagrams. A revision of the GIF standard in 1989 added support for transparency (one of the "colors" in the image could actually be "transparent") so that, when used on a web page, the background could show through regions of the image. Simple animations can also be stored in GIF files.

BMP (*bee-em-pee*) is a bitmapped (pixel-based) image file format developed on the Windows platform and essentially used only on the Windows platform. It is an uncompressed full color image format, so preserves image quality, but at the cost of large image files. The file extension is .bmp

The Tagged Image/Interchange File Format or TIFF (*tiff*) is a widely used, flexible file format for bitmapped images. The name comes from the fact that "tags" within the file describe the image data, therefore allowing greater flexibility. There is no limit to the size of the image which can be stored in TIFF files, which can even support multiple pages. Although used across platforms, the file format standards are not always the same on all platforms, and not all tags are universally recognized. Most imaging programs can adapt to these differences, but some cannot and therefore a TIFF image may not be readable in all environments. TIFF files (extension is .tif) support a different type of compression algorithm known as LZW (stands for Lempel-Ziv Welch) which can be lossless and therefore preserves image quality, but results in files only a little smaller than the uncompressed versions. LZW compression and decompression is also time consuming. The TIFF format is popular within production-graphics and printing organizations. Despite their cross-platform "compatibility", TIFF images are not supported by most web browsers. If you have a digital camera which allows you to take an uncompressed high resolution image, actually using the 2 or more "megapixels" which they advertise, that image is likely to be a TIFF image.

The Portable Network Graphics or PNG (*ping*) image file format is a relatively new standard and is slowly replacing the use of GIF images for web pages. It is cross-platform and can support more color information than GIF images. Unlike GIF, it is not a patented format. It also allows for compression and brightness control. Transparency is supported, but animation is not. PNG image files (file extension .png) can also store, in the file header, textual information which is not displayed, such as the title and author of the image.

JPEG 2000 is another standard developed by the Joint Photographic Experts Group. Despite the similarity in name, there is no relation to the

JPEG file format. JPEG 2000 (file extension usually .j2k, although I have also seen .jp2 used) uses a completely different method of image compression which is reportedly more efficient. A lossless option exists. It can support enormous images and 256 channels of color information (unlike JPEG which supports only 64K x 64K images and 3 color channels) as well as seamless quality and resolution scalability, meaning it will be possible to "request" from the file a portion of the image at any desired resolution, without having to load the entire file into memory. Although JPEG 2000 has not become very popular yet, it is likely to make a big impact in the field of medical imaging, especially wide-field microscopy.

PICT (pronounced *picked*, short for "picture") is an object-based image file format originally developed for the Macintosh, and although still used on that platform has not become popular on other platforms. Multiple version of the PICT standard have been developed, and its capabilities have increased. Although originally purely a vector image format, PICT files acquired the ability to store raster images, either as the entire file or as an object within a vector file. Because of the comprehensiveness of the file format, it is still used on the Macintosh as the preferred format for storing image information on the clipboard. The most common extension for PICT files is .pct.

WMF for Windows Meta File is a vector-graphics file format which, as its name implies, is used only on the Windows platform. It supports both vector and bitmapped graphics, and is used to exchange images between Windows applications.

There are no good, cross-platform vector image file formats, but the one that comes the closest is EPS (*eee-pee-ess*) for Encapsulated Postscript. This is based on the PostScript language, the industry standard for desktop publishing which is used by many printers. Like the later PICT formats, it can support both pure vector graphics as well as raster graphics as objects within an object-based image. In fact, any combination of text, graphics, and images can be used. The operating system and printer must both be able to support PostScript in order to be able to use this file format.

Chapter 4

NETWORKING AND THE INTERNET

A computer network was originally defined as two or more computers connected by a wire which allowed exchange of information. That definition has been generalized to two or more devices (at least one of which is a computer) connected by some medium (wired or wireless) which allows exchange of information. The purpose of networking is to allow sharing of resources (printers, CD-ROM drives, disk drives), information (files, electronic mail, web pages), and sometimes software (program sharing, distributed processing).

Most pathologists will never have to deal with the details of network communications, and for that we can be grateful. Unfortunately, networks and networking issues have subtly worked their way into our daily lives. Almost every desktop computer is connected to the internet, and many pathologists use the internet on a daily basis for things such as electronic mail and literature searches. Successfully connecting to the internet requires that the desktop computer be properly set up and configured, and that requires some basic understanding of networking. In addition, many pathology information systems use a distributed processing configuration known as client-server. In this configuration, network communication is fundamental to the functioning of the system, and network performance issues will directly impact the performance of the pathology information system. Thus, an understanding of network terminology and logic can be important in understanding and addressing issues which will impact the workflow in the pathology laboratory.

Networks are loosely classified by their size, both with respect to number of attached devices and geographical distribution. The smallest is referred to as a Local Area Network or LAN (rhymes with *can*). This covers a relatively small area, perhaps a department, a home, or even just the floor of a building, and generally has less than 200 devices, although in many instances it can be far less: as few as two or three. Communication between devices on a LAN typically is homogeneous; that is, everyone uses the same communication protocol (this term will be discussed in more detail later). LANs are usually owned and maintained by a single entity. In contrast, Wide Area Networks or WANs (also rhymes with *can*) cover a larger geographic area: an institution, town, or even state. WANs are usually made up of interconnected LANs. As such, they are often owned and maintained by multiple organizations. Each connected LAN, referred to as a "subnet" of the larger network, typically has a single entry/exit point to the rest of the network, sometimes referred to as the "gateway" or "router" for the LAN. The technology by which devices are connected to the network make possible the concept of a virtual local area network or V-LAN (*vee-lan*). This represents a group of devices which are physically quite separated from each other, but appear to the networking software to be on the same subnet of the network.

Network Topologies

The term "topology", with respect to a digital communication network, refers to the physical layout of the cabling for that network. The topology describes how the devices in a local area network are connected to each other. There are three basic configurations: star, ring, and bus. Each carries different implications about how the machines can communicate, and each will be discussed separately below. However, these three basic topologies can then be combined in different combinations, creating star-wired rings or starred-busses, etc., so the ultimate topology of the wide area network, and sometimes even the local area network, can be more complex than these models.

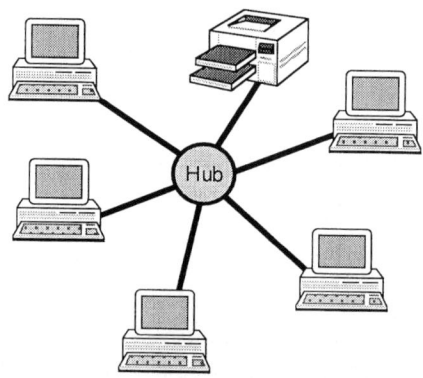

Star Network

In a star network (Figure 4-1), each device is connected to a central connection point, known as the concentrator or hub. There are two types of star networks, which differ in the capabilities of the hub. In a "passive star" network, the hub has

Figure 4-1: Star network. All of the devices are connected to a central point.

no intelligence. It simply takes each message it receives and broadcasts it to all of the connected devices. The data is transmitted to everyone, with the understanding that only the intended recipient will accept the message and respond to it. The second type of star network is an "active star". Here, there is an intelligent device at the hub location, usually a dedicated computer. As each message is received, the hub determines which device it is intended for, and transmits it only to that device. The hub is responsible for the flow of information within the network, and represents a single point at which network communication can be managed. If two devices on the network try to talk at the same time, it is the responsibility of the hub to handle this conflict.

For this topology, the overall performance of the network is dependent upon the efficiency of the hub, and upgrading the hub can improve network performance. The network is also resistant to node failure: if one of the connected devices fails, the others can continue to communicate. It is, however, sensitive to failure of the hub, which will bring down the entire network. Adding new devices to the network requires running a new connection to the hub, and for intelligent hubs may require reconfiguration of the hub.

Ring Network

In a ring topology (Figure 4-2), each device is connected to two other devices on the network, in such a way that the aggregate of all the connections forms a ring. Communication on a ring network is sequential and unidirectional. Each machine speaks to only one other machine, and listens to only one other machine. When one device wants to communicate with another, it transmits a message to the next device on the network. That device receives the message and determines if it is intended for itself. If so, it removes the message from the network and processes it. If not, it transmits the message, unaltered, to its neighbor. This process continues until the message reaches its intended recipient.

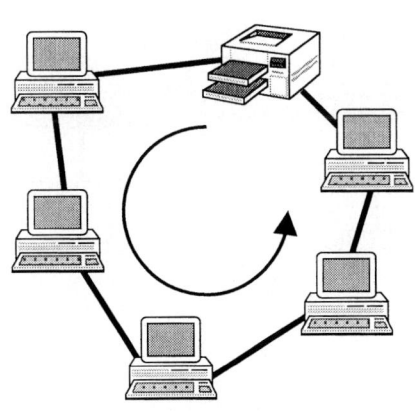

Figure 4-2: Ring network. Each device is connected to two other devices, forming a ring.

The ring topology uses less wire than a star configuration. In addition, it is relatively easy to add a new device to the network, especially if that device is going to be located near an existing device. One simply removes one of the wires from an already connected device, plugs it into the new device, and then places a new cable between the new device and the one from which the wire was disconnected.

In a ring network, everyone has equal and fair access to the network. No dedicated central administrator is required, and each member of the network shares the administrative responsibility of propagating messages within the network. Since communication on a ring network is unidirectional, multiple messages can, theoretically, travel simultaneously on the network. However, the more devices which are connected to the network, the slower the communication rate. The process of having each machine in the network read the message, determine whether or not it is the intended recipient, and then forward it if not, is inefficient and time consuming, resulting in a "propagation delay". Although at first is might seem like the communication rate with an adjacent downstream machine would be much faster than communicating with an adjacent upstream machine, in reality both take the same amount of time, because each message sent must be acknowledged by the recipient back to the sending device, so a full circuit is required in either case.

One of the major shortcomings of ring networks is that they are very susceptible to node failure. If one node goes down, the entire network goes down. "Going down" could be something as simple as someone turning off their computer before going home. Therefore, ring networks are generally not used for office desktop computers but rather for machines which are on all the time, like servers.

Bus Network

With a bus network, all of the devices are connected like leaves on a stem to a central "backbone" (Figure 4-3). This would seem to be easier to wire than a star network, but not as easy as a ring network. In reality, however, the backbone is usually in a central location, and the wire runs to that location are quite comparable to that of a star network.

Bus networks are often referred to as broadcast networks,

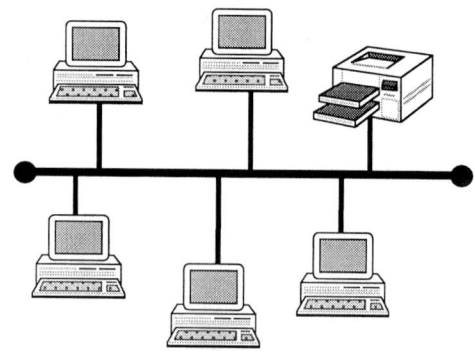

Figure 4-3: Bus network. Each device is connected to a central backbone, often a fiber optic (high bandwidth) cable.

because when a device has something to say, it places the message on the network backbone, and all connected users hear it. The message is supposed to be ignored by everyone except the intended recipient. Since digital "talking" on a network means voltages on a wire, and since a wire can only carry one voltage at a time, two devices trying to talk at the same time creates a situation known as a "collision" (both devices are trying to "drive" the voltage of the backbone to a different value), and the result is that neither message gets through.

A bus network does not have the propagation delays of a ring network, nor does it require a central administrative device like a star network. A bus network is very resistant to node failure, and devices can be connected to or disconnected from the network while the network is running without any interruption of communications. Each device must understand the rules for communication on the network, but those rules can be relatively simple.

At low levels of usage, either because of few connected devices, or because the majority of the devices are only occasional communicators (referred to as "casual users"), a bus network can be very efficient. However, as usage levels increase, the number and percentage of collisions rises exponentially, and eventually no communication can occur. In addition, this network configuration is very susceptible to a phenomenon known as "streaming" or "babbling", in which one device "talks" all the time (either because of failure of it's network interface card, or because the device with which it is trying to communicate is not available and none of the messages are acknowledged). When this occurs, it can be very difficult to determine which device is responsible for the streaming, and diagnosing this or other problems often requires systematically removing each device from the network until normal network function is restored.

Communication on a Network

To get information from one computer to another, often of a different type, on a network, a number of tasks need to be accomplished. There needs to be an interconnecting medium, such as a wire, and way of representing digital information on that medium. The information needs to be broken down into transmissible "packets". Rules need to exist for identifying the intended recipient, and for sending and routing the information to the recipient. Mechanisms need to be in place to manage the network and user access to it. Communication errors need to be detected and corrected. Message receipt needs to be acknowledged, and missing packets need to be re-requested. The recipient must be able to reassemble the received packets of information into the correct order, and then interpret the reconstructed message.   The details of the procedures, rules, and materials used to communicate on a network are collectively referred to as a network communication protocol.

Network Protocols

A network communication protocol is a set of rules which govern how computers and other devices (e.g. printers) communicate over a network. It includes both hardware and software specifications.

Since networking procedures developed independently among multiple computer vendors, there were initially a large number of different communication protocols, none of which could speak with each other. The increasing need for devices from different manufacturers to be able to communicate was first met by each manufacturer designing their equipment to understand and use a number of different protocols. To achieve this, the rules of the protocols needed to be clearly defined, and standards for the more popular communication protocols began to emerge. The International Standards Organization (ISO) developed a layer-based reference model for computer networking known as the "Open Systems Interconnect" (OSI) model (Figure 4-4). It divides the rules for a complete networking standard into seven distinct layers. The lowest layer, the physical layer, specifies the wires, voltages, cabling, and connectors. The data link layer addresses transmission of data frames,

7	Application Layer
6	Presentation Layer
5	Session Layer
4	Transport Layer
3	Network Layer
2	Data Link Layer
2a	Logical Link Control
2b	Media Access Control
1	Physical Layer

Figure 4-4: The Open Systems Interconnect (OSI) model. Network communication is modeled as seven layers of protocols, with different issues addressed at each layer.

and includes rules for adding packets of data to the network (media access control) as well as rules for higher level layers to access the data (logical link control).   The network layer addresses fragmentation, routing, and reassembly of data packets. The transport layer monitors the quality of the connection and contains procedures to assure data integrity. The session layer controls when users can and cannot send or receive data. Presentation rules govern character translation, data conversion, and any compression or encryption which may be used. Finally, the seventh layer, the application layer, addresses program level access to the network, for operations such as electronic mail, file exchange, and web browsing.

Needless to say, the seven layer OSI model is rather complex. A more simplified, three layer model is used by some. The lowest layer, the "technical layer" specifies the cabling, hardware, addressing, and digital data representation rules, combining the lowest three layers of the larger model. The middle layer or "logical layer" governs who can talk when and for how long. The highest layer or "software access layer" addresses how computer programs put data on the network, get data off, and manage the network.

Bandwidth

Essentially all network communications protocols use a serial (rather than parallel) method of data representation (see the discussion in Chapter 2 on desktop computer hardware for a more detailed description of the differences between these two approaches). For purposes of this discussion, we will consider wire as the transmission medium and voltage as the data representation scheme, but the discussions would be equivalent for radio, light, or sound data representation.

Digital communication, as its name implies, consists of a series of ones and zeros. On a wire, this is most commonly represented by the flipping of voltages between one of two states with time (Figure 4-5). By convention, the higher voltage, usually about 5 volts, represents a "zero", and the lower voltage, close to zero, represents a "one." Although this seems opposite what one might predict, it is most likely related to the fact that pin voltages in many integrated circuit chips, unless driven to a specific voltage, tend to float toward the power voltage of 5 volts. In order to use this serial method to send digital data along the wire, both the sender and the receiver must know what the time spacing is between each bit of data; that is the only way to tell if a constant five volts, for example, represents one zero or two zeros or three zeros, etc. The more reliable the conductive medium and the more protected the transmission is from external interference and noise, the closer together (in time) the individual bits of data can be packed, resulting in more data being transmitted in any given block of time. The maximum rate at which the data can be sent reliably is referred to

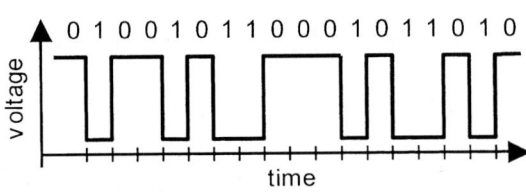

Figure 4-5: Digital data transmission on a wire. Binary information is represented as a series of "high" and "low" voltages, which change with time.

as the bandwidth of the connection. Note that this is not the same thing as the bandwidth of a radio or television broadcast. Digital bandwidth, expressed in bits per second (bps) or simply hertz, is more accurately a measure of the fidelity of the transmission, and therefore how tightly together (temporally) the data can be sent. It has nothing to do with the actual speed that the electrons move along the wire. The maximum bandwidth obtainable is determined both by the transport medium used and by the communication protocol employed.

There are three different types of cabling used for networks: unshielded twisted pair, coaxial cable, and fiber optic cable. Each will be discussed briefly.

Unshielded twisted-pair (UTP) copper cabling is by far the most common network cabling used. It consists of two or more insulated braided copper wires wrapped around each other in an insulated, but not shielded casing. It is thin and flexible, and therefore easy to install. Unshielded twisted pair cabling is rated by the number and gauge of wires into a numeric category. Category 3 cable can support a bandwidth of 16 Mbps, Category 4 a maximum of 20 Mbps, and Category 5 a maximum of 100 Mbps. Category 5e, an expanded version of Category 5 cable (same cable, but connected in a different fashion such that pairs of wires are used) is formally rated up to 340 Mbps, but can support a 1 Gbps bandwidth. Category 5 or 5e is the most common networking cable currently being installed. Category 6 cable is recommended for 1 Gbps communication.

The greatest drawback of unshielded twisted-pair cabling is that it is unshielded and therefore subject to noise/interference from surrounding

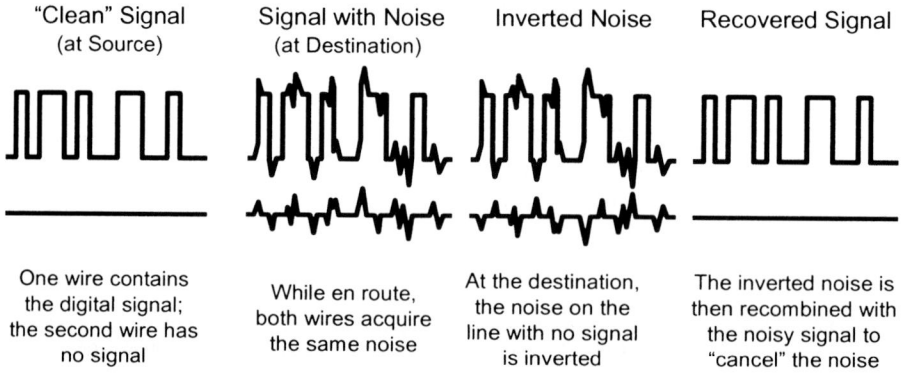

"Clean" Signal (at Source)	Signal with Noise (at Destination)	Inverted Noise	Recovered Signal
One wire contains the digital signal; the second wire has no signal	While en route, both wires acquire the same noise	At the destination, the noise on the line with no signal is inverted	The inverted noise is then recombined with the noisy signal to "cancel" the noise

Figure 4-6: Signal recovery in unshielded twisted pair cabling. Both the signal line and the "ground" reference line acquire similar electronic noise. The noise on the ground line can be inverted and added back to the signal line to recover the original signal.

electrical wires. This noise degrades the quality of the signal received at the destination. Although the data is carried over only one of the wires in the cable, the noise is acquired by all of the wires. The presence of noise on a non-signal wire can be used to recover the signal quality on the signal wire. The theory is that the signal and non-signal wire are likely to acquire similar noise. At the destination, the noise on the non-signal wire is inverted and then added back to the signal wire, recovering the original signal (Figure 4-6).

Coaxial cable consists of an inner copper conductor with a surrounding outer metallic shield, separated by an insulator. The foil-like shield is kept grounded, which shields the inner conductor from interference from nearby electrical currents, markedly decreasing the amount of noise acquired. Coaxial cable is relatively inexpensive, but is more difficult to install since the cable is stiffer and cannot make sharp turns as is often required in building installations. Coaxial cable supports a maximum bandwidth of approximately 350 Mbps.

The highest bandwidth conductor is fiber optic cabling. Fiber optic cable consists of a glass or plastic core fiber surrounded by a protective sheath. Data is transmitted in the form of pulses of light. Fiber optic cabling is expensive, requires special skills to install and connect, and cannot make sharp turns. However, it is a high fidelity conductor which is immune to electrical interference. Early fiber optic cabling supported a minimum bandwidth of 7 Gbps, but terabit-per-second fiber optic standards exist. In addition, fiber cannot be tapped or otherwise monitored, so transmission is more secure.

Network Communication Logic

Although the cabling used for communication on a network limits the maximum rate at which data can be transmitted, the communication logic determines how close, in practice, one can come to achieving that rate. Communication logic addresses the rules which determine when members of the network can transmit data, and how long they can talk. All network communication protocols include fragmentation/segmentation of large messages into smaller packets, rather than sending an entire message all as one data stream. This serves multiple purposes. One main reason is to prevent one user from monopolizing the network, just because he/she has a lot to say. Another is that random communication errors do occur. When they occur, the message is discarded at the destination and re-requested. If an error occurs in a single long message, the entire message needs to be re-transmitted. This is very inefficient. By breaking up the message into smaller segments, only the segment containing the error needs to be re-transmitted. Other reasons exist which are protocol specific.

The topology of the network can have a significant impact on the communication logic employed. The full details of network communication logic are complex and beyond the scope of this discussion. However, a few illustrative examples will be presented, one for a ring network, and then a few for a broadcast network.

Token Passing Logic

A common communication protocol used for ring networks is referred to as Token-Ring, which is based on "token passing" communication logic. The fundamental concept is that an electronic token is passed from node to node on the network. Only the holder of the token can add a message to the network. If a node has something to say when the token arrives, and if the token is available, that node marks the token as busy, attaches its message, and sends it on to the next node in the ring. The next node will then examine the message, determine whether or not it is intended for itself, and if not forward it to the next node on the network. Once the token and message reach the intended recipient, the message is taken off, and an acknowledgement message is attached to the token, which is then sent on its way. When it reaches the initial sender, the sender accepts the acknowledgement, marks the token as available, and then passes the token to the next node. If the sender still has more to say, it has to wait until the next time the token comes around and, if it is still available, it can take possession of the token at that time. This gives each other node, in turn, an opportunity to send a message.

This communication logic has some definite advantages. It is an extremely stable communication protocol, since there are no issues associated with more than one node trying to talk on the network at the same time. Therefore, messages essentially always make it to the recipient on the first attempt. No central administrator is required, but each node has to be relatively intelligent. The disadvantages include the propagation delays associated with passing the message from node to node, continually involving nodes which have nothing to say, and this delay increases with the number of nodes on the network. Another major disadvantage is that the communication is very susceptible to node failure. Adding or removing a node from the network requires internal reconfiguring to be sure that everyone has a chance at the token.

Communication rates of 16 Mbps are routinely achievable with a token ring network. Greater communication rates can be achieved by using multiple tokens via a procedure called "early release of the token", but this requires greater intelligence of the nodes and collision monitoring (to make sure one token does not catch up to another).

Token passing logic has also been used for other networking protocols, such as the Fiber Distributed Data Interface protocol (FDDI), which uses token passing logic on fiber optic cabling to interconnect different networks to each other.

Broadcast Networks

Broadcast networks, using either a star or more commonly a bus topology, include all networking models in which any message placed on the network is communicated to all of the nodes on the network, with the understanding that only the intended recipient will pay any attention to the message. The fundamental problem complicating this design is message "collision": two nodes talking at the same time, each trying to "drive" the network signal to different voltages, resulting in neither message being received in an interpretable fashion. Therefore, the various communication logics employed for broadcast networks all must address how collision is managed. A variety of solutions have been achieved. Each of the examples presented below are based on a simple, four computer network. In each case, machine 1 will have a lot to say, machine 3 will have a little to say, and machines 2 and 4 will have nothing to say. For simplicity, acknowledging receipt of the messages will not be specifically considered, but this is still an important part of the functioning of the network, because failure to receive an acknowledgement is the only way a "sender" can know that the message was not received by the recipient.

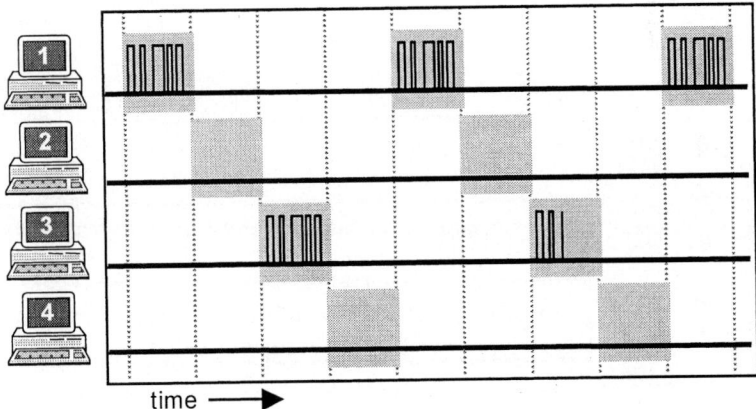

Figure 4-7: Time sharing protocol. Each networked device is given, in turn, a fixed block of time to communicate on the network. If a device has nothing to say, that time is wasted.

A simple communication logic for broadcast networks is proportional time sharing (Figure 4-7). In this approach, each node on the network is given, in turn, a fixed, predetermined block of time to access the network. The nodes are allowed to transmit only during their allotted time periods. This approach has a few advantages. There is very little overhead associated with this communication logic. There is no risk of collision, since only one node can speak at a time. In addition, the amount of time it will take to transfer a given amount of data can be very reliably predicted, once one knows the number of nodes on the network and the amount of time in each time block. The disadvantages of this approach are rather obvious: a lot of time is wasted on nodes which have nothing to say, which will be the case most of the time. As more and more "occasional" users are added to the network, the fraction of time available for any given node progressively decreases, and the communication rate becomes slower and slower.

A modification of this proportional time sharing logic is a polled logic. In this approach, a designated "administrator" polls each node in turn (Figure 4-8). If that device has something to say, it is given a block of time to say it. If not, the administrator moves immediately to the next node. The administrator could be a dedicated computer, or simply one of the devices on the network. Again, since only one node is allowed to talk at any given time, there is no risk of collision. Since nodes with nothing to say are not given any more time than is needed to respond to the polling of the administrator, significantly less time is wasted on nodes which have nothing to say. Therefore, a large number of occasional users can be added to the network with only minor impact on the overall network performance. But time is still spent polling machines which don't have anything to say. Also,

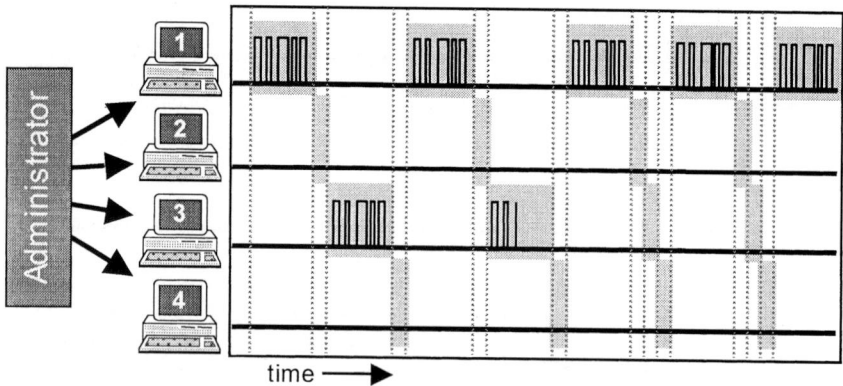

time ⟶

Figure 4-8: Polled communication protocol. Each node, in turn, is "asked" if it needs access to the network. If so, a block of time is given. Less time is wasted on nodes which have nothing to say.

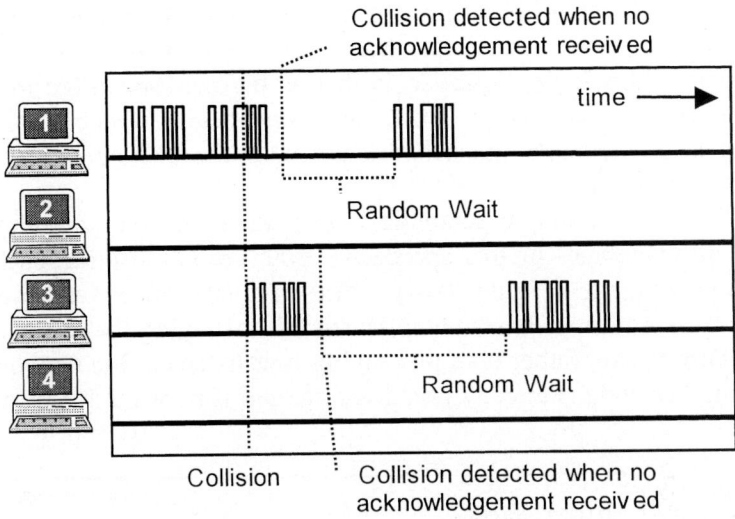

Figure 4-9: Contention protocol. In this model, any device which needs to transmit on the network just transmits. When a collision occurs (two devices talk at the same time), the lost packet of information is retransmitted after a random wait period.

as seen in the example with the second packet transmitted by node 3, the block of time allotted is fixed, not dependent on how much the node has to say, and therefore some network time is wasted here as well. Finally, a central administrator is required, and this represents a vulnerable point for total network failure.

A third approach to communication logic on a broadcast network is known as contention. In this model, there is no allotment of time to individual nodes to use the network. When a node has something to say, it simply says it (Figure 4-9). Most of the time, the message will get through, and an acknowledgement will be received. However, if two nodes try to talk at the same time, neither message will be interpretable by either intended recipient, so neither sender will receive an acknowledgement. When this happens, each of the senders waits a random period of time, and then retransmits. A random wait period is employed because if a fixed waiting period were used by both senders, this would guarantee that another collision would occur.

An obvious advantage of contention logic is that it is very simple, requiring very little administrative overhead. In addition, absolutely no time is wasted on nodes which have nothing to say. Therefore, at low network usage levels, this communication logic allows for very rapid communication. Some time is still wasted after a collision occurs, because both transmitting nodes have to finish their messages and wait for an acknowledgement to not arrive before either realizes that there was a problem. The greatest disadvantage of this logic, however, is that as the network usage increases due to increasing numbers of users, collisions begin to occur far more frequently, and eventually the network becomes deadlocked such that no messages get through.

A modification of simple contention logic was developed to address the two main disadvantages of this approach. Both are based on good human conversation etiquette (Figure 4-10). The first is "carrier-sense/multiple access" or "CSMA", which is a complicated way of saying that when a node has something to say, rather than just saying it, it listens to the network first to see if another node is already broadcasting, and if so waits for it to finish

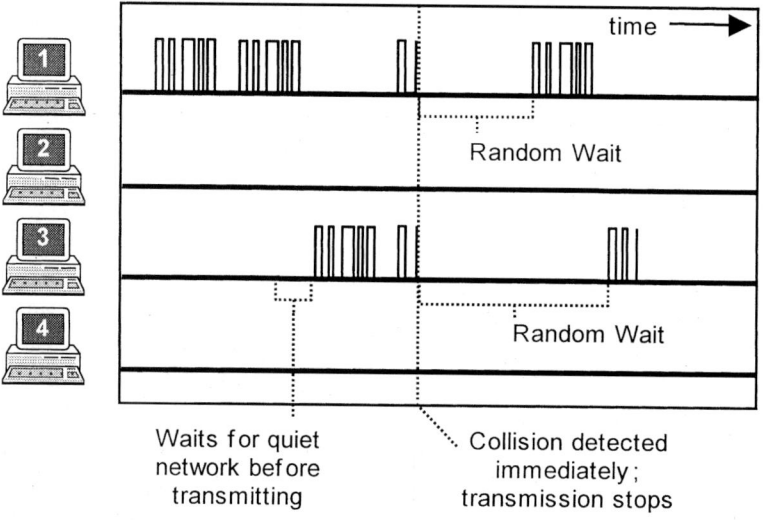

Figure 4-10: Contention with CSMA/CD. This protocol, the basis for Ethernet communication, decreases the frequency of collisions as well as decreases the amount of time wasted when a collision occurs.

its packet before transmitting its own message. The second enhancement is known as "collision detection" or "CD". When a node is talking, it also listens to the network. If a collision is detected (two nodes try to talk at the same time), both speakers stop transmitting immediately and enter their random wait period. It is unnecessary to wait for failure of the acknowledgement to arrive. These enhancements to simple contention logic require more intelligent nodes (perhaps explaining why this does not always work for human conversation). However, the number of collisions is markedly decreased, most occurring immediately after a transmission is completed. The end result is that by using this communication logic, it is possible to achieve 70-80% of the theoretical hardware bandwidth of the network. This communication logic, known as "contention with CSMA/CD", is the underlying logic used by the Ethernet networking protocol.

Ethernet

Ethernet is the most common networking protocol used by desktop computers and within most healthcare environments. Essentially every manufacturer of desktop computers and every operating system supports Ethernet networking. By convention, "Ethernet" is usually capitalized, although not everyone follows this convention, especially when using the term as an adjective (e.g., "ethernet cable"). This communication standard for broadcast networking is based on contention with CSMA/CD logic, and was first published in 1982 as a joint effort of Xerox, Digital Equipment Corporation, Intel, and 3Com. The standard was later adopted by the Institute of Electrical and Electronic Engineers as IEEE 802.3. As part of the standard, each device which wishes to communicate using Ethernet must have a globally unique identifying number, known as the media access control address or MAC (*mack*) address (sometimes referred to as the hardware address). This 48 bit number is usually expressed as 6 pairs of hexadecimal digits, each hexadecimal digit representing 4 bits. No two networking devices in the world are supposed to have the same MAC address. The first 3 pairs of digits (the first 24 bits) identify the manufacturer of the network interface card and are assigned by the IEEE. The remaining are assigned by the manufacturer. MAC addresses are used not only by Ethernet networking, but also in token ring networks and wireless networking communications.

A number of different "versions" of Ethernet networking are available, each with different cabling requirements and transmission rates (Table 4-1). The one most commonly in use currently is "Fast Ethernet" or 100BaseT, which communicates at 100 Mbps over category 5 unshielded twisted pair cabling. The maximum cable run is 100 meters. Many networks are beginning to switch to gigabit Ethernet, at least for communication between servers.

On an Ethernet network, information is transmitted in packets known as data frames. Each data frame starts with an 8 byte preamble (identifying the frame as an Ethernet frame), followed by the 6 byte (48 bit) destination MAC address, followed by the 6 byte source MAC address, a two byte type code, and then the actual data payload, between 38 and 1492 bytes long. A four byte data integrity trailer is added at the end. Thus, the maximum size of an Ethernet data frame is 1500 bytes. Ethernet has a minimum size, so

Table 4-1: Version of the Ethernet standard.

Official Name	Nickname	Bandwidth	Cable	Connector
10Base2	Thinnet	10 Mbps	0.2 inch Coax	BNC
10Base5	Thicknet	10 Mbps	0.5 inch Coax	DIX
10BaseT	Twisted-Pair	10 Mbps	Cat 3 UTP	RJ-11
100BaseT	Fast Ethernet	100 Mbps	Cat 5 UTP	RJ-45
1000BaseT	Gigabit Ethernet	1 Gbps	Cat 5e/6 UTP	RJ-45
10GBase	10 Gigabit Ethernet	10 Gbps	Fiber	(varies)

Each version has specific requirements for cabling and connectors. (Mbps = megabits per second; Gbps = gigabits per second; Coax = coaxial cable; Cat = category; UTP = unshielded twisted pair cabling)

the data is padded as needed to achieve that size. The minimum size is needed to allow for proper collision detection to occur.

Network Interconnectivity Devices

For communication among a small number of devices, the devices themselves can administer the network. This is handled by capabilities built into the network interface cards. As the networks grow larger and larger, however, additional devices are needed to propagate signals and improve efficiency. This section will briefly introduce some of those devices.

Network Interface Cards

At the desktop computer level, all of the local tasks of network communication are performed by the computer's network interface card (see the Chapter 2 on desktop computer hardware for more information). The network interface card takes a stream of data from the computer bus, breaks it down into segments or packets, adds an addressing header and tail, and places the resulting data frame on the network. The same process, in reverse, is used to take data off the network. Most network interface cards contain on-board memory and a dedicated processor to buffer messages and to allow the network communications to occur without having to draw upon the central processor of the computer.

Repeaters and Hubs

As network transmissions travel along the wires of a network, the signal strength will deteriorate due to resistance inherent in all wires. If the signal becomes too depleted, the voltage difference between a "1" and a "0" becomes blurred, and the signal can no longer be interpreted. A repeater takes a depleted signal and boosts it, re-establishing the strength of the original signal. A hub is simply a repeater with multiple ports. Any signal received on any of the ports is amplified and sent out along all of the other ports. Hubs are sometimes referred to as concentrators. Both hubs and repeaters are said to operate at layer 1 (the physical layer) of the OSI networking model, since they only concern themselves with voltages and cabling, and do not "see" the network messages as anything more than voltages.

When multiple devices are connected to a network via a hub, those devices are sharing the bandwidth of that network connection. Since transmissions from any one of the devices are sent to all the connected devices, including the network, only one of the connected devices can actually be using the network at any given time.

Bridges

Bridges are far more sophisticated than hubs, and are used to interconnect two similar local area networks to each other. Bridges are dedicated computers with two network interface cards, each connected to a different LAN. The bridge builds an internal address table, keeping track of the MAC addresses of the devices on each of the two networks. It uses this information to filter messages and segment the networks from each other (Figure 4-11). If a device on network A transmits a message intended for a machine on network B, the bridge will receive the message from network A and retransmit it to network B. In this way, the bridge acts like a repeater. However, if a device on network B transmits a message intended for another

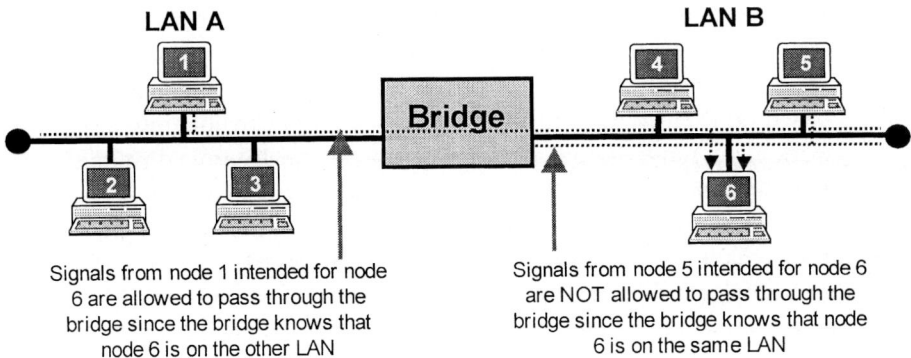

Figure 4-11: Network bridges. Bridges interconnect two local area networks. Only communications intended for a device on the other network are passed through the bridge, minimizing unnecessary use of network bandwidth.

device on network B, the bridge will recognize that the message does not need to pass to network A, and filters out the message so that network A remains available for other communications. To accomplish this, the bridge needs to be able to read and interpret the addresses in data frames, and thus operates at layer 2 (the data link layer) of the OSI networking model. Bridges also have the ability to amplify signals and to buffer them (buffer means that the bridge can receive a message from network A which needs to be passed to network B, but if network B is currently unavailable, the bridge will hold on to the message until network B is available, and then retransmit it onto network B.

Bridges can segment a large local area network into two smaller LANs, decreasing the number of collisions in each segment and thereby improving overall network performance. Both of the connected LANs must be using the same communication protocol.

Switches

Whereas a bridge has two ports and can connect two networks, a switch accomplishes the same tasks but has many more ports (typically from four to forty-eight) and can support multiple simultaneous transmissions. Like a bridge, the switch builds an internal address table, keeping track of the addresses of the devices connected to each port. When a message is received from one port, that message is forwarded only to the port to which the intended recipient is attached. This forwarding occurs with very minimal delay (low latency), since the switch has the ability to read the address while the message is being received and to connect it very rapidly to the correct output port. In addition, the switch can simultaneously be receiving data from another port and forwarding it to a different output port. This process is known as "packet-switching" and is the primary function of a switch. Typical switches can process about a million packets per second.

Switches can operate at different layers of the OSI networking model. "Low-end" switches operate at layer 2 (the data link layer) and switch packets based on their MAC address. Higher-end switches operate at layer 3 (the network layer) and switch packets based on the Internet Protocol (IP) address (see discussion below). Layer 4 (the transport layer) switches also exist, which can incorporate more information into the packet switching decisions such as the communication protocol being used.

In the typical configuration, most of the ports on a switch will have a single device attached. One of the ports will be connected to the larger network. Although physically the wiring of the connections is similar to connecting multiple devices to a hub, the performance is significantly better. Switches are both faster and port specific, allowing multiple simultaneous transmissions. Therefore, to the extent to which communication is occurring between two devices connected to the same switch, rather than the connected machines sharing the available bandwidth, each has full access to the total bandwidth. In addition, switches are more secure, since the message is only forwarded to the port containing the indented recipient, decreasing the risk of electronic eaves-dropping.

Gateway

A gateway is similar to a bridge in that it connects two local area networks to each other, and can filter, buffer, and amplify data packets. However, unlike a bridge, the two networks connected to a gateway can use different communication protocols. When a data frame is passed from one network to another, the gateway translates the data frames appropriately for the new network protocol. Since this requires the gateway to be able to interpret and reformat the data frames, gateways operate at layer 4 (the transport layer) or higher of the OSI networking model.

Gateways are most commonly used to connect a local area network to a much larger network (such as the internet). In this way, they represent the "doorway" (hence the term gateway) into the larger network. Security functions such as "firewalls" which control what types of communication are allowed to pass in and out of a LAN are typically associated with gateways.

Routers

Routers (first syllable rhymes with *cow*) are similar to bridges but with multiple ports interconnecting multiple networks and directing data frames only to the segment of the network which will ultimately lead to the final destination. Routers can direct traffic among a small number of devices such as within an institution, or among a very large number of devices such as the internet.

Routers build and maintain dynamic internal routing tables, which keep track of where to forward traffic destined for any computer on any connected network anywhere in the world. This is accomplished not only by learning the addresses of devices connected directly to it, but by talking to other routers on the network and learning what devices are connected to those. By working together, the routers pass data frames between themselves until they reach the router connected to the network containing the intended recipient. Routers are what make the internet possible. The addressing tables are constantly updated, and adjust automatically should a portion of the internet become congested with too much traffic.

Routers operate at layer 4 (the network layer) of the OSI networking model, and use Internet Protocol (IP) addressing (see discussion below) to determine the destination of the data frame. As the packet passes through each router, the addressing headers are stripped off and new ones are added to appropriately re-address the packet to its final destination. Since routers typically interconnect more than two networks, a "web" of interconnected routers (note the foreshadowing) is created. As a result, there are generally multiple possible routes for getting from one device on the internet to another. If a large message is broken up into many data frame packets, each of the packets could potentially follow a different route to the destination.

The Internet

The internet is an international network of computers and other electronic devices spanning the entire globe. Each device is connected to a local area network, and that network is then connected via one or more gateways or routers to the backbone of the internet. Since April 1995, the backbone of the internet has been owned and operated by major commercial telecommunications companies and internet service providers, including MCI, Sprint, GTE, and America Online. No one knows for sure how many devices are connected to the internet. As of 2004, it is estimated that over 800 million people, more than 12% of the total world population, use the internet on at least an intermittent basis[1]. Approximately 25% of this use was in the United States, where nearly 70% of the population are considered internet users.

The internet has so deeply and extensively penetrated our daily lives that it is difficult to imagine that it did not exist as little as forty years ago. The amount of information which is available, literally at our fingertips, is staggering, and has forever changed the way mankind will think of "looking something up". Whether one is checking the daily news, accessing the text of a rare book, trying to find the show times for a movie at the local cinema, submitting comments to the federal government about new proposed healthcare regulations, researching the most recent prognostic information for breast cancer, buying Christmas presents, or simply catching up with old friends, many of us cannot even conceive of how we might accomplish these tasks without the internet.

In addition to the obvious data gathering activities, the internet has undoubtedly changed our lives in ways we do not even appreciate. As a small example, let me quickly contrast the old and new approaches for researching a topic. In the not too distant past, if one had to learn about a topic in order to write a paper, for example, this involved numerous hours in the library looking through books and journal articles, gathering the small

---

[1] Statistics from www.internetworldstats.com

pieces of data which would ultimately be used to build an argument or a thesis. Simply trying to figure out where to look for the data was often the rate limiting step in gathering the needed information. In the process, however, one was forced to learn more about the larger field of which the desired data was a part. An appreciation for the depth, complexity, and nuances was a natural by-product of the data gathering process. In contrast, with the internet, the scope of information available to us has increased by orders of magnitude. No longer are we restricted by the collections of material comprising the local library, and sources of information which formerly were not accessible at all are now just keystrokes away. What's more, the information is available at such a granularity, that we can easily jump right to the information we are looking for, without having to wade through pages of background information. While on the one hand this is incredibly efficient, the information can also be gathered in such a superficial way that we cannot hope to do anything meaningful or significant with that knowledge. In essence, the internet has made it possible for someone to either learn more about a topic then was ever before possible, or to correctly answer a highly detailed question on a topic which they know nothing about – and still know nothing about even after having answered the question. Will the long term affect of this be a more highly educated population efficiently achieving greater accomplishments and advancing society, or a collection of superficial hackers passing themselves off as experts in a field without the fundamental knowledge needed to address any of the real underlying problems? Only time will tell.

A Brief History of the Internet

In the early 1960's each branch of the United States Military awarded, separately, the contract for development of their computer system to a different branch of the military. The Army went with Digital Equipment Corporation, the Air Force with IBM, and the Navy with Unisys. Although army computers could talk to other army computers, they could not talk to air force or navy computers, and vice-versa. Toward the end of that decade, the department of defense was charged with developing a "network of networks" to interconnect these systems. In 1969, the Advanced Research Projects Agency (ARPA, pronounced *are-pah*) developed ARPANet, the first "internet".

In 1971, the File Transfer Protocol (FTP) was introduced as a consistent way of transferring data files from one system to another. With proper passwords, a user on one computer could "log-in" to another computer, obtain a list of files, and either "get" files (transfer files from the remote computer to the local computer) or "put" files (transfer files from the local computer to the remote computer). The following year, the National Center for Supercomputing Applications (NCSA) introduced telnet, a protocol whereby one computer could, over the network, connect to a mainframe computer as if it were a terminal directly connected to that mainframe. This allowed a full range of operations rather than simply viewing files.

In 1973, ARPANet extended to include the University College of London and the Royal Radar in Norway, making it an international network. By the following year, 62 computers worldwide had been networked together in ARPANet. This network continued to grow over the next decade, with the addition of several university computer centers.

TCP/IP (Transmission Control Protocol/Internet Protocol; see below for more details) was introduced in 1983 and became the standard for communications between networks. By adopting this standard as the only standard for communicating on ARPANet, any network which could speak TCP/IP could be connected to ARPANet. This allowed rapid addition of new networks to the network of networks. That same year, the military decided, for security reasons, to segregate its computers to a different network, so ARPANet was split into a military network (MILNet) and a civilian network, the "Internet". The National Science Foundation created NSFNet to interconnect the nation's supercomputing centers together and to the civilian network. The backbone speed for the internet at this time, 1986, was 56 Kbps, or the speed of the dial-up modems in use today (less than 20 years later). Additional academic, government, and commercial agencies joined the internet, which by 1986 had grown to over 5,000 connected computers. That number doubled by the end of the following year, and passed the 100,000 mark two years after that in 1989.

The 1990s marked the explosion of the internet, which was already growing exponentially. The backbone speed had been upgraded to 44.7 Mbps by 1991 (nearly a 1000 fold increase in speed in five years). By 1993, the number of host computers connected to the internet passed the 2 million mark. Essentially all of the communication on the internet used the File Transfer Protocol for exchanging data.

In 1993, the European Laboratory for Particle Physics (CERN) introduced the HyperText Transfer Protocol (http), a way of transferring text documents which could be viewed from a local application called a browser. These documents could contain internal links which would connect the user to other http documents on the same or any other computer in the world. Since documents could contain multiple links, all of these documents across the world were interconnected in a complex web-like fashion, and the World Wide Web was born. The ease of use of this method of data exchange led to another wave of host computers joining the internet. Initially, "web" (http) traffic accounted for less than 1% of the total internet traffic, but this grew at a rate of 350,000% annually, and within two years (1995), web traffic had surpassed FTP traffic as the largest volume protocol used on the internet. The 5 million connected computers mark was passed in 1996, 10 million in 1997, 20 million in 1998, and 50 million in 1999.

TCP/IP

As mentioned above, as of 1983, all communication on the internet used the TCP/IP (*tee-see-pee-eye-pee)* communication protocol. This actually represents a combination of two layered protocols (one inside the other). TCP or Transmission Control Protocol is responsible for the fragmentation, transmission, and reassembly of the information, where as IP or Internet Protocol is responsible for the routing of the data frame to the proper destination. Each protocol adds a header to the data in the message. Sandwiching a TCP/IP message into an Ethernet message adds an additional header and a footer (Figure 4-12).

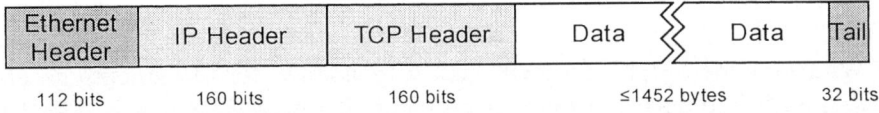

Ethernet Header	IP Header	TCP Header	Data	Data	Tail
112 bits	160 bits	160 bits	≤1452 bytes		32 bits

Figure 4-12: Structure of an Ethernet data frame. Ethernet data frames have a maximum length of 1500 bytes. This includes a 14 byte Ethernet header and 4 byte tail. The header and tail sandwich the message while it is on the local area network. At the router, the Ethernet header and tail are removed, and replaced with a header appropriate for the communication protocol on the portion of the internet backbone being used. The IP header is replaced as the message moves from router to router.

Transmission Control Protocol

TCP, as its name implies, controls the transmission of the data. The message is broken up into fragments called "datagrams" of a size appropriate for the local area network communication protocol being used (such as Ethernet). Since each message is likely to have multiple datagrams, and there is no way of knowing the order in which the datagrams will arrive at the destination, each datagram must be identified with the message to which it belongs and its sequence number within that message. There also needs to be a mechanism for checking the integrity of the datagram when it is received, known as a "checksum" (more on this in a second). On the receiving end, TCP procedures reassemble the datagrams to rebuild the original message. The TCP protocol also includes procedures for acknowledging receipt of each datagram, and for resending datagrams which were lost or corrupted in transit. All of this occurs "automatically" in the network interface card.

The "checksum" is a common approach to verifying data integrity following transmission, and several algorithms exist for doing this. Basically, one performs some mathematical operation on the digital representation of the data (for example, simply adding up the bytes). This is done initially at the transmitting end, and this sum is sent along with the message to the destination. At the destination, the same mathematical operation is performed on the data, and the result compared to the checksum value received with the message. If they don't match, the recipient knows that something happened during transmission which corrupted the message, so it is discarded and re-requested.

In a TCP datagram, all of the information about datagram sequence, the checksum, as well as the source and destination "ports" (which identify the message) are stored in a 160 bit TCP header which is added to the beginning of the data. The data with the TCP header is then passed to the Internet Protocols (IP) for addition of an IP header.

Internet Protocol

Whereas the TCP protocol is responsible for fragmenting and reassembling the data, the internet protocol (IP) header (which is added in front of the TCP header) is responsible for routing the data to the correct destination. The IP header is also 160 bits long, and is used by gateways and routers along the way to get data to its ultimate destination. Routers traditionally will strip the IP header off incoming messages and create a new IP header, readdressing the message to the next router in the path. The IP procedures do not care about the content of the data contained within the payload of the message, only the addressing information.

The IP header contains, in addition to the IP address of the source and destination computers, length bytes, internal quality control checksums (to verify the integrity of the header, not the data), and an expiration time. The expiration time, in my humble opinion, was a clever addition. Because of the dynamic nature of internet traffic routing, one could conceive of a message traveling in circles endlessly, constantly being re-routed due to congested traffic or simply because the recipient machine is no longer available. Without some way of dealing with this, the internet would eventually be full of messages going nowhere. The expiration time is used to filter these messages off the internet. When a message is received at a router, if the expiration time has passed, that message is simply discarded.

Every internet connected device is identified by a 4-byte (32 bit) IP address, usually expressed as four decimal numbers from 1 to 254, separated by periods (eg. 10.85.123.16). "0" is used for devices which don't know the value for a particular byte, and "255" is used for broadcasts, indicating that the message is intended for all devices matching the other bytes in the address. The four bytes are hierarchical, with each successive byte representing greater resolution. Thus, in the example above, 10.85.123.16 would be device #16 in subnet #123 of the 10.85.x.x network, etc.

IP addresses worldwide are assigned by a central agency. In 1993, this responsibility was awarded to InterNIC (www.internic.net). In 1998, assignments were regionalized to four Regional Internet Registries, of which the American Registry for Internet Numbers (ARIN) handles North American and Sub-Sahara Africa. The Internet Assigned Numbers Authority (IANA) coordinates the activities of these registries.

Why create a whole new addressing system when, as discussed above, each network interface card already has a unique media access control address? The reason is one of routing. MAC addresses are assigned at the time of manufacturing, but there is no way to tell, in advance, where in the world that piece of hardware might end up. Devices with sequential MAC addresses could be on opposite ends of the world. To route messages based on this address, the routing tables in the routers would have to contain the address of every machine in the world. Keeping that updated would be cumbersome and slow, as would searching such a table. The hierarchical nature of the IP address allows regional addressing. Therefore, a router in Germany, for example, only needs to know that all of the IP addresses that start with "207" are in the United States to be able to send a message on to the next router. Once the message gets to the United States, the routers will have higher resolution data for that group of addresses. This allows for much smaller routing tables and much faster routing of traffic.

When the IP addressing system was originally developed in 1983, no one conceived of the possibility that the four billion possible IP addresses allowed by this 32 bit system would not be sufficient. However, maintaining the hierarchical nature of IP address assignments is not very efficient, yielding "wasted" IP addresses, and the result is that there are simply not enough IP addresses to uniquely assign one to every device which would like to be connected to the internet. Three solutions have been developed to deal with this problem. The first is to simply create a new addressing system. IP Version 6 was developed in 1999 and uses a 128 bit address (that should keep us going for a while!), but most of the networking devices in use today do not support version 6. The vast majority of internet users are still using the 32 bit version.

The other two solutions are based on the fact that although many devices may need to connect to the internet, on occasion, they do not all have to be connected at all times. Dynamic Host Configuration Protocol (DHCP) is a mechanism for managing a pool of IP addresses. This is the process used by

Internet Service Providers (ISPs), commercial organizations which sell internet connections to end users. Basically, when a user connects to their ISP (via a modem of some sort), they are assigned an IP address from the pool, and use that address as long as they are connected to the internet. When they disconnect, that IP address goes back into the pool and is available for another user. If the same user connects again, they are more likely than not to receive a different IP address from the pool. In this way, thousands of users can share a pool of hundreds of IP addresses, because all of the users are not using the internet at the same time.

A second solution to the limited number of available globally unique IP addresses is to use IP address translation. This is based on the fact that an IP address does not really need to be unique world-wide, it only needs to be unique on the network it is being used. For organizations with many networked computers, most of the network traffic is between computers within the organization. Therefore, each device is assigned a local IP address, which is unique within the organization, but might be the same as a local IP address used within a different organization. (A specific subset of IP addresses are used for these "private" addresses.) When a device needs to communicate outside of the organization on the real internet, their local IP address is translated, at a gateway, into a globally unique public IP address for communication with the rest of the world. This process is known as Network Address Translation, or "NAT-ing". Since only some of the devices will need to communicate with the internet at any given point in time (and some of the devices, like printers, will never use the internet), a small pool of globally unique IP addresses can serve a large number of networked devices.

Note that while dynamic IP address assignment works fine for client users who are browsing the content on the internet, it will not work for server devices which are providing the content; servers need a fixed or static IP address so that other servers will always know where to find them. NAT-ing protocols can be set up such that certain devices on a private network are always given the same public IP address, creating a static address assignment.

The Domain Name System

Although the IP address uniquely identifies a particular device on the internet, it can be rather cumbersome to remember that if I want to go to a particular web site, I have to type in, for example, 10.85.123.16. The domain name system (DNS) allows each machine on the internet to also be given a textual name, known as the domain name. Domain names are a variable number of alphanumeric strings, separated by periods. Like IP addresses, domain names are hierarchical, but in a reverse fashion, such that the most specific element, the host name, comes first, and the most general element, the top-level domain name, comes last. Thus, domain names are of the format hostname.subdomain.top-level-domain. An example would be "www.yalepath.org". Domain names must be globally unique. This require that a system be in place to make sure two people do not try to assign the same domain name to two different machines. The "Internet Corporation for Assigned Names and Numbers" or ICANN serves this role. It oversees not only the assignment of unique domain names, but also the resolution of those names into unique IP addresses.

When a user wants to send a message to a device by using its domain name, that name needs to be translated into its corresponding IP address. This is done by looking up the domain name in a domain name server. How does the internet find a domain name server? There are 13 root servers scattered about the world, all containing the same information. Each serves as a backup for the others and they are continually synchronized. These root servers contain the IP addresses for all of the "top-level-domain" registries. Also scattered about the internet, usually in association with internet service providers or larger organizations, are thousands of domain name resolvers. These maintain an internal table of recently used domain names. These computers respond to requests to resolve a domain name by first checking their internal tables, and if no entry can be found, request a resolution from the appropriate top-level-domain registry.

Initially, there were a relatively small number of top-level-domains. Table 4-2 shows the ones originally in use. However, the initial restrictions for use of these domains have been softened, and a number of new top-level-domains have been established, so this list is not as important or meaningful as it once was. There are also a number of national top-level-domains.

Table 4-2: Original "top-level" domains.

Domain	Type of Organization
.com	Commercial organizations
.edu	Educational institutions (4 year colleges)
.gov	US government agencies
.int	Organization established by international treaties
.mil	US military
.net	Network providers
.org	Non-profit organizations

TCP/IP Ports and Sockets

Most of the readers will have had the experience of using a web browser on their computer and having more than one browser window open at a time. When you request a new web page and receive it through the internet connection, how does the browser know which in window to display the page? Also, how is it that you can receive electronic mail while you are "surfing the web" if you only have one internet connection with one IP address? This is made possible by something known as TCP ports. Ports are the equivalent of different virtual channels for a single receiver. Just as your television can receive different programs on different channels, in the same way the network interface card on your desktop computer, which has only one IP address, can receive different data on different ports. The port number is a number from 0 to 65535 (a 16-bit number) which can be specified after an IP address, separated from the IP address with a colon. For example: 10.85.123.16:80 would represent TCP port 80 for IP address 10.85.123.16. In most cases, you will not have to specify the port number; the software in the computer takes care of that automatically.

A "socket" is an abstraction of a single connection between an IP address and port on one computer and an IP address and port on another computer. It is a connection between two applications. Each connection requires a new "socket", and each socket is owned by exactly one application on each end of the communication connection. However, an application (like a web server or browser) can own multiple sockets at the same time. Once a socket is established, data can pass back and forth bidirectionally between the two applications. The network interface card keeps track of which applications are using which sockets and therefore which port numbers, and when a transmission is received, it is passed off to the appropriate window in the appropriate application.

Port numbers 0 - 1023 are reserved for specific uses. Some of the more commonly used ones are listed in Table 4-3. Values greater than 1023 are available for use at the end-user's discretion, and are often assigned dynamically. When you open a window in your browser, that window will

Table 4-3: Commonly used reserved port numbers.

Port	Use	Port	Use	Port	Use
0	Ping	37	Time server	110	POP3
21	FTP	53	DNS	137	WINS
23	Telnet	80	http	143	IMAP3,4
25	SMTP	109	POP2	514	HTTPS

be assigned a port number. A socket will be set up between that port on your computer (a process known as binding) and port 80 on the web server to which you are connecting. The server sends its information back to the browser using that socket. Each open window would have its own unique socket with its own unique port number.

The World Wide Web

The World Wide Web, usually referred to simply as the "web", is not a separate communication system than the internet, but rather a method of communicating over the internet. As with all internet communication, the web uses TCP/IP as its base protocol. The data transmitted, however, adheres to a higher level protocol referred to as the HyperText Transfer Protocol, or HTTP.

Information on the web is divided into pages. Each page corresponds roughly to a document sitting on some web server somewhere in the world. Web pages are uniquely identified by their Uniform Resource Locator or URL (*you-are-el*), which identifies both the web server which the page is on and the name of the document file which corresponds to that page. These documents are written in hypertext markup language, or HTML, and can support not only text but also graphics, images, and sound. A key feature of HTML documents is that they contain links, referred to as hyperlinks, to other HTML documents. The user browsing the web simply clicks on one of these links and they are presented with that new document. Since each document frequently contains links to several other documents, and since most documents can be reached from several other documents, a complex interconnecting web of information is created allowing non-linear browsing of information.

To understand how the web works, it is essential to understand the concept of a web client and a web server. A web server is an internet connected computer with a fixed IP address (and often a DNS name) which is running a program called a "web server application". That server also contains a collection of HTML files and supporting images (web pages), and these, together with the web server application, constitute a web site.

Any internet connected computer running a web server application can be a web server. The web server application constantly monitors its network line, specifically port 80, for requests for one of its pages. The client, on the other hand, is a different computer running a different program called a "web browser" (examples include Netscape, Internet Explorer, Safari, and Firefox). When the user of a client computer clicks on a hyperlink in their web browser, that hyperlink has a corresponding URL identifying a particular web server and a particular web page on that server. A request is

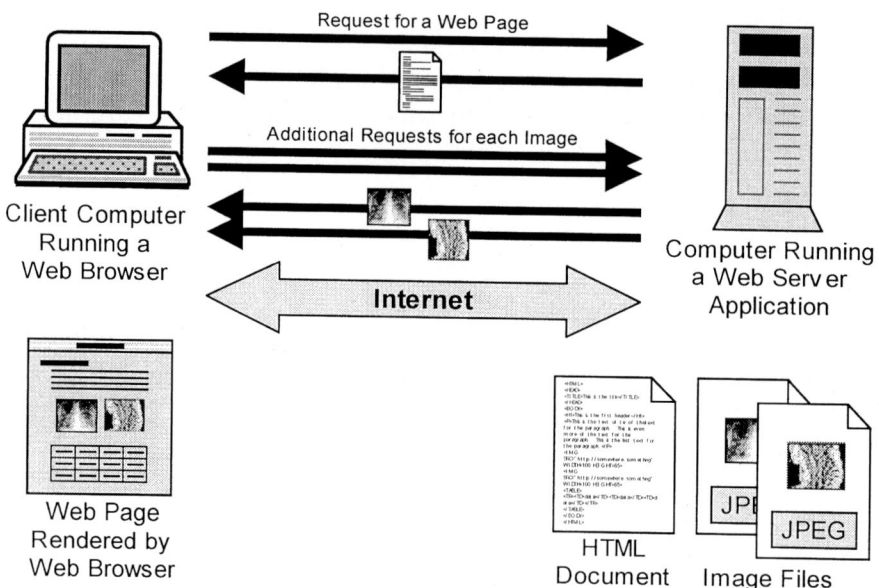

Figure 4-13: Viewing a web page on a client web browser. When the client user clicks on a hyperlink, a request is sent, over the internet, to a specific web server for a specific web "page". The server responds by sending the appropriate HTML document back over the internet to the client computer. The client browser, while interpreting the HTML and "rendering" the page, identifies other page elements it needs and places separate requests for each of these.

sent, through the internet to port 80 on the web server identified in that link, requesting the specific web page (Figure 4-13). The web server application running on the web server computer receives this request, and sends the HTML document requested back to the browser application running on the client computer. The hypertext transfer protocol handles the issues of identifying the document and sending it with the appropriate header to the appropriate window on the client computer. Once received, the web browser application interprets the hypertext markup language commands embedded in the document and "renders" (i.e., draws) the document in a window on the client computer. As the browser interprets the document, it may discover that it needs additional files, such as images, to render the page. Separate requests are sent back to the web server for each of these additional page elements.

Hypertext Markup Language (HTML)

Hypertext markup language has evolved significantly from its initial conception. The original thought behind this "language" was to create a method by which information could be distributed to other computers independent of the type of operating system present on those computers. The author of the document would "markup" the various parts of the document such as "this is a header", "this is a paragraph", "this is a list", "this is a table". Marking-up is done with "tags", special text enclosed within less-than and greater-than signs. One tag marks the beginning of a marked portion of the document, and another tag

```
<TABLE>
  <TR>row1</TR>
  <TR>row2</TR>
  <TR>row3</TR>
</TABLE>
```

Figure 4-14: HTML. A portion of an HTML document illustrating the use of nested tags to build a three row table.

(usually the same text preceded by a forward slash) marks the end. Thus, "<TITLE>This is the title</TITLE>" indicates the title of the document. The web browser, when it renders the page, knows to put this text in the title bar of the window. Tags can also be nested within each other (Figure 4-14). For example, the tags for each row of a table should be nested between the opening and closing tags for the table.

Using markup-tags, the author of the web page determined the content of the page and defined what each part of the page represented, but would not specify any of the details about what a header or a paragraph or a list or a table were supposed to look like. The browser application on the client machine would have settings whereby the user could specify "I want to use this type-face and this font size for paragraphs, and I want headers to be in bold and two font sizes larger, ..." etc. Thus, depending upon the settings of the client browser, the same web page could look very different on two different client computers, and this was considered a good thing, since the user could control the look while the author of the page controlled the content. With the explosion in popularity of the web, however, this separation of the look from the content did not hold up. To attract users to their web sites, authors of web pages wanted more control over how the pages were actually going to look, not simply what information was going to be in them. In addition, authors wanted to be able to create interactive and dynamic web pages, rather than simply displaying static content. To meet these needs, HTML, web browsers, and web servers evolved.

Authors of web pages obtained greater control of the look of their pages when rendered on a client browser by the addition of new capabilities to HTML. This was in the form of new tags, new attributes for existing tags, and style sheets. The details of this are beyond the scope of this discussion, but suffice it to say that the authors could now specify fonts, colors, etc. This "capability" has come at a cost. Not every client computer will have the fonts the author of the web page has chosen to use. In addition, these new capabilities were implemented by web browsers before they were standardized, so not every browser on every operating system platform uses these in the same way. The end result is that not only do the pages still not look the same on every client machine, but now some pages simply do no work on some client machines, depending upon what version of which browser the client is using. Although some standardization has occurred, this continues to be a problem for more complex web pages.

Client-side and Server-side Processing

To add interactivity for the user, such as something happening when the user clicks on a button, or pop-up help windows appearing and disappearing, authors of web pages needed to be able to write small programs which could be embedded within web documents and with which the user viewing the web page within his/her browser could interact. Two solutions were introduced to handle this, which are actually quite different solutions with, unfortunately, very similar names. JavaScript is an interpreted object oriented language which can be run within most of the more sophisticated web browsers. The HTML document which comprises the web page has, embedded within it inside <SCRIPT> tags, the source code for small programs. As the web browser is rendering the web page, it recognizes the <SCRIPT> tags as indicating areas where there are JavaScript programs, and since the web browser has a built in interpreter (see the discussion in Chapter 3 on desktop computer software under "Computer Programming"), these lines of source code are converted to machine language and executed. JavaScript allows defining variables as well as small routines (functions) which can be executed when the user clicks on a button or mouses over an image. The second solution to add interactivity to web pages is Java Applets. Despite the similarity in name to JavaScript, these are completely different. Java Applets (applet = small application; it has nothing to do with apple the fruit or Apple the computer company) are written in advance and precompiled into bytecode (again, see the "Computer Programming" section in Chapter 3). The precompiled bytecode is stored on the web server as a file, and sent with the web page to the client. However, the client's web browser cannot directly execute the Java Applet, but rather has to hand it off to a Java runtime library which must also be present on the client computer for all of this to work. This is much more complicated than JavaScript, both for the author and for the setup of the client computer, and the possibility of incompatibilities is greater. However, unlike JavaScript, Java is a full computer language, allowing greater control of the user interface and more complex operations.

JavaScript and Java are two examples of "client-side-processing", because the ultimate execution of the programs occurs on the client computer, allowing greater interaction with the user. However, the content of the web pages was still static. The user on the client computer always received a pre-made web document which, although it might have a lot of bells and whistles (literally!), always had the same content. There needed to be a way to provide custom content, to make possible such things as reporting search results, on-line shopping, and on-line banking. This functionality requires "server-side-processing", small programs which run on the server computer and produce a custom HTML document containing the desired information. There also needed to be a way for the user on the client computer to send information to the server which could be used by the server-side programs to gather the requested information. "Forms" have been implemented in HTML to allow users on a client machine to send information to the server. The user fills in blanks or selects elements from a drop down list, or checks check-boxes, and then presses a submit button. This sends the information back to the web server, which makes the data available to programs running within the web-server application. These server-side programs can then use this information to search a database (see Chapter 5 for more information) or look up files, and then package that information in HTML format and return it to the user. More intelligent web server applications are required to achieve this capability.

Several options exist for server-side-processing and programming. Among the first was Common Gateway Interface or CGI, a method to pass information from a form on a client computer to a program on the web server, usually a Perl script. Microsoft developed Active Server Pages (ASP) to address server-side-processing. This solution runs only in Microsoft's web server, which can only run on Microsoft's operating systems, but is nonetheless widely used. PHP is an open source solution which can run with a variety of web server applications on a variety of platforms. (PHP is actually a recursive acronym which stands for "PHP: Hypertext Preprocessor".) Finally, just to make things a little more confusing, Java programs can also be embedded within web pages to be run on the server (Java Server Pages or JSP). JSP source files are processed by the JSP container of the web server into Java source code for server-side-processing, called servlets, which are compiled into a Java class and executed when requested. The combination of server-side-processing and client-side-processing allows the creation of fully functional web applications.

Electronic Mail

Very few pathologists have never used electronic mail, or "email", for short. The speed, convenience, and (at least for now) low to no cost make this an invaluable tool. Email is often a more effective communication tool than the telephone since the recipient does not have to be available at the same time you are available to send information. Thus, the email can remain in the recipient's box until it is convenient for him/her to answer it. Unfortunately, email can be more easily ignored than a phone call.

A basic understanding of electronic mail is helpful in allowing you to more effectively manage your email account. In order to send or receive email, you need an email account on a computer which is connected to the internet and is running mail services. This computer, known as the email server, is responsible for sending your messages to their addressees, and for receiving and holding messages addressed to you until you can read them. Electronic mail travels from email server to email server around the world via the internet.

Although it is possible to read your email by logging into the email server directly and viewing your email there, it is much more common to use an email client program on your local desktop computer. That program communicates over the network with your email server. Examples of dedicated email clients are Eudora and Outlook. Web browsers also have the ability to act as an email client and access accounts on an email server.

New messages you receive (and any associated attachments) reside on the email server under your account, where they take up disk space. It is important to know that all email servers limit the amount of space your mail can take up on the server. If you exceed your storage capacity on the server, any new messages sent to you will be rejected by the server.

Simple Mail Transfer Protocol (SMTP)

In much the same way as web traffic on the internet uses the hypertext transfer protocol (http) on TCP port 80, electronic mail is sent over the internet using simple mail transfer protocol on TCP port 25. Originally defined in 1982, SMTP (*ess-em-tee-pee*) is by far the most popular method for sending email messages between email servers. A few other protocols exist, but they are only minimally used. The SMTP protocol includes the necessary capabilities to forward mail from server to server until it reaches the appropriate destination. Computers known as name servers allow the various email servers around the world to translate your email address into the address of the email server on which you have your email account.

It is often useful to attach documents and other files to an electronic mail message. Since SMTP was designed only for transmitting ASCII text data, most servers will encode non-text messages (images, sound, executable code) using a coding system known as Base64, which converts the files to ASCII files. The attachments are decoded when received. This encapsulation process is known as Multipurpose Internet Mail Extensions protocol or MIME (rhymes with *time*). To allow each computer to know what type of file is being transported, the files are designated with a MIME type. Examples of MIME types include "text/html" and "image/jpeg".

SMTP is not only used to send email between email servers; it is also the method used to send email from your email client to your email server. Checking your email, which involves connecting your email client on your local desktop computer to your email server to see if any mail has arrived there for you uses one of two different protocols, and each has some advantages and disadvantages.

Post Office Protocol (POP)

Post Office Protocol is the most popularly used method for an email client to connect to an email server, and most commercially available dedicated email application software uses POP (pronounced like what you might do to a bubble). With this protocol, the user intermittently connects to the server, looks for any mail which may have arrived, downloads that mail (with attachments) to the local desktop computer, deletes the email from the server, and then disconnects from the server. Then, any reading of the mail and/or attachments is done locally with the email client. Since the original messages are typically deleted from the server, they (and more importantly any attachments) are no longer taking up space on the server, so your account is "free" to receive more messages. The downloaded messages remain on your local machine (where you have "unlimited" storage space) until you delete them. Most email client software allows you to create a variety of storage mailboxes in which you can file mail messages which you wish to save.

When using POP to check your mail from an office desktop computer, the email client software is usually configured to automatically check for new mail on a regular basis, such as every 15 minutes. If any is found, it is downloaded, deleted from the server, and then you are notified that you now have unread mail in your local IN box, where the mail can sit until you have the opportunity to read it. If you traditionally use a laptop computer, or a home computer which is not constantly connected to the internet, then you decide when you want to log in to check your mail.

Since the only time you are connected to the email server is when you are checking for and downloading messages, and all of the managing of your email is done from your local computer, Post Office Protocol is often referred to as an "offline" protocol. It has undergone some revisions since initially introduced in 1984. The current version, POP3, uses TCP port 110.

Internet Message Access Protocol (IMAP)

In contrast to POP, the Internet Message Access Protocol is an "online" protocol. With IMAP (*eye-map*), the user uses their email client to connect to the email server. There, they can view the mail in their mailbox, read the mail, delete it if desired, or simply mark it as read. The mail remains on the email server unless the user chooses specifically to download a message and/or attachment to their local machine, and even then the original remains on the server until specifically deleted. IMAP supports multiple mailboxes (unlike POP), so the user can transfer mail into storage mailboxes if desired. In addition, IMAP can support simultaneous access to a common mailbox from multiple client locations, and all connected users will constantly receive updated information about the contents of the mailbox.

When one uses capabilities built into a web browser in order to check ones email, that web browser almost always uses IMAP to access the email account. In addition, most email servers allow IMAP based web access to your email account ("webmail") by simply directing your browser to an appropriate log-in window. When accessed in this way, you are not actually using the email capabilities of the web browser, so no configuration or set-up is required. This is ideal for checking your email from someone else's computer.

IMAP is currently at version 4, and uses TCP port 143 for communicating on a network.

Is POP or IMAP better for me?

The main differences between POP and IMAP is that with POP, the time you spend connected to the email server is minimal, and all of the messages are downloaded to and managed on your local desktop computer. With IMAP, the message remain on the mail server, and you manage them there, requiring longer connection times.

Whether POP and IMAP is better for you depends upon how and where you read your email. For example, say you usually read your email at work, but occasionally read it from home. In addition, lets assume both the work and home email browsers use POP. Before leaving work, you check your mail and find you have 20 unread email messages, and not enough time to read them, so you shut down your computer and go home. Later that evening, from home, you log in to the email server and check your email. However, the 20 unread messages you downloaded at work aren't on the server any more, so you can't read them from home. You will be able to see any new messages that have arrived since you turned off your computer at work. However, if you download those to your home computer, they will not be available to you at work the next day, because they will have been removed from the server and reside only on your home computer. In addition, if you forgot to turn off your computer at work before going home, and your work email browser is set up to automatically check your mailbox, it will continue to download your mail to your work computer, and when you log into the server from home you will always find an empty mail box.

Similarly, if you do not have a dedicated computer at work, but tend to use any of a number of computers to check your email, then using POP protocol will be problematic, since your email will rapidly become scattered across multiple computers. IMAP would keep all your email on the server, so it would all be available to you no matter where you are when you access it. IMAP is also useful for keeping the client computers "data-less", since email is not automatically downloaded. This tends to work best for multi-user computers as might be found in a laboratory or signout area.

On the other hand, with IMAP, your connection time to the server is prolonged. If you have a slow internet connection, or a heavily used email server, even reading your email can take a long time. If you pay for your connection by the minute, you are paying while you are reading, and it would be cheaper to download the messages and read them "offline". IMAP does, however, allow you to see what is in your mailbox without having to specifically download everything. If you notice that a message has a 3 MByte file attached to it, you can choose to not download the file until later when you have more time or a faster internet connection.

The main disadvantage of IMAP is that since all your messages and attachments remain on the email server until you delete them, they are constantly taking up space there. Most email accounts place a limit on how much space you can use (some even charge based on the amount of space used). If you get many messages or even a few large attachments, you will rapidly reach your storage capacity on the email server and effectively shut-down your email account, since the server will accept no more messages for you. Therefore, careful management of your email storage is necessary.

If for some reason the email server were to go down or be unavailable, users of IMAP lose all access to their mail, whereas POP users can still access any email they have downloaded.

One final note: the differences between POP and IMAP are starting to blur. For example, POP email browsers can be configured to leave a copy of the email on the server. If you do this, deleting a message from your local computer does not automatically delete it from the server (unless you activate that option as well). Traditionally, when one sets up a POP mail server to be more IMAP-like, one sets parameters like "delete any read mail from the server after xx days".

Each user must find the solution that works best for them. We have found that for our faculty, who each have a dedicated computer in their offices and who do most of the electronic mail management from their offices, a POP email client works best, and one has been installed on every faculty machine. It automatically checks and downloads email on a regular basis. When that faculty member is traveling out of town, they are instructed to shut off their office computer to prevent the downloading, and then can use any web browser to check their email while away using the IMAP based webmail interface. In contrast, for our residents, who share a set of computers, these computers use an IMAP based method for checking their email, since they never know which machine they will be using next to access their email account.

Remember that both POP and IMAP protocols are for reading email only. Your email client software still uses SMTP to send email to the email server. Therefore, your local email client application will need to be configured for SMTP as well as for either POP or IMAP.

E-mail and Security

Because email travels from the sender's computer to the recipient's computer via the internet, it is generally not possible to predict the route that the message will take through all the various internet lines. Therefore, it is possible for "sniffer" programs to intercept and read the email. For this reason, email is not generally considered a secure form of communication, unless encrypted. This needs to be kept in mind when composing an email message. In particular, **email messages should not contain any personally identifiable protected health information about patients**. Indirect references to a patient with information which is sufficiently vague as to make it impossible to determine the patient in question is acceptable.

However, within an institution, if all of the users are using the same email server, and that server is located within the institution, the email may never actually make it out onto the internet, so patient communication may be allowed. Check with your email administrator and institutional security policies. However, even if your intra-institutional email is secure, beware of members of your institution who may have multiple email accounts, and may have sent you email from a public email server, before simply hitting the "reply" button and including protected health information in your response.

On the subject of security, a brief mention should be made of email viruses. Electronic mail is, by far, the most common method by which computer viruses are spread. Computer viruses are small programs, often embedded within other files, which, when executed, "hijack" your computer's CPU and can do anything from annoyingly changing the system date to devastatingly erasing the contents of the hard disk. As a general rule of thumb, do NOT open executable files or archives from anyone you do not know, and always keep viral protection software running on any machine which is internet connected.

Chapter 5

DATABASES

As with so many other disciplines, the storage and maintenance of data is fundamental to the practice of pathology. Whether one is talking about specimen results, physician addresses, or patient history, it is difficult to imagine the practice of pathology, or medicine for that matter, without some electronic access to historical information on patients. Building a patient history is a fundamental functionality in any pathology information system. All of this history, all of the information about patients and specimens, all of the dictionaries listing billing codes and ICD-9 codes, all of this data is stored in databases. The practicing pathologist may feel they don't need to know anything about electronic databases since they don't use them, but in reality, pathologists uses electronic databases on a daily basis, often without even realizing it.

In its most general sense, a database is any collection of information about anything. Therefore, a stack of books constitutes a database, as does a filing cabinet full of files, or a pile of index cards, of a disk full of computer files. However, that is not a very useful definition. So, let's consider some properties of a database, and for purposes of this discussion let's consider only electronically stored databases. The database should be non-volatile. Although technically one could have a database which is erased whenever the computer is shut down, that is not a very useful database. The database should be a repository for data which has some inherent meaning. Therefore, I will exclude things like an index, or a thesaurus, or a dictionary, from our concept of a database. A database should be designed, built, and populated for at least some purpose, although it may be for several purposes, and may be used for several things which were not considered in the initial design and population. A database should store multiple instances of some type of information: for example information about multiple specimens, or multiple patients, or both. The number of instances allowable should be large, and each instance should be essentially as important or significant as any other instance. Finally, the database should store similar details about each instance of the information. A database in which one stored only the name of one patient, and only the address of another patient, and only the phone number of a third patient, would not be a very useful database.

Taking these properties together, a better definition of an electronic database would be something like "a non-volatile, structured collection of similar information about a variable number of instances of some entity."

Database Terminology

Databases have been around for a long time, and a number of different models have been developed to describe and refer to databases. They have been depicted as index cards, tables, trees, objects, etc. Some of these models will be described later. However, with each model, a unique terminology developed to refer to various parts of the model. Of course, these models all described the same concepts, and as a result, multiple different, somewhat model specific terminologies developed to refer to these concepts. Thus, almost every concept in database structure has two or more terms used to refer to it. What makes this even more confusing is that since most "database people" are familiar with various models, there is a tendency to mix and match the terminology from multiple different models, treating the different words for the same concepts as synonyms. This can make it difficult for them to communicate with "non-database people".

To describe and define these various terms, it is helpful to have a specific example to refer to. Rather than diving up front into the complexity of a database for a pathology information system, let's start with a simple database as our example: an address book. Everyone has kept an address book of some sort, paper or electronic, so the pitfalls and problems of some approaches will be easier to understand.

In our sample address-book database, we will store, for each entry, a last name, first name, street address, city, state, zip code, and phone number. One model which can be used for this database is a stack of index cards (Figure 5-1). Under this model, each index card stores information about one name and address. The name and address is considered the "entity". Each instance of the name and address is considered a "record". An important concept about databases is that each record is supposed to be independent of every other record. The informational elements stored about each record (not the data itself, but the place holders for the data) are referred to as the "fields". The actual information is referred to as the values for the fields, or the data. In this model, the fields determine the structure of

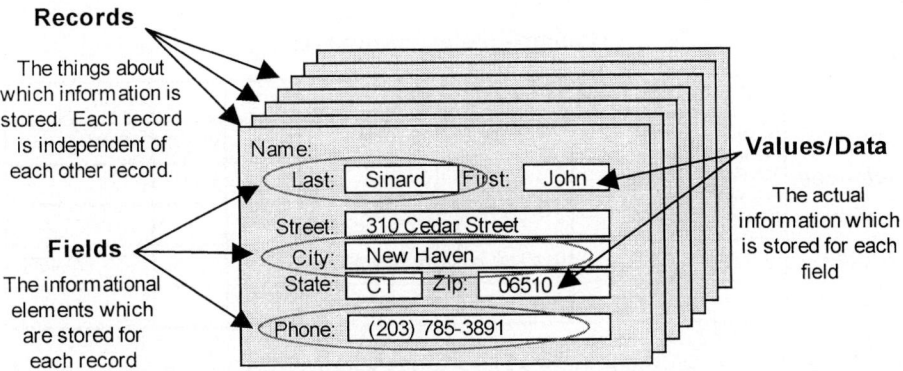

Figure 5-1: Sample address book database modeled as a set of index cards. A database can be thought of as a collection of index cards, each containing similar information about a different instance of some entity. Each card or instance is a "record", each item of information stored is a "field", and each data element is a "value".

each record, and therefore the structure of the data. Different fields can hold different types of data: for example, some may hold textual data whereas others may hold numeric data.

Another model which can be used to represent the same data is a table rather than a stack of index cards (Figure 5-2). In this model, the table itself represents the "entity". The columns of the table represent the fields, also known as the "attributes" ("attributes" is a particularly common term when using the object model to depict the entity). The rows represent the "instances", or records, sometimes referred to as "tuples" (although I must admit I have heard very few people use this word!) In the table model, each cell in the table contains the actual data, also referred to as the "value" or the "data elements". The number of columns is sometimes called the "degree" of the entity, whereas the number of rows is referred to as the "cardinality" of the entity.

The table model is commonly used to conceptualize a simple database. It highlights the fact that a spreadsheet is actually a form of database. More complex databases are similarly often thought of as collections of tables. This conceptualization allows the designer to abstract (separate) him/herself, somewhat, from the details of how the data is stored in the database. As will be seen below, this abstraction process is not only theoretical, but is also the usual practice, since database management systems generally handle the details of data storage.

The process of retrieving data from a database is referred to as "reading", whereas putting data into the database is called "writing". Adding new data

Columns (fields, attributes)

	Last Name	First Name	Street	City	State	Zip	Phone
Rows	Sinard	John	310 Cedar St.	New Haven	CT	06510	(203) 785-3891
(instances,	Mouse	Mickey	Disney World	Orlando	FL	32300	
records,	Potter	Harry	4 Privet Drive	Little Whinging	Surrey		
tuples)	Torrance	Jack	Overlook Hotel	Sidewinder	CO	80200	(303) 123-4000

Figure 5-2: Sample address book database modeled as a table. The same data represented by the index card model of Figure 5-1 can also be represented as a table, where each row is an instance (a card) and each column is a field. This is one of the most commonly used models for conceptualizing a database. Spreadsheet software can be used for a simple database.

is frequently referred to as "inserting", especially for databases with a table-based model. Removing data is "deleting", and changing existing data is "updating".

Database Architecture

Database architecture is a vague term used to describe, for the most part, how one conceptualizes the database. It may or may not have any direct relationship with how the data is actually stored, but it does speak to the underlying rules for data access and update. The theory behind the design can place constraints on how the user can view the data, and how searching of the database can be performed.

Single Table Databases

The greatest advantage of a single table database is that it is simple to conceptualize. Essentially anyone can imagine a two dimensional grid with columns representing the different types of data and rows representing the different instances of the data. This type of database also has many options for implementing it electronically, including simply using a spreadsheet. However, the world is generally not that simple, and few real world situations can be effectively handled, even in a purely abstract way, by a single table.

Nonetheless, a simple, single table database is worth discussing since it will illustrate some of the reasons for using more complex databases. Two issues which illustrate the shortcomings of a single table database are repeating fields and redundant fields.

Repeating Fields

Repeating fields are one or more attributes which can occur multiple times for a single instance of an entity. In our sample address book database, examples of this would include the fact that a person can have more than one phone number, or more than one people can live at the same address. Let's just consider the multiple phone number problem. How can this be incorporated into our database model? To keep a single table database, we need to add additional columns to handle the additional phone numbers (Figure 5-3). Of course, this raises a few additional questions. How many phone number slots are needed? Is three enough? After all, a person could have a home phone number, a fax number, a cell phone number, and a beeper number. To store all the phone numbers one might want to store, there have to be enough slots in each row to accommodate the needs of the one row (instance) with the greatest number of phone numbers.

Last	First	Street	City	State	Zip	Phone1	Phone2	Phone3
Sinard	John	310 Cedar St	New Haven	CT	06510	(203) 785-3891	(203) 137-1234	(203) 785-3644
Mouse	Mickey	Disney World	Orlando	FL	32300			
Potter	Harry	4 Privet Drive	Little Whinging	Surrey				
Torrance	Jack	Overlook Hotel	Sidewinder	CO	80200	(303) 123-4000		

Figure 5-3: Repeating fields. Repeating fields are two or more columns (attributes) storing similar information for a single instance (row) of an entity (table).

When multiple repeats of the field are included in a table, one then needs to consider whether or not all the repeats are equivalent, or if the position of the repeat carries some inherent meaning. If there are three phone numbers stored, and the first one is deleted, do the other two stay in positions two and three or should the remaining two phone numbers be shifted to positions one and two? If "Phone2" is always a beeper number, one should not move the numbers around. If they are all equivalent, will the search routine which finds no phone number in position one continue to check positions two and three? This logic needs to be determined up front, before any data is stored.

A potential solution to the significance of the position of the phone numbers is to add a second repeating field which identifies what each phone number represents (Figure 5-4). While the meaning of each phone number is now clear, even more "wasted space" is present in rows which don't use all of the allotted phone number slots.

Last	First	Street	City	State	Phone1	Tp1	Phone2	Tp2	Phone3	Tp3
Sinard	John	310 Cedar St	New Haven	CT	(203) 785-3891	W	(203) 137-1234	B	(203) 785-3644	F
Mouse	Mickey	Disney World	Orlando	FL						
Potter	Harry	4 Privet Drive	Little Whinging	Surrey						
Torrance	Jack	Overlook Hotel	Sidewinder	CO	(303) 123-4000	H				

Figure 5-4: Paired repeating fields. When repeating fields are used to store multiple similar attributes for a single row, it is often necessary to add a second repeating field to describe how each of those attributes differ from each other.

Redundant Fields

Redundant fields are attributes or groups of attributes which have the same values over multiple instances of an entity. The fact that multiple people can live at the same address was mentioned before. That could be addressed by adding more name columns to the database table, as was done for phone numbers. Alternatively, one could add additional rows for each additional person, and simply duplicate the data which is the same for the new instances (Figure 5-5).

Last Name	First Name	Street	City	State	Zip	Phone
Simpson	Homer	742 Evergreen Terrace	Springfield	KY	40069	(800) 555-1234
Simpson	Marge	742 Evergreen Terrace	Springfield	MO	65850	(800) 555-1234
Simpson	Bart	742 Evergreen Terrace	Springfield	MA	01150	(800) 555-1234
Simpson	Lisa	742 Evergreen Terrace	Springfield	GA	31329	(800) 555-1234

Figure 5-5: Redundant fields. Data which is shared by multiple instances of an entity (e.g., multiple people living at the same address) can be handled by repeating the data values across multiple rows of a table. However, this creates an opportunity for data inconsistency.

A consequence of this approach is that a lot of database space can be used storing the same data multiple times. This approach also creates the potential for inconsistencies in the data. In the example above, we know that all of the Simpson's live in the same house in the town of Springfield, but there seems to be some confusion as to what state Springfield is in. Whether this inconsistency arises from data entry error or true ambiguities in the data, inconsistent data across the rows is something that can and will occur, and procedures need to be developed to address this. Even if careful data entry results in consistent data, the redundancy needs to be considered if the data is ever edited because of real changes to the data. If the Simpson's decide to move to Shelbyville, data has to be updated in multiple rows to maintain internal consistency.

Multi-table Databases

The shortcomings of a single table database, illustrated above, came about because the sample database which we were trying to model as a single table really contains more than one entity. Entities are best thought of as independent real world objects, rather than just descriptive details which are solely dependent upon the instance of those objects. The actual process of determining what are the entities in any data storage system is far from trivial, and will be discussed in more detail below under "database normalization". However, our sample address-book database can be thought of as consisting of three discrete entities: people, addresses, and phone numbers. City, state, and zip code are not entities per se, but rather further details or attributes of the address entity. Similarly, first name and last name are attributes of the "person" entity.

A common approach used when considering the relationships between entities is to divide those relationships into one of three categories: one-to-one, one-to-many, or many-to-many. Most homes have only one home phone number. In this case, there is a one-to-one relationship between the address and the home phone number: the address has only one home phone number, and the home phone number belongs to only one address. Attributes which hold a one-to-one relationship with each other can often be expressed as columns within the same table. If we consider only primary residences in our address-book database, then a potential one-to-many relationship exists between addresses and people. Each person has only one primary address, but an address can be the primary address for many people. Note that even if most of the addresses in our database have only one person living there, the potential for multiple people makes this a one-to-many relationship (unless we decide up front that we will not allow that to occur, at least not in our database). The most complex relationship to tackle is the many-to-many relationship. Our address-book database is being designed to store any phone number, not just the home phone number. Therefore, we know that one person can have many phone numbers. Also, the same phone number can belong to multiple people. A similar situation holds in the medical profession: patients often have more than one physician, and most physicians have more than one patient, so this is a many-to-many relationship.

The problems we encountered with our single table database, in particular the repeating fields and redundant fields, came about because a single table database does not provide a good mechanism for dealing with anything beyond a one-to-one relationship. As a result, more complex, multiple entity databases have been developed to handle this multiplicity. A few examples will be discussed.

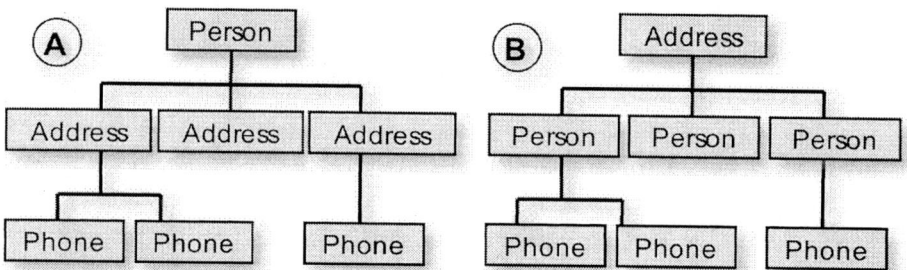

Figure 5-6: Hierarchical databases. The design of a hierarchical database determines the relationships between the entities. In example A, the primary point of view is the person. Each person can have multiple addresses. In example B, the address is at the top of the hierarchy, and each address can be associated with multiple persons.

Hierarchical Databases

One-to-many relationships can be effectively represented by a hierarchical database design, in which the relationships of the data entities to each other are represented by an inverted tree structure. In an inverted-tree hierarchy, each "parent" can have one or more children, but each "child" can have only one parent. The choice of the hierarchy determines the viewpoint of the database, and has implications for searching the database and updating it. For example, our address-book database could be modeled, hierarchically, in a couple of different ways (Figure 5-6). In model A, the primary point of view is the person. This model recognizes that a person can have multiple addresses (work, home, vacation home), and that each of those addresses can have one or more phone numbers. If we are really only interested in a single person at each address, this might be an effective model for our database. However, if we want to keep track of all the people at each address, using model A would require redundant address entries. If this occurs a lot, then model B might be better suited to our purpose. This eliminates redundancy at the address level, but introduces redundancy at the phone number level. In addition, model B would be a more difficult database to search by person.

Hierarchical databases have many advantages. They can easily deal with one-to-many relationships, allowing an entity to have as many "children" as necessary. Also, when searched from the viewpoint by which the database was designed, searches can be very fast. It is also relatively easy to add data to a hierarchical database, and even additional hierarchies can be added after the initial conception of the database without significant consequences.

The file system on the hard disk of your computer is another example of a hierarchical database. Each "folder" can have many children (files or other folders in the folder), but can have only one parent (a file/folder can be in only one folder at a time).

However, as illustrated even in our simple address-book example, a major limitation of this architecture is that each entity can have only one parent, so a choice has to be made up front as to which viewpoint one is going to use. Subsequently searching the database from a different viewpoint is not easy (for example, I have a phone number, and I want to find out to whom it belongs), and often requires a sequential search of all the data in the database. In addition, the hierarchical model does not support relationships which violate the hierarchy. For example, consider a person with a cellular telephone. We would like to associate that phone number with a person, but it doesn't really make sense to associate it with a single address. Under model A above, the only way to enter a phone number into the database is to associate it with an address. A final disadvantage of the hierarchical database structure is that it frequently requires a significant amount of programming to access and update the data, especially if one attempts to address the shortcomings discussed programmatically.

Despite these limitations, hierarchical databases are frequently found in medical information systems. This is primarily due to the fact that the highest level in medical record databases is a well defined entity: the patient. The next level often represents some sort of encounter, such as an admission to the hospital, or an outpatient visit, or an emergency room visit. Laboratory data can then "hang off" of the encounter data. Unfortunately, if the pathology laboratory gets specimens on a patient which did not come from an institutional encounter, as is often seen in laboratories with an outreach program to community physician offices, one is often forced to "invent" encounters so that one has a place to put the laboratory data. This hierarchical approach also does not readily support quality assurance and/or research programs which may, for example, want to find all of the patients with a particular diagnosis.

Network Databases

The difficulty in representing anything other than sequential one-to-many relationships in a hierarchical database led to a different database architecture in which any type of relationship could exist between the entities. A Network Database allows complex interrelationships between data entities, and in particular emphasizes many-to-many relationships (people can have many addresses, addresses can house many people, people can have many phone numbers). In addition, "multiple inheritance" is allowed, meaning that a given child entity can have multiple parents, with different types of relationships with each. In our example (Figure 5-7), phone numbers could be related to addresses (like home phone numbers) or could be related directly to people (like cellular telephones and beepers). A network database can also be "entered" at any point (not just the top level hierarchy), and from that point one can navigate to other entities.

However, the down side of network databases is that, due to their complexity, all of the entities, attributes, and relationships must be pre-defined in a database schema. This makes it difficult to add new entities or attributes

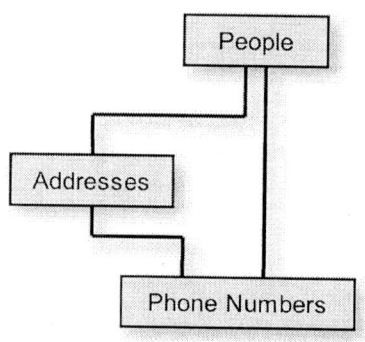

Figure 5-7: Network database. In a network database, each entity can have multiple parents. There is no primary point of view.

once any data has been entered into the database, and it can be very difficult to define new, ad-hoc relationships at the time of a query.

Object Oriented Databases

Object oriented databases use the "object model" developed in many programming languages to express and access data within the database. Part of the advantage it offers is a data representation interface similar to the programming interface, where database elements are modeled as objects with properties and instances, thereby integrating seamlessly into the programming routines used to access and manipulate the data. Like object oriented programming languages, object oriented databases allow object inheritance. Our simple address-book database is not sufficiently complex to adequately illustrate the concept of object inheritance, so let's deviate from that example for a moment. In an inheritance model, one defines first a "base object", which has properties common to all instances of the object. For example, a generic person object could have properties for name, date of birth, and social security number. Another more specific object, say employee, would inherit from the generic person object, and would thus inherit the base properties of name, date of birth, and social security number, but then would supplement these with descendent specific properties of date of hire, division, and salary. Similarly, a client-contact object might also inherit from the base person object, but instead supplement the base properties with the descendent specific properties of client name and date of first order.

Although any database, even simple ones, can be expressed using an object model, the advantages of the object oriented approach are realized only with complicated objects like images and sound, requiring tight coupling with the underlying programming which manipulates those objects. Object oriented databases are more commonly used for applications such as computer aided design and civil, electrical, or structural engineering.

Shortcomings of Non-relational Database Architectures

The major limitation of the three database architectures discussed, hierarchical, network, and object-oriented, is that the "viewpoint" of the user is inherently reflected in the pre-defined design of the database structure. Data is searched or otherwise processed by following links from pre-defined entry points to other data entities. Adapting to other, unanticipated viewpoints is difficult, and often requires scanning the entire database to locate the desired information. For small databases, this is not likely to be a problem. However, as databases become large, as is invariably the case with medical information systems, including millions of instances of some entities, complete database scanning can be both very time consuming and compromise the performance of the database for routine daily use. Adding to this complication is the fact that as the database becomes more complex, it becomes more and more difficult to predict, ahead of time, how users will want to access the data.

A need arose for a database architecture in which the data could be stored simply as data, with the relationships definable either initially or dynamically at the time of the query, and where the details of the data stored could be changed or updated without compromising any application code already written to access the data. This is the need that relational databases were designed to meet.

Relational Databases

Essentially all major "modern" databases in use in the healthcare industry today are relational databases, and as such understanding the basics of their structure and use will provide insight into nearly every medical information system you are likely to encounter in your career.

In a relational database, all of the data is stored in tables; that is to say, there is no separate schema which predefines the entities or their relationships. Each table in the database represents an entity, and as described above (and in more detail below) should correspond to some real-life concept, such as, in our address-book example, a person, an address, or a phone number. Each entity (table) has attributes (columns), the values of which further define a particular instance (row) of that entity. For example, attributes of a person table might include first name, last name, date of birth, and gender. Attributes of address would include street, city, state, and zip code. Within a table, each instance of the entity (each row) is defined uniquely by the values of its attributes. That is not to say that two instances cannot have the same values for some of their attributes, but it does say that two instances cannot have the same values for all of their attributes. This is an important concept, because if follows from this that the order and/or location of the rows in the database is unimportant, and rows can be changed, moved, added, deleted, swapped, or sorted without any consequence.

Relationships between instances of different entities (rows of different tables) in a relational database are defined by data (the values of an attribute or attributes) which are common between the two tables. This will become more clear once the concept of a "key" is introduced.

Primary and Foreign Keys

The primary key for an entity (table) is an attribute (column) or combination of attributes for which every instance (row) of the entity (table) has a unique value. To use some examples from the anatomic pathology domain, the accession number for a specimen would make a fine primary key for the specimen table, because each specimen must have a unique accession number. However, for the block table (the table which has one row for every histology block), the accession number would not be sufficient as a primary key, since multiple blocks may have the same accession number. Block number would also not be a good attribute to use as a primary key, because essentially every specimen will have a block 1. In fact, for the block table, one has to combine the specimen accession number, the part number, and the block number to uniquely identify a particular block. When a combination of attributes (columns) is used as a key for a table, it is referred to as a composite key.

Most tables in a relational database will have a primary key defined, although some database systems do not require this. In general, however, it is a good idea to define a primary key for each table, since a primary key might be needed at a later date. When the table is created in the database, if the database is "told" what column or combination of columns constitutes the primary key, the database will enforce the uniqueness of that key (that is, it will not allow you to enter two rows with the same value for the primary key).

Choosing an appropriate key cannot be done simply by looking at the data in the database for a column which seems to be unique. One must have an appropriate understanding of the real-world concepts which the attributes represent, referred to as "domain knowledge". For example, in our address-book, a quick perusal of the data might suggest that a combination of last name and first name would make an appropriate primary key for the person table. However, understanding how names get assigned to people, we know that it is very possible for two different people to have the same first name and same last name, so from our understanding of the real-world concepts that first name and last name represent, we realize that even the composite of these two columns would not make a good primary key. Not only must the primary key be unique for each row, but ideally it should be a value which will not change, ever, once it is assigned. This is because the primary key of the table is likely to be "pointed to" by the foreign key in another table (more on that in a moment), and if the value of the primary key were to change, the link to the other table would be broken. Thus, this is another reason why a combination of first name and last name would not make a good primary key for the person table, since a person's name can change with time (such as through marriage or a legal name change). Similarly, phone number, which might seem like a fine primary key since it must be unique, would not be ideal since a phone number might change (for example, the telephone company might assign you a new area code).

An appropriate choice for a primary key can also depend on the environment in which the database will be used. For a small pathology practice serving only a community hospital, for example, the medical record number might make a fine primary key for the patient table. After all, the medical record number is supposed to uniquely identify the patient, and each patient should have only one medical record number. However, what happens if the pathology practice decides to start accepting outreach specimens, that is, specimens sent in from physician offices outside the community hospital for evaluation, like skin biopsies or prostate biopsies? Some of these patients may not have been seen at the community hospital, and may not have a medical record number. Since the primary key is a required field for each row in the table, the pathology practice in this example would have to assign medical record numbers to these patients in order to include them in the database.

Depending upon the entity, it may be impossible to identify an appropriate primary key from the attributes of the table. In our person table example, where we store first name, last name, date of birth, and gender, we have already decided that neither the first name nor the last name, nor the combination of the two, would make an appropriate primary key. Similarly, date of birth would not do it, since two people can have the same birth date, and gender certainly would not. One could combine all four values into a big composite key, and although the chances of a duplicate are now much smaller, we know from our understanding of the concepts which those attributes represent that it is still possible for two people born on the same date to have the same name and gender. When no attribute or combination of attributes will suffice as a primary key, we have to create a new, artificial attribute such as a sequential "person identifier" to serve as the primary key. We simply assign each person a unique number, for example, and use that number (within the database) to refer to that person. Since the number is arbitrary, we can make sure that it is unique. Even if the person's name should change, the number does not. Since this identifier has no real-world concept which it represents, it is generally referred to as an "internal identifier" for the row. It is always possible to add an internal identifier column to every table and use that as the primary key, and some database designers do that, because then one does not need to understand what the other columns of data really represent. The disadvantage of that approach, however, is that this identifier takes up space in the database, and any programs which add data to the database must have the ability to generate a unique value for this column when a new row is added.

A foreign key in a table is an attribute (column) which defines a relationship between two entities (tables). The related rows are identified by the value in the foreign key column of one table matching the value in a column (often the primary key) of another table. In the histology block table example, having a column in the block table for the specimen accession number establishes a link to a specific row in the specimen table, the row which has the same value in its specimen accession number column, and associates that block with a specific specimen. The specimen accession number field in the block table is a foreign key which "points to" the specimen accession number field in the specimen table, which could be the

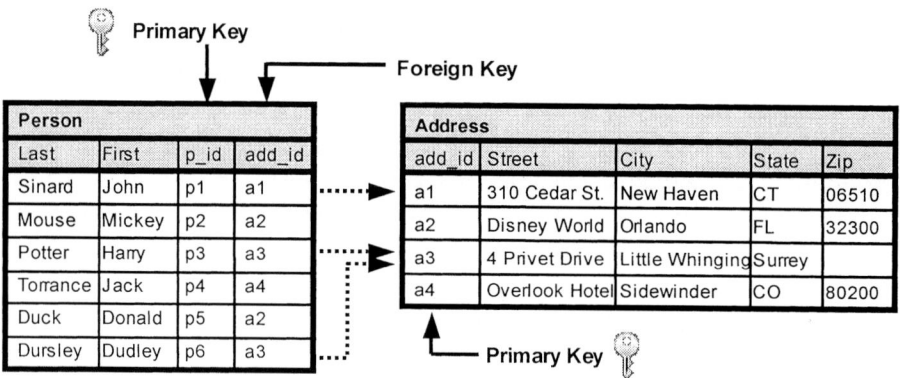

Figure 5-8: Primary and foreign keys. The primary key uniquely identifies each row in a table. Tables can also have foreign key columns, which define the relationships of an instance of one entity with an instance of another entity. The add_id column in the person table is a foreign key which "points to" the primary key column of the address table. This relationship indicates that "John Sinard" has "310 Cedar Street" as an address, and that both "Harry Potter" and "Dudley Dursley" live at "4 Privet Drive".

primary key for that table. Depending upon how the foreign keys are set up and used, they can support one-to-one, one-to-many, many-to-one, or even many-to-many relationships. For example, let's go back to our address-book database (Figure 5-8). We already decided we needed to add a column to the person table to be the primary key. Let's say we name that column p_id for person_id. Similarly, let's create a column in the address table called add_id to be its primary key (since none of the other columns make a particularly good primary key). We can then add an "add_id" column to the person table as a foreign key, which links people to addresses. In the example shown in Figure 5-8, the value "a1" in the "add_id" column of the "Person" table links person "p1" (John Sinard) to the address in the "Address" table which has the value "a1" in the "add_id" column of that table. It was not necessary to use the same column name, "add_id", as the name for both the primary key in the address table and the foreign key in the person table, but that convention is often used to suggest the foreign-key:primary-key relationship. Placing a foreign key in the person table allows multiple people to be linked to a single address, establishing a many-to-one relationship, as shown for the two inhabitants of 4 Privet Drive. Alternatively, we could have placed a foreign key in the address table, referencing the p_id column of the person table, and this would have allowed us to assign multiple addresses to a single person. If we want to be able to do both, that is, to create potential many-to-many relationships, a third table is required with two foreign key columns, one related to the p_id column of the person table, and one related to the add_id column of the address table. Such a table is often called a linkage table. Entries in the linkage table establish which people are to be associated with which addresses. The two columns together can form a composite primary key for the linkage table.

Entity-Relationship Diagrams

The process of designing a relational database, including defining the tables, the attributes for the tables, and the primary and foreign keys, can be complex. Tools have been developed to assist in this process. A common tool used is referred to as an "entity-relationship" diagram. These diagrams do not contain any actual data, but rather specify the various entities (tables), their attributes (columns), and some sort of symbolic representation of the relationships between these entities. A variety of different formats exist, two of which are shown in Figure 5-9.

A possible entity relationship diagram for our sample address-book database is shown in Figure 5-10. In this example, a foreign key has been added to the person table which points to the address table's primary key, allowing multiple people to be assigned to the same address. This model

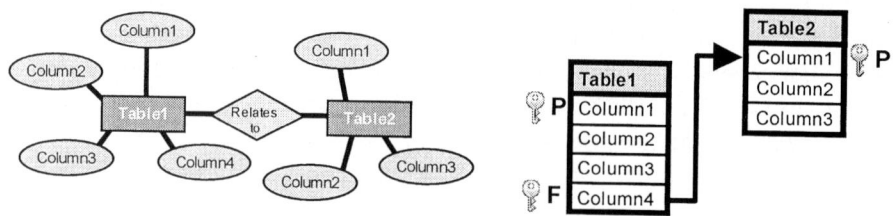

Figure 5-9: Entity-relationship diagrams. The entity-relationship diagram is a tool used in designing relational databases. They contain no actual data, but rather describe the entities, the attributes associated with each entity, and the relationships between the entities.

does not support multiple addresses for the same person. For the phone table, two foreign keys have been added, one pointing to the primary key of the person table, and one to the primary key of the address table. This allows phone numbers to be assigned to either a person or an address, or both. The former would be used for beepers and cellular telephones, whereas the latter would be used for a home phone, a business phone, or a fax. Although, for the reasons discussed above, the actual phone number column does not make an ideal primary key (it will be unique, but it might change with time), we have elected to make it the primary key in this model since it is not pointed to by a foreign key in any other table, and therefore any changes will not result in broken links. Maintaining links between primary and foreign keys in a database is known as referential integrity, a topic which will be discussed in greater detail below.

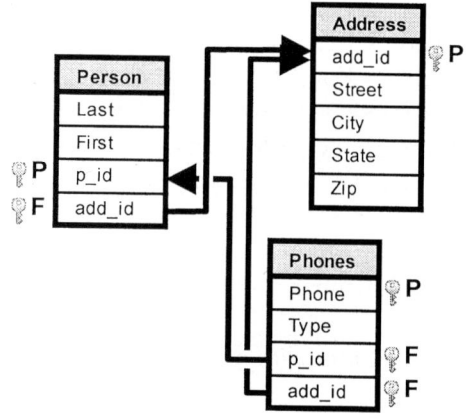

Figure 5-10 Entity-relationship diagram for the address-book database. In this example, two foreign keys in the Phones table allow a phone number to be associated either with a Person, an Address, or both.

Database Normalization

Databases are built to store information which represents instances of concepts. When designing a database, the process of determining which of those concepts constitute discrete independent entities (and therefore belong in their own tables) and which are further details or attributes about those entities (and therefore are best represented by columns in the tables) is known as database normalization. This is a formalized design process for a relational database, addressing the structure with particular attention to the handling of repeating and redundant fields. The goal is that a given piece of data should only be represented once in the database. Database normalization improves data storage efficiency, data integrity, and scalability. This process is not as straightforward as one might think. It requires a thorough understanding of not only the names of the types of information which will be stored, but also an appreciation for the real-world concepts that those fields represent, and an understanding of the interrelationships between those concepts. This domain knowledge includes understanding how the concepts usually interact, as well as the unusual interactions which might occur. The scope of the data to be stored also must be considered, since that can have a significant effect on the normalization process. Finally, one must consider not only the current data storage needs, but likely future needs as well.

Some of the basic rules have already been mentioned. Each table should represent a single entity (do not store information on tissue blocks and glass slides in the same table). The columns define the attributes of that entity. The order of the columns should be irrelevant. Each column, for each row, should have a single value (do not have a column like "parts"). All of the values for a given column should be of the same kind for all of the rows. Stated another way, you should not store one type of data in a column for one row, and a different type of data in that column for a different row. (If a specimen table has a column for "patient location", do not store the ward name for specimens from inpatients and a pointer to the client for outreach specimens – this will complicate ad hoc searches as well as on-the-fly relationships). Each row in the table must be unique, and the sequence of the rows should be irrelevant.

After these basic rules have been addressed, one then removes any repeating or multi-valued attributes to a child entity. For example, since a specimen may have one or many parts, part information should not be stored in the specimen table, but rather should be put in a separate "parts" table. When this has been done for all repeating attributes, the database is said to have achieved "first normal form".

Second normal form requires that a table be in first normal form, and that additionally each column in the table be dependent upon the entire primary key for that table, not simply a portion of it. It follows, therefore, that a table must have a composite key in order to not be in second normal form. In our anatomic pathology example, part information is placed in its own table, not in the specimen table. The parts table would likely have a composite primary key, consisting of the specimen number and the part number, since these two together uniquely identify a part. It would be a violation of second normal form to place a column like "signout date" in the part table, because the pathologist does not sign out only one part at a time; he/she signs out the entire case. Since signout date would be dependent only upon the specimen number and not on the part number, it does not belong in the part table, but rather should be placed in the specimen table.

Third normal form requires that the table be in second normal form, and that all of the columns in a table be dependent upon ONLY the primary key, and not on any other non-key columns. In our address-book example, we created an address-table, to which we added the primary key "add_id". The street address is dependent only upon the primary key, as is the zip code. However, the state, and perhaps the city, are really dependent upon the zip code. Since zip codes do not cross state boundaries, the zip code uniquely determines the state (city is a little more complicated, since some cities can share some zip codes). Therefore, to achieve third normal form, state should be moved to a separate table, whose primary key would be the zip code, and then the zip code in the address table would become a foreign key.

In any database design process, it is not uncommon to intentionally violate normalization on occasion. Normalization clearly can increase the complexity of the database. The disadvantages created by this complexity need to be weighed against the advantages achieved through the normalization process. Let's examine the example of achieving third normal form in our address table by removing the state column to a table with just the zip-code and state. If most of my addresses are in a relatively few zip codes, I will save space in the database, because rather than storing the state for each row of the address table, I only need to store the state for each unique zip code in the zip-code/state table. However, if my addresses are scattered across many zip codes, I may use more space storing the zip code twice (once as the primary key in the zip-code/state table and once as a foreign key in the address table) than I would use by storing the state abbreviation with each address. Of course, is zip-code really a good primary key? I know from real life experiences that zip-codes occasionally change. In addition, there are instances where I may know what state someone lives in, but don't know their zip code. Finally, not all foreign countries use zip-codes. For all these reasons, I would probably intentionally elect to violate third normal form for my address table.

Fourth and fifth normal forms also exist, but are generally not applicable to medical databases and therefore will not be discussed.

Entity-Attribute-Value Data Models

In some cases, there may be a large number of possible attributes for a particular entity. However, any given instance of that entity may have values for only a small number of those attributes. When this is the case, it can become inefficient to define each possible attribute as its own column, since, for any given row, most of the columns will be empty. Which columns actually contain values will vary from row to row. When this situation exists, it might be more efficient to store the data in a different way. The entity-attribute-value (EAV) model is one such way. This approach removes the entire collection of attributes to its own table. The EAV table has three columns, one each for the "entity", "attribute", and "value". The "entity" value refers to the row or instance of the entity to which the attribute applies. The "attribute" value defines which attribute is being recorded, and the "value" column contains the value of that attribute for that instance of the entity. (The terminology is a little unfortunate, because it might have made more sense to refer to this model as the "instance-attribute-value" model.)

For example, consider a database which stores the admission test results from a group of patients. A large number of possible tests could be ordered on these patient, but it is likely that only a relatively small number will be ordered on each patient. Which tests are ordered will be tailored to that patient's condition, and therefore are unlikely to be the same for each patient. Although one could create a table (Figure 5-11, AdmissionTests1) in which each possible test represents its own column in the table, that will result in a large number of unused storage locations. Alternatively, using the

AdmissionTests1									
p_id	BP	Pulse	Resp	Hct	WBC	Plts	Na	K	Glu
p1	120/80	60		42.2	3.4		139		120
p2		80	23					3.4	
p3	140/90						141		
p4				39.0					110
p5									

AdmissionTests2		
Entity	Attribute	Value
p1	BP	120/80
p1	Pulse	60
p1	Hct	42.2
p1	WBC	3.4
p1	Na	139
p1	Glu	120
p2	Pulse	80
p2	Resp	23
p2	K	3.4
p3	BP	140/90
p3	Na	141
p4	Hct	39.0
p4	Glu	110

Figure 5-11: Entity-attribute-value transformation of data. In the traditional approach (AdmissionTests1), attribute information (test results) about each instance of an entity (patient) are stored in separate columns. However, when many of the attributes are unvalued for many of the instances, it can be more efficient to store the data in a different format (AdmissionTests2) in which each row stores the value (result) for a particular attribute (test) of a particular instance of the entity (patient).

EAV approach (Figure 5-11, AdmissionTests2), each test result could be stored as its own row in a "value" column, with "entity" and "attribute" columns defining the patient and test, respectively. In both of these formats, exactly the same information is stored, it is simply stored in a different way.

As already mentioned, in cases in which many of the possible attributes for an instance of an entity are likely to remain unvalued, the EAV data storage model can be more efficient. Different combinations of attributes can be stored for each instance of an entity. This approach also has another extremely important advantage, namely that one can store values for attributes which one did not know about when the database was initially designed. Returning again to Figure 5-11, consider what would have to happen if, for patient p5, we wanted to store the result of a chloride level. When we created AdmissionTests1, we didn't think about storing chloride results, and therefore did not create a column for it. In order to store this result, we would have to either alter the table structure (something which can be done with relational databases, but requires administrative privileges in the database) or add another table for the additional result. However, with the EAV model (AdmissionTests2), we simply would insert a new row in the table with values of "p5", "Cl", and the result. No changes need to be made to the structure of the database.

Of course, there are some disadvantages to the EAV approach. If a particular attribute has data values for the majority of the instances of an entity, it is actually more efficient to store the data in a column rather than as a row in an EAV table. This is because as a column, only the value has to be stored, whereas in the EAV table, the entity and the attribute also have to be stored. Data stored in the EAV format is also less efficient to retrieve. In the most common use, one would like to retrieve all of the test results for a particular patient. When the data is stored in the column format, all of the data about that patient is stored in the same place, and can be more rapidly retrieved. In an EAV table, the data for a given patient is likely to be scattered throughout the table, resulting in slower retrievals. Also, if one wants to do aggregate data analysis such as looking at the average admission glucose level for all the patients, all of this data is stored in a single column with the traditional approach and therefore can be easily averaged. With an EAV table, one first has to find all of the glucose values before one can average them.

Database Management Systems

So far, we have only really considered databases as stand-alone entities. In reality, databases are used through computer applications (programs) which allow us to look up information in the database, display that information, and perhaps edit that information. Many of the rules as to who can do what, and what are allowable values for various fields, are imposed not by the database itself but rather by the application programs which access the database.

Application Access to Databases

When initially developed, computer programs accessed databases directly. This meant that the program had to directly build and maintain the contents of the database. The programmers had to know about the structure of the database, including the specifics of what data was stored where and how it was stored. The computer programs would generally have a set of database routines which dealt with the actual data storage and retrieval steps (Figure 5-12). To speed-up access to the data in the database, each database table routinely had a number of indices. Each index was a partial duplication of the data in the table, sorted, however, in a particular order, thereby allowing the program to search the index rapidly to find a particular instance (row) rather than having to look through the main table one row at a time. Database routines were also needed to maintain any indices which might be built on the data tables, and still more routines were needed to make sure two programs were not trying to change the same data at the same time. These, or similar, routines needed to exist in every application which accessed the database. Any application which tried to short-cut these

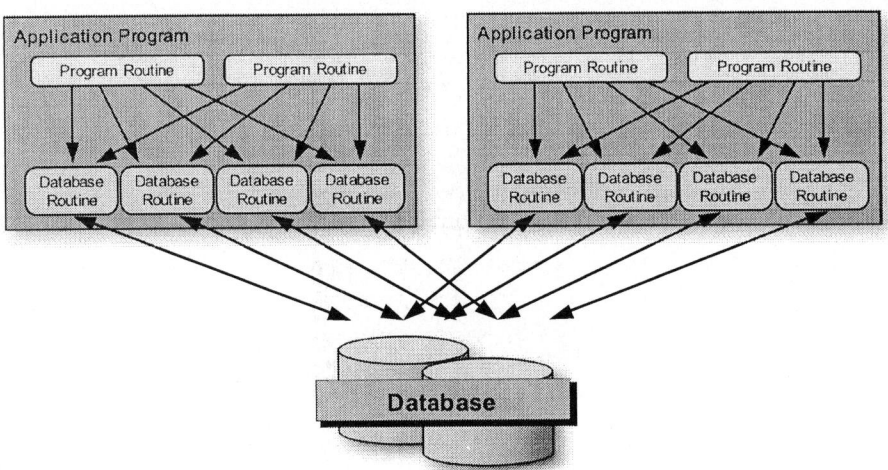

Figure 5-12: Direct program access to databases. With direct application program access to databases, each application program must have all of the routines necessary to access and update the data in the database.

routines could corrupt the integrity of the database. Therefore, application programs which built and maintained databases were quite complex. In addition, any change in the structure of the data stored usually required extensive modifications to all of the applications which accessed the database.

The inefficiency and complexity of developing computer applications under these rules led to the development of database management systems. A database management system, often abbreviated simply as DBMS, is a type of "middle-ware" which sits between the applications and the database (Figure 5-13). All access to the database by the application programs must go through the DBMS, and the routines which actually read and update the data in the database are all consolidated into the DBMS. This has tremendous advantages. Applications which need to access the database can now share the routines which manage the store data, and the management of simultaneous program access is now centralized at the point of access. Functions which are purely internal to the database, like updating and maintaining indices, are fully performed by the DBMS, and do not have to be considered in the application programs at all. Beyond the decreased redundancy in programming, however, is the physical and philosophical separation of the routines which "create" and "use" the data from the routines which store the data. It is no longer necessary for the application programs, and thus the application programmers, to know any of the physical details about how the data is stored. The application simply

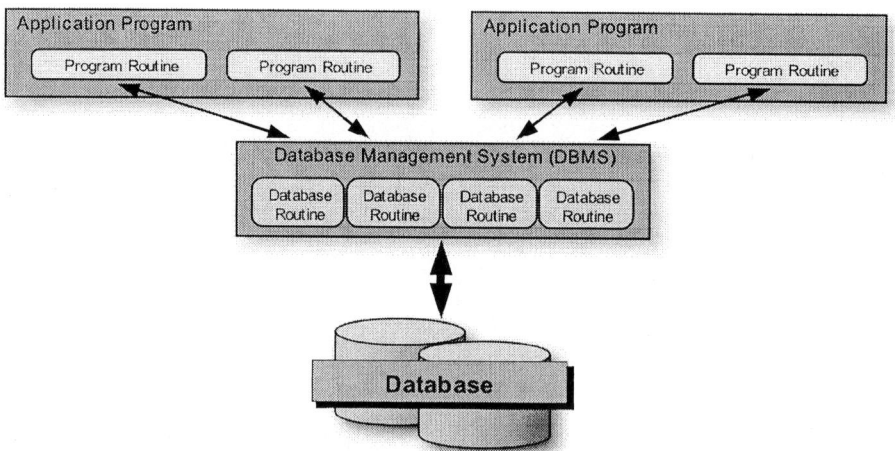

Figure 5-13: Database management systems (DBMS). A database management system is a series of routines which lie between the application programs and the database. All access to the database goes through the DBMS. The DBMS manages all of the details of data storage and index maintenance.

communicates its "needs" to the DBMS using a language understood by both sets of routines, and the DBMS deals with the details of data storage and retrieval. If a common language is used to communicate with the DBMS, then a completely different database system can be substituted without requiring any modifications to the application routines.

The example used in Figure 5-13 assumes that the programs accessing the database and the database itself are on the same computer. In fact, most large databases, to be really useful, need to be accessible to multiple users on multiple computers at the same time. To achieve this, the database management system is split into two parts, a "front end" which runs on each user's computer (the client), and a "back end" which runs on the computer housing the database (the server) (Figure 5-14). The program routines submit their requests to the DBMS front-end (often called a "driver") on their local machine. This front-end communicates over the network to the DBMS back-end. The back-end interacts with the database and processes the requests of the front-end(s). Results are returned to the appropriate client computer, where the DBMS front-end hands the data off to the application program. This "client-server" model is the most common method of data distribution in institutional environments, including essentially all health care settings. This will be discussed in a little more detail in Chapter 6.

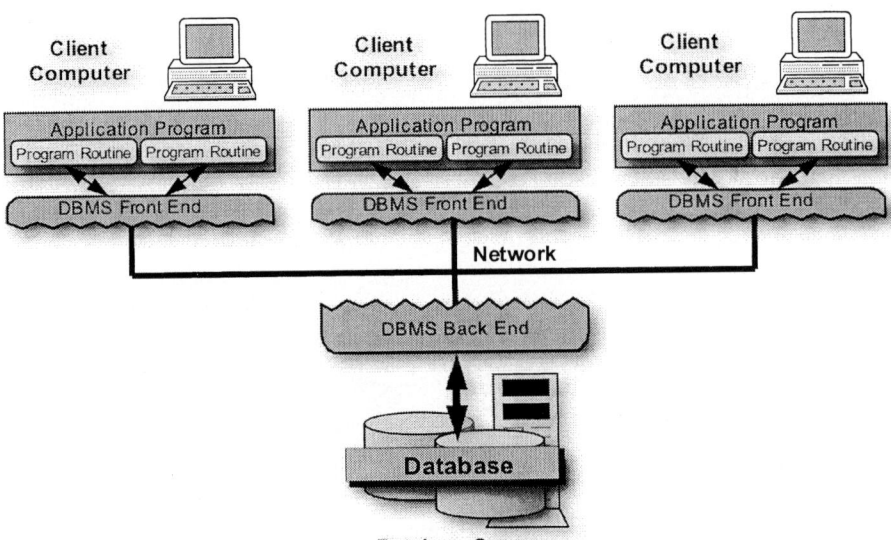

Figure 5-14: Client-server database management systems. In most deployment situations, the database resides on a server, and multiple clients connect to the database over a network. In this situation, the DBMS is split into a "front end" which resides on each client machine and a "back end" which resides on the server containing the database.

Database Abstraction

The separation of the routines which address the physical storage and retrieval of data in the database (the routines which comprise the DBMS) from the application routines which use and create that data is known as "database abstraction". This has tremendous implications beyond simply the reusability of computer code. It allows the database designer and the application programmer to conceptualize the database in whatever model is desired, and to design their programs around that model. It becomes the responsibility of the DBMS to handle the particulars of disk space allocation, free space consolidation, index management, etc. The separation of responsibilities made possible through database abstraction is further illustrated in Table 5-1.

Table 5-1: Database abstraction.

Concerns of the Database Designer and Application Programmer	Concerns of the Database Management System
What type of data is stored in the database?	How and where on the disk is the data stored?
What are the entities and their attributes?	How is free space in the database managed?
How are the fields in the database related to each other?	How is the storage of data adjusted as new rows are added or existing rows are deleted?
What data needs to be retrieved?	
What data should be indexed, based on how the data is most frequently requested?	What changes need to be made to an index to accommodate a change in the data?
	What is the best way to find the data requested?
	How is simultaneous access by multiple users managed and accommodated?

Conceptual Data Model

Physical Data Model

Capabilities of a "Full-Featured" DBMS

As databases grew in size and complexity, database management systems were drawn upon to take on more and more responsibilities. Current high-end commercial databases use very sophisticated DBMSs to manage the data and to facilitate solution development by application programmers. The major capabilities which a full-featured database management system should include are in Table 5-2. Several of these features are discussed in the following sections.

Table 5-2: Capabilities of a full-featured DBMS.

- Handling all of the details of the physical storage of data
    - Support for multiple data types with different storage needs
- Automatically maintain indices and keys
- Support the addition, updating, and deletion of data
- Support changes in the conceptual database design
- Allow for client/server distribution and multiple simultaneous user access
- Provide security, authorization protocols, and user privilege definition and enforcement
- Preserve data integrity
    - Referential integrity
    - Transaction processing and data concurrency
- Allow for data recovery
    - Database backups
    - Transaction logs
- Address data locking
    - Deadlock management
- Support a standardized query language and standardized application interfaces

Data Types

To allow the data in the database to be stored accurately, indexed correctly, and sorted properly, each column of each table in the database must be assigned a data type, indicating what type of data will be stored in that column. Setting the data type often requires also defining the amount of space to be reserved for data storage. Selecting an appropriate data type requires understanding something about how different types of data are represented and stored digitally. Many of the details of how this is done have been previously discussed under the section entitled "Non-executable software" in Chapter 3 on "Desktop Computers: Software". This discussion will assume the reader is familiar with the contents of that section.

Setting the data type determines what data is valid or invalid, and how that data will be treated. For example, if one were to attempt to store a word into a column defined as an integer, this would represent invalid data and generate a "data-type mismatch" error. In contrast, one could store a "7" in a column defined as an integer column or in a column defined as a string column, because "7" is also a string. However, the "7" will be treated differently based on the data type definition for the column, and this difference becomes apparent when one sorts the data. In a numeric data-type sorted in ascending order, a "7" will sort to a final location before a "12", because 7 is less than 12. However, if the same values are stored as string data, the "12" would sort before the "7", because strings are sorted one character at a time, and the "1" character of the "12" has a lower ASCII value than the "7" character.

Different database management systems offer slight variations in how the different types of data are stored, but a representative example will be discussed here. The basic data types are integers, decimal numbers, date/time, strings, text, and blobs.

Integers are stored in their strict binary representation. The range of possible numbers which can be stored is determined by the number of bytes used to store the integer. Some DBMSs allow the user to specify the number of bytes to use at the time the column is defined. Others use a set of pre-defined data-types such as "tinyint", "integer" or "short", and "long", for example, to represent 2-byte, 4-byte, or even 8-byte integers.

Decimal numbers are handled by databases in one of two ways: as approximate values or as exact values. Approximate value variables typically use four bytes of storage space for standard or "single" precision values, and eight bytes for "double" precision values. It is important to remember that these are approximate values. For example, if one stores the result of one divided by six in a single precision column called "data" for a row, and then selects all rows where "data * 6 = 1" (value of "data" multiplied by 6 is equal to one), the row may not be selected. This is because "data * 6" might evaluate to "1.000000001", which is not equal to one. Doing the same thing with a double precision column might cause the row to be selected, since there will be less round off error. "Exact" value columns are possible in databases, and usually go by names like "decimal" or "real", as opposed to single or double. The exact data types require the user to specify the precision and scale of the column at the time it is defined. Precision is the maximum total number of digits allowable in the number, and the scale is the number of those digits which can be to the right of the decimal point. A number stored in an exact decimal column is stored exactly as entered, often as text. However, not all possible values can be stored. For example, the result of one divided by six cannot be exactly expressed with any number of digits, so will be stored only as "exact" as the precision and scale specified will allow.

Date and time can be stored in databases, and frequently are stored together in a single variable called "datetime", usually requiring eight bytes of storage. Some databases store this information with a precision of one second, and others with a precision as high as one millisecond. It is important to realize that the precision with which the date/time is stored may not be the same as the precision with which the date/time is displayed. For example, if one asks for the value in the "when_accessioned" column for a particular specimen, one might get back "Dec 15, 2004 9:24AM". However, if one asks for all specimens where "when_accessioned" equals "Dec 15, 2004 9:24AM", that specimen might not be matched. This is because the actual value stored is probably something like "Dec 15, 2004 9:24:18AM", and you have asked for "Dec 15, 2004 9:24:00AM". Therefore, when selecting data based on time, it is usually a good idea to specify a range.

Textual information is stored in databases in a few different ways. "Strings" are used for small amounts of text, less than 256 total characters. They can be stored either as fixed length character strings ("char") or variable length character strings ("varchar"). One specifies the maximum length for the string when creating the column. Fixed length strings always take up the same amount of space in the database, even if much of that space is not being used. Variable length strings have the advantage that only the amount of space needed to store the value is used, but storing and retrieving the data takes a little bit longer. For textual information longer than 255 characters, a different type of storage is used, These columns often are called "text" columns, to distinguish them from "strings". What is actually stored in a text column is a pointer to a special part of the database where the text data is stored, usually as "pages" of a size predetermined by the particular database, traditionally on the order of about 2K bytes (2048 bytes). Pages are allocated as needed, and a single text field can use as many text pages as needed, but these must be allocated in whole page increments. Therefore, a text field which is 300 characters long will take up 2K bytes of storage. A text field which is 1900 characters long will also take up 2K bytes of storage. However, a text field which is 2100 characters long will take up 4K bytes of storage.

Some database management systems have been designed with the understanding that the user may want to store information which does not fit well into the limited concepts of text and/or numbers. The most common example of this in anatomic pathology would be an image, but similar situations include a sound file, video, or compiled code for an application. Rather than try to handle all of the details of the various things a user might want to store, databases with this capability simply store the data as a large object of binary data. These "Binary Large OBjects" or "BLOBs" are stored in pages similar to text, but the database makes no attempt to interpret the data as anything other than a collection of bytes. It is up to the application program which reads the data to make sense of that data.

A special value to be considered when dealing with databases is the pseudo-value known as "NULL" (rhymes with *dull* and is commonly written in full capital letters). NULL is more of a concept than a value, in much the same way that infinity is a concept. If one thinks of a database table as a set of columns and rows, NULL is used to indicate that, for a particular column in a particular row, the value of the data is unknown. NULL is not the same thing as zero, and is not the same thing as an empty string. The concept of NULL is best illustrated with a couple of examples. Consider a sample database table which stores the temperature in three different cities at a particular time each day. This table could have one datetime column to store the time, and three decimal columns to store the temperatures in city A, city B, and city C, respectively. Now, let's imagine that on a given time of a given day, the thermometer in city C is broken. I have the temperature for cities A and B, so I can enter those, but what do I put in the column for the temperature of city C? I don't know that value. It would not be appropriate to enter a zero, because that means something very different. It would also not be appropriate to say that I cannot store the temperatures for cities A and B simply because I do not know the temperature in city C. This is a case where the value for the column containing the temperature for city C would be set to NULL. Now consider a table which contains three string columns for first name, middle name, and last name, into which we want to enter the names of three United States presidents: Kennedy, Lincoln, and Truman. "John Fitzgerald Kennedy" is not a problem. What about "Abraham Lincoln"? I know that he had no middle name. Then there is "Harry Truman". I can't remember his middle name. (OK, so his middle name is simply "S", but let's say I don't know that). There should be some way I can indicate that Abraham Lincoln does not have a middle name, but that I simply don't know Harry Truman's middle name. This could be done by entering an empty string "" for the middle name of Mr. Lincoln, and entering NULL for the middle name of Mr. Truman. The empty string, expressed as a beginning quote immediately followed by an ending quote, is also known as "nil". NULL and nill are NOT the same thing.

NULL values can lead to interesting results when used in expressions and conditionals. If any of the components of an expression has a value of

NULL, then the entire expression evaluates to NULL. Thus, if the value of "data" is NULL, the value of "data + 7" is NULL. This makes sense. If I don't know how many of something I have, giving me seven more of them will not help me figure out how many I have. Any conditional in which one of the expressions is NULL evaluates to FALSE, by definition. For example, lets say I have five rows in a table which has a column "data" of type integer with the following values for the five rows: 3, 2, 3, NULL, 4. If I ask for all rows where "data <= 3" (the value of "data" is less than or equal to "3"), I will get back three rows. If I as for all rows where "data > 3", I will get back only one row. The row with the value of NULL for data is not retrieved in either case, because NULL is not less than or equal to three, and NULL is not greater than three.

When creating a database table, one often has to tell the database whether or not each column in the table is allowed to contain NULL as a value.

Index Maintenance

One of the biggest advantages of database management systems is that they will automatically take care of any index you decide to create. Indices are created on tables to allow more rapid searching. Without an index, if one asks the database to find all rows in which a particular column has a particular value or range of values, the database has to look at each row in the table to see if it satisfies that criteria. This is known as a "table scan". That approach may be fine if the table is my personal phone book, but the specimen table in an anatomic pathology database can have over a million rows. Even with a very fast computer, it might take 30 minutes to look through a million rows. If it took the database 30 minutes to find a specimen every time I enter a specimen number, that would not make a very useful database. Therefore, when the specimen table is created, I would also create an index on the specimen number column. The specimen number index is kept sorted, and contains pointers to the actual rows in the specimen table. Every time I add a new specimen, the DBMS automatically makes a new entry in the index, and keeps the index sorted. When I ask for a particular specimen by specimen number, the DBMS knows there is an index on the specimen number field, looks up the specimen in that index (since it is sorted, it does not have to look at each row, and in fact can find the correct entry in less than a second, even if there are a million entries), and then uses the corresponding pointer to find the specimen I am looking for.

Of course, I might also want to look up a specimen by the patient identifier. Therefore, I need another index for that column. I might also want to look up a specimen by the date that it was accessioned, so let's create an index on that column as well. It is not uncommon to have several indices for each database table. Of course, for every index one adds, more space is needed in the database, and the process of adding or updating a row takes longer, because every one of the indices also needs to be updated. Therefore, if one rarely looks up a specimen by, for example, the billing type, then it would be better to not create an index for that column. In a typical anatomic pathology database, it is not uncommon for the indices to take up as much disk space, or more, as the actual tables being used to store the data.

Relational databases typically support two types of indices, referred to as "clustered" and "non-clustered". For a clustered index, the rows of the actual database table are kept sorted by the value of the indexed column. This is possible because, as discussed above, in a properly normalized relational database, each row is determined wholly by the values of its attributes, and the order is not important. Of course, the rows can only be sorted in one order, so a given database table can have only one clustered index. The advantage of a clustered index is that it does not take up any extra space in the database. However, one has to carefully choose which index to make the clustered index for a table, since one would rather not have to re-sort the specimen table every time a new specimen is added. Therefore, one traditionally picks, for a clustered index, a column for which each new row will have a larger value. For the specimen table, "when_accessioned" makes a good choice, since each new row will have a larger value in that column (assuming it is a datetime column and not simply a time column!) than all of the previous rows, so the new row will always go at the end. Not all tables will have a column which increases with each new row. A patient table would be an example of this. Therefore, to prevent having to re-sort the patient table every time a new row is added, one would make all of the indices on the patient table non-clustered.

Just as primary keys can represent a combination of columns, an index can also be created on a combination of columns. Most tables have at least one index for the primary key, especially if that key is pointed to by a foreign key in another table.

Query Optimization

A very important feature of any database management system is how it fulfills requests from application programs for data in the database. The database abstraction which is made possible by DMBSs offers many advantages for the programmer, but one mixed-blessing is that the application programmer, who knows what data he/she needs at a particular point in the application, does not necessarily have any idea how best to get that data. A request is simply submitted to the DBMS for the data, and it is up to the DBMS to figure out the most efficient way to retrieve that data. I call this a mixed blessing because the DBMS does not understand the meaning of the data it is holding, and therefore does not always make the best decision about how to retrieve the data.

When the DBMS receives a request for data, it has to figure out how to find the data before it can retrieve it. The query request often involves several tables, each with a different collection of indices and different data distributions. The DBMS has to decide which approach it will use to find the data. Do I search table A first, using index A2, and then find the corresponding rows in table B, or do I search table B first, using a table scan, and then find the corresponding rows in table A? Let's use a more concrete example: Pretend I am a DBMS, and I have been asked to find all of the specimens accessioned within the last year to any patient named "John Sinard" with the word "carcinoma" in the final diagnosis. There are several ways I could do this. Not knowing anything about the concept of what a patient is, what a specimen is, or how many specimens a patient is likely to have in a given period of time, I could, for example, decide to 1) first find all the specimens accessioned in the last year, and then go through each one of those to see if the patient name was "John Sinard", and then check each one of those to see if the word "carcinoma" appears in the diagnosis. Even worse, I could 2) find all of the specimens in the system with the word "carcinoma" in the diagnosis, and then throw out any which were not accessioned in the last year, and then see how many belong to "John Sinard". Alternatively, I could 3) find all of the patients named "John Sinard", find all of the specimens accessioned to them, throw out any not accessioned in the last year, and then check the remaining ones for the word "carcinoma." The overall efficiency is most affected by how many matches I find in the first thing I look for. If my first lookup yields only three or four matches, it takes no time whatsoever to determine if each of those meets the other criteria. On the other hand, if my first lookup returns 10,000 matches, I have to go through each one to test the remaining criteria, and that will take a lot longer. If I were a pathologist (remember, right now we're pretending I'm a DBMS), I would know that we get about 140,000 specimens a year, that there are hundreds of thousands of specimens with the word "carcinoma" in the diagnosis, but there are probably only one or two patients named "John Sinard", so option 3 would be the best choice. Also, were I a pathologist, I would also know that I might take a different approach if I were looking for patients with the name "John Smith" and the phrase "xanthogranulomatous pyelonephritis" in the diagnosis. However, as a DMBS, I do not know in advance how many instances of a particular value are likely to occur for a particular attribute of a particular entity. Instead, I rely on knowing which attributes (columns) of which entities (tables) are indexed. Also, as I have been updating these indices, I have been keeping track, roughly, of some statistics about the data, like how evenly it is distributed and how many times, on average, each value occurs in each index. I use that information to make <u>my</u> best guess about how to retrieve the data. I know I will not always make <u>the</u> best guess.

The process by which a database management system decides how to fulfill a query is known as query optimization. The rules which a DBMS uses to make this decision are often proprietary, and directly affect the overall performance of the database.

Referential Integrity

Relationships between tables in a relational database are created by having a value in a column (the foreign key) of one table match the value of a column in another table (usually the primary key). The row(s) in the table with the foreign key is often called the child, and the row in the table to which the foreign key "refers" is called to as the parent. Preservation of referential integrity means making sure that a child row is not orphaned by deleting the corresponding parent row. Let's go back to our address book database. In the example shown in Figure 5-15, the Person table has a foreign key column, add_id, which refers to the primary key column add_id in the Address table. In this model, the Person is the child of the Address

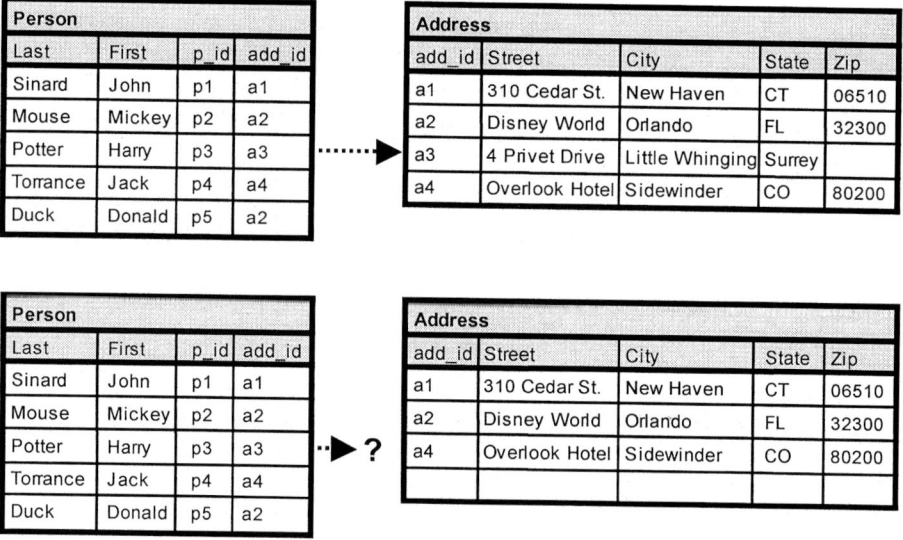

Figure 5-15: Referential integrity. The add_id column in the Person table is a foreign key pointing to the add_id column in the Address table. Thus, each row in the Person table is a child of the related parent row in the Address table. If a referenced row in the Address table is deleted (top pair of tables), the foreign key now points to a row which no longer exists (bottom pair of tables). Referential integrity is lost.

which is the parent. In particular, Harry Potter, in the Person table, refers to 4 Privet Drive in the Address table, and therefore the Harry Potter row is a child of the referenced 4 Privet Drive row. If one were to allow the row in the Address table for 4 Privet Drive to be deleted, then Harry Potter's row in the Person table would be pointing to an address which no longer existed. If this were to happen, Harry Potter would be said to have been orphaned (again!), and there would have been a loss of referential integrity.

Referential integrity can be preserved in one of two ways. With "declarative referential integrity", the database is told, at the time the tables are created, that the add_id column in the Person table is a foreign key referencing the add_id column in the Address table (Figure 5-15). When an attempt is made to delete the row from the Address table with an add_id of "a3", the DBMS, knowing about the relationship, would first check to see if any rows in the Person table had an add_id value of "a3". Finding one, it would not allow the row in the Address table to be deleted, generating an error. The advantage of this approach is that an application developer does not need to do anything other than define the relationship to the DBMS in order to preserve the data integrity. However, the application would have to be able to respond to the error. In addition, if one actually wanted to delete "4 Privet Drive" from the Address table, one would have to either delete the child rows from the Person table first, or at least change the value of the add_id column in the Person table for Harry Potter to NULL or some other value before attempting to delete the referenced row from the Address table.

Since developers may not want to have to deal with addressing all of the child rows both separately and in advance before a parent row can be deleted, an alternative approach called "procedural referential integrity" can be used. Special small programs called "triggers" are created and attached to database tables. Whenever the contents of the table is changed (a new row is inserted or one is deleted or updated), the "trigger" is executed. This trigger can then handle whatever changes are needed to maintain referential integrity. For example, a trigger could be put on the Address table which, when an address is deleted, automatically deletes any rows in the Person table which point to that address. Alternatively, it could simply change the pointers in the add_id column of the Person table to NULL. Triggers give the application developer greater flexibility than declarative referential integrity, but require that the developer write the correct triggers to properly address any referential integrity issues.

When properly written, triggers can make it much easier to preserve referential integrity than the declarative approach. Consider an example in the anatomic pathology domain. A specimen can have many parts, so the parts table would be a child table of the specimen table. A part can have many blocks, so the blocks table would be a child table of the parts table. If one wanted to delete a specimen, one would not want to leave any of the parts or the blocks behind. If these relationships were defined to the DBMS via declarative referential integrity, the DBMS would not allow the specimen to be deleted as long as it has any part rows pointing to it. Likewise, the DBMS would not allow a part to be deleted as long as there were any block rows pointing to it. To delete the specimen, the application would first have to delete all of the blocks, then all of the parts, and then would be allowed to delete the specimen. With the procedural approach, one would create a trigger on the specimen table which would delete any associated parts. One would also create a trigger on the parts table which would delete any associated blocks. Once this is done, if the application program wants to delete a specimen, it simply deletes the row from the specimen table. The DBMS has not been told about any foreign-key relationships, so it lets this happen. However, the DBMS does run the trigger on the specimen table. This trigger deletes the related rows from the parts table. As each row in the part table is deleted, the trigger on the parts table deletes the blocks associated with that part from the blocks table. By using triggers to perform these "cascading deletes", a single command to the database to delete a row from the specimen table will automatically remove all of the associated parts and blocks.

Data Concurrency

Another important concept in data integrity is known as "data concurrency", which means that all of the data in the database represents the same point in time. This becomes an important issue for relational databases, since related information is not all stored in one place but rather in a number of tables within the database. For example, let's consider an inventory system. An order is entered for items which are in the inventory. When the order is marked as shipped, the shipped quantities are billed and added to a log of sales. This makes updates to the order table, the shipping manifest table, and the sales table. However, suppose that when the database goes to deduct the items from the inventory table, that table is not available (perhaps it is locked by another user), so the deduction cannot be made. Now, the value in the inventory table is no longer correct. But the order has been marked as shipped. If we re-mark it as shipped to try to get the inventory value corrected, this will trigger a duplicate shipping, duplicate billing, and duplicate entries in the sales log. The data in the database no longer represents the same point in time. Data concurrency has been lost. This problem is relatively unique to relational databases, because related data tends to be stored in different places, and not all of those places will always be available at all times.

To maintain data concurrency, modifications to the database are performed in groups known as transactions. A transaction is a set of modifications to the database which must be completed as a group with an "all or nothing" logic. If any one of the modifications within a transaction cannot be completed (either due to an error, a locked table, insufficient privileges, etc), then any of the modifications which were made are undone ("rolled back"); NONE of the modifications are made, and the entire transaction errors. This assures that data in the database is always internally consistent with itself. Transactions can also be used to help preserve the integrity between foreign keys and primary keys, and, as will be seen below, can be important in data recovery.

Data Backup and Recovery

In most large databases, but particularly important in medical systems, the existence of the data must be preserved. Computer disk drives are mechanical devices with moving parts, and like all mechanical devices they can malfunction. If the malfunction is a physical one, it is possible that the surface of the disk storing the contents of the database could get destroyed, and the data would become unrecoverable. To protect against this, the contents of the database are "dumped" on a regular basis to an alternate storage device, usually magnetic tape. This backup tape should not be stored in the same physical location as the database, since a disaster such as a fire or explosion could destroy both the database and the backup tape.

More sophisticated databases can perform this data dump in the background while the database is still in use. However, there can be significant degradation of the overall performance of the system while this is occurring, so it is generally done at low usage times such as overnight. Writing to a magnetic tape can be relatively slow, so in some configurations, the data is dumped rapidly to another disk device to free up the production database, and then copied from this alternate device to a backup tape.

Backups of clinical data are routinely done once a day, usually overnight. This is fine, but imagine a situation in which an irreversible event causes a database failure at about four o'clock in the afternoon. If the hardware is under a two-hour repair agreement, or better yet if backup hardware is immediately available, the database hardware can be relatively quickly restored to operation, but the contents have been lost and need to be restored from a backup tape. The backup tape can return the database to the state it was in at the time the backup tape was made, namely the previous night. This means that everything which was done in the computer system since then will need to be redone. This includes not only every new accession, but every histology block entry, every stain order, every final diagnosis entered, every report printed, every interface message sent or received, every log closed or status change, not to mention any edits, amendments, or addendums. Reproducing even a days worth of work, assuming everyone can remember what they did, can be a daunting task. Even if backups were performed twice a day rather than once a day, one would still have to reproduce a half a day's worth of work. In addition, until the old data is restored, new work cannot begin, and this can be even more of a problem.

A solution exists to this problem, and it is made possible by the transaction processing used by large databases. Transaction processing was introduced in the previous section as a way of preserving data concurrency by assuring that grouped modifications to the database are all completed as a group. In fact, all modifications to the data in the database is performed as transactions. This is true whether the modification is the addition of a new row of data, deletion of an entire table, or simply changing the value of one column in one row. To enable "up to the minute" data recovery, the details of each transaction are stored in a "transaction log", an electronic log maintained by the database on a different physical device than the one which is used for the database (a different disk drive, or at least a different surface of the disk drive). This transaction log is cleared each time the database contents are dumped to a backup. Therefore, the transaction log contains only those transactions which occurred after the last backup was created. As a result, this log contains the instructions on how to convert the database "state" from the way it was at the time of the backup to the current state.

Consider the example (Figure 5-16) of a database in state A (this refers to the content of every column of every row of every table). At this point in time, the database is dumped to a backup tape and the transaction log is cleared. Then, while the database is in use, each modification to the data is recorded in the transaction log. When the database is in state B, an "incident" occurs on one of the devices used to store the data in the database – for example, a failure of the drive head which scrapes across the surface of the magnetic storage platter making its contents unreadable. At this point, the backup tape contains information about the contents of the database in state A. The transaction log, hopefully on a device not destroyed by the above mentioned "incident", contains information about how to convert the database from state A to state B. The transaction log is identified and copied to a secure location. The recovery process involves first repairing the damaged device, and then using the backup tape to restore the database to state A. Then, the transaction log is "replayed" back into the DBMS, instructing the DBMS to repeat each of the steps, in turn, which were used to convert the database from state A to state B. The database is now fully recovered to the point in time at which the incident occurred.

Unfortunately, a major "incident" like an explosion or fire is likely to destroy both the database and the transaction log. When this occurs, it is not

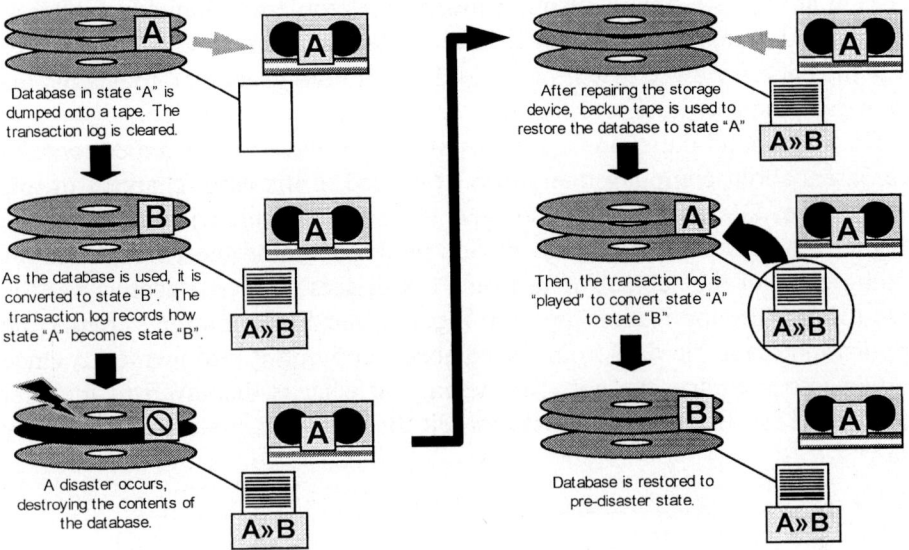

Figure 5-16: Backup tapes, transaction logs, and data recovery. In this example, the backup tape records the database contents in state A, whereas the transaction log records the details of how to convert state A to state B. If a device failure occurs, the backup tape is used to restore the database to state A, and then the transaction log is used to convert state A to state B, as the database existed just before the device failure.

possible to do any better than recover the database to state A from the hopefully offsite backup tape.

Although a little off track, this seems like an appropriate place to comment on the fact that, although probably every pathology practice backs up its data on a regular basis, few have ever actually tested whether or not they can successfully restore their data from a backup tape. This is sort of like not knowing whether or not your spare tire has any air in it. However, if your car gets a flat and you don't have air in your spare tire, plan B is to call a tow truck. If you are unable to restore your production database from a backup, there is no plan B. Ideally, this "test" should be performed on parallel equipment (you don't want to destroy your working production database to test to see whether or not you can restore it from a backup, and then find out you can't!)

Data Locking

Any time that a database can be used simultaneously by different users, it is possible that two users may try to access the same pieces of data at the same time. If they only plan to look at the data (read only), that is not a problem. If one of them plans to change the data, but the other one is just looking at the data, that is also not much of a problem. Granted, the "view only" user is looking at data which is about to become obsolete, but the next time the data is viewed it will be up-to-date. If both users plan to change the same data, then we have a problem.

To understand the source of the problem, we have to remember some of the basics about computer operations discussed in the early chapters of this book. The data in the database, that is, the data which is stored on the magnetic or other mass storage device which contains the contents of the database, it not the "actual" data which a user sees. When a user access the data through an application program (eg. a clinical information system), the application reads the data from the database, copying it into memory. Once copied into memory, the copy in memory is what is displayed to the user (Figure 5-17). If the user chooses to edit the data, it is the copy in memory

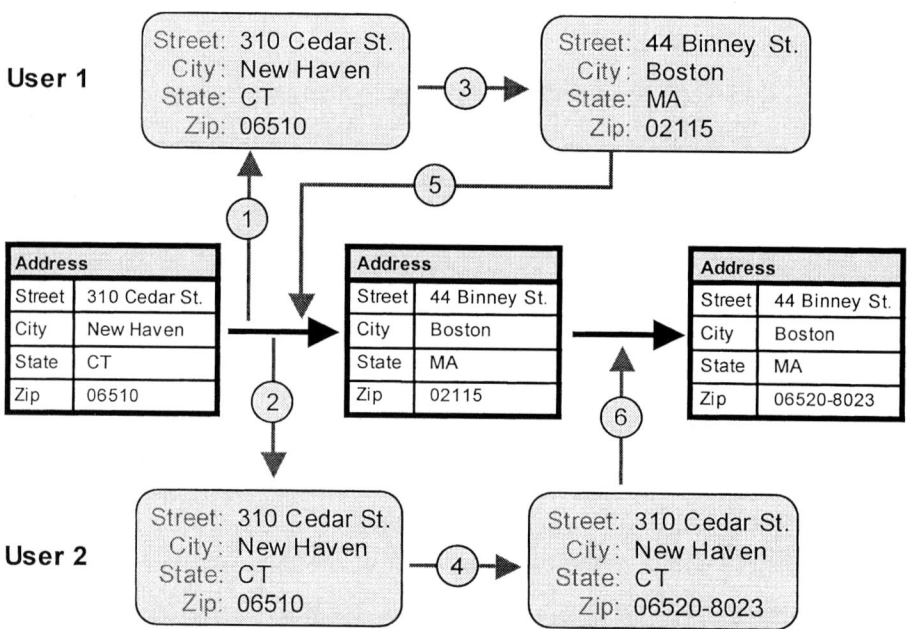

Figure 5-17: Simultaneous data modification without record locking.
1. User 1 reads the address into memory. He plans to completely change the address to a new one.
2. User 2 reads the address into memory. She plans to correct the zip code.
3. User 1 changes the address in the memory of his computer.
4. User 2 changes the zip code in the memory of her computer.
5. User 1 writes his changes back to disk. The database now contains the new address.
6. User 2 writes her changes to disk. In this example, since only the zip code has changed, only the zip code is written, replacing the zip code in the database with the corrected version of the old zip code.
At the end, the data in the database is internally inconsistent, representing parts of the information entered by each of the users.

which is being changed. The copy in the database is not changed until the user requests that the modifications be saved, at which time the data in the database is overwritten by the new data.

Now consider a second user who reads the same data into his computer's memory as was read by user 1 above, and reads it before user 1 commits his changes to the database. Now, user 2 has in his computer's memory a copy of the original data, as does user 1. They each make changes to the data, possibly different changes to the same data. User 1 finishes first and commits his changes to the database. Then user 2 finishes. When user 2 commits his changes, they overwrite the changes made by user 1. User 1 may think he has updated the data, but any changes he made are not reflected in the database. The details of what happens depends upon the design of the application, and whether all of the data read by user 2 is written back to the database, or just the values which have been changed. If the latter, the resulting data will be a mix of the changes made by both users. The situation can also be more complicated in a relational database where the data is likely to be stored in different tables. If the changes made by user 1 involve a different table than the changes made by user 2, there could be loss of data concurrency.

To prevent this from happening, database management systems employ a procedure known as data locking. Data locking is designed to prevent users of a multi-user database from modifying data in memory which is no longer representative of what data is stored in the database. When an application program requests data from the database, it requests it in one of two modes. In "read-only" mode, the DBMS places no restriction on the access, and will provide the data as it currently exists in the database, with the understanding that the user is not going to change the data. Alternatively, the data can be requested in "read with intention to write" mode. The DBMS checks to see if anyone else has read the same data with intention to write. If not, the data is locked and then transferred into memory. The user can then modify the data in memory as needed. If another user attempts to read the same data in read-only mode, they get an "old" copy of the data. If that other user attempts to read the same data in read-with-intention-to-write mode, the DBMS refuses the request because that would require locking the data and the data has already been locked by the first user. The second user must wait until the first user finishes editing the data and then writes it back to the database and releases the lock. Then, the second user can get a lock on a "fresh" copy of the data in the database. It is important for the user holding the lock on the data to remember to release the lock, even if the data is not going to be changed, or no one else can modify this data. Of course, in the real world, one often does not know whether or not they are going to modify the data until after they see the data. Therefore, most clinical information systems are written in such a way that all reads from modules which have the ability to change the data are done with the intention to write. This is why, when accessing an active case in the clinical information system, one might get an error message indicating that another user is currently accessing the case.

Data locking can be managed either by the application or directly within the database management system. Within the DBMS, locking can occur at the level of the table, the record (row), or the field (column). Locking at the level of the table is easiest to administer, but generally way too restrictive. It would mean that if any user were modifying information on any specimen, no other user could modify information on any other specimen. This would simply be absurd. Locking at the field (column) level allows the greatest access to the data for reading and modifying, but is very difficult to administer. This would allow one user to modify the histology information for a particular specimen while another user modifies the final diagnosis for that same specimen. Most databases use record (row) level locking for user tables, but table level locking for indices, since modifications to an index often require multiple rows to be modified as part of the same transaction.

Transaction Deadlocks

The combined features of multiple updates within transactions, triggers, and data locking create the possibility for an irresolvable conflict. Consider the following example: user 1 modifies data in table A. It locks the data in table A, modifies the data, and writes it back out to table A. A trigger on table A needs to modify the data in table B, as part of the same transaction (transaction 1). At essentially the same time, user 2 is modifying data in table B. It locks the data in table B, modifies the data, and writes it back out to table B. A trigger on table B needs to modify the data in table A, as part of the same transaction (transaction 2). Transaction 1 cannot finish because table B is locked by transaction 2. So transaction 1 goes into a wait state, waiting for transaction 2 to finish and release its lock on table B. At the same time, transaction 2 cannot finish, because table A is locked by transaction 1. Transaction 2 waits for transaction 1 to finish and release its lock on table A. Now, transaction 1 is waiting for transaction 2 to finish, and transaction 2 is waiting for transaction 1 to finish. Neither can finish. This is referred to as a "transaction deadlock". At this point, the database management system detects the conflict and steps in, selecting one of the two transactions as a "deadlock victim". That transaction is rolled back, releasing any locks it is holding, which allows the other transaction to finish. The "victim" transaction errors out and is not restarted, because the state of the underlying data is now different than when that transaction was originally started, and it may no longer be a desired transaction.

Transaction deadlocks are relatively rare, and usually require high levels of user access, or one user which is constantly accessing the database and modifying many tables. In the pathology information system at my institution, we see transaction deadlocks only occasionally, and those are almost invariable associated with our admission-discharge-transfer interface which is running constantly. Transaction deadlocks can be minimized by avoiding complementary triggers (triggers on two different tables, each of which modifies the contents of the other), and by updating a sequence of tables in a consistent order.

SQL – A Database "Language"

Thus far, we have discussed mostly issues which are internal to the database management system. However, as mentioned when the concept of a DBMS was introduced above, application programs need a mechanism to communicate with the DBMS. This communication language, ideally, should have a number of capabilities. It needs to be able to support the creation of tables and indices, as well as the modification of those tables later without destroying the contents of the tables (dynamic data definition). It needs to support the description of queries for data retrieval, including defining on-the-fly relationships between tables. Finally, of course, the language must support the insertion, deletion, and updating of data.

The industry standard "language" for communication between programs and relational databases is SQL (most commonly pronounced *ess-cue-ell*, although some still use the older pronunciation of *see-kwell*).

In the 1970's, IBM developed the concept of a relational database and the first incarnation of a database query language called "SEQueL", which stood for "Structured English Query Language". For legal reasons, it was forced to change the name, and changed it to "SQL", but still pronounced it "*see-kewll*". The American National Standards Institute (ANSI) formed a SQL standards committee in the early 1980's, and in 1986 they released a standard for SQL, which was ratified by the International Standards Organization (ISO) the following year. The US Government Federal Information Processing Standard adopted a standard based on SQL in 1989, which became known as SQL-89. Because, as will be discussed in a moment, SQL was originally designed as a non-procedural language, it was limited in what it could do, so various manufacturers of database management systems began to add features to their implementations of SQL, creating a variety of "dialects" for which the core commands were still compatible across databases but the additional features were not. Somewhere in the late 1980's, the pronunciation of SQL changed from *see-*

kwill to *ess-cue-ell*, presumably in relation to the realization that SQL and especially many of its derivative dialects did a lot more than simply query. ANSI released a revised standard in 1992, known as SQL-92 or SQL-2, with expanded descriptions, attempting to re-unify various vendors implementations of these additional features, but this has not happened, no commercially available database is fully SQL-92 compatible, and there has not been another version of an SQL standard released.

Most computer programmers cringe a little bit when the word "language" is used to refer to SQL. This is because SQL is not a complete programming language (which is why you will frequently find quotation marks around the word "language" when used in conjunction with SQL). It was designed to be completely non-procedural, in that the statements specify to the database management system what to do, but not how to do it. It is up to the DBMS to figure out how. Since true SQL is non-procedural, it does not support the definition of variables, and there are no flow control statements like "IF" or "GOTO", and no loops like "FOR" and "DO". For access to the database from within an application program, this is not a problem, because the application program can provide all the flow control necessary, and the program only needs to interact with the database to get the data. However, some complex queries cannot be performed with a single statement, and it became desirable to be able to assemble a sequence of SQL statements together, perhaps with some flow control logic which determined which statements were to be performed and in which order, and then store the resulting aggregate of statements in the database so that it could be executed as needed. It is precisely for this reason that individual vendors decided to enhance the language, adding variable definition and flow control. This allowed programmers to author "procedures", a group of SQL statements which could be executed in succession and with logic based on values of data provided to the procedure or data obtained from the database. It is in the syntax of these procedures that compatibility between different vendor implementations of SQL breaks down. Even with these enhancements, however, SQL is not a stand-alone language like C, Pascal or BASIC. No one would (could) write a stand-alone program in SQL. It does not compile to machine code, and in fact it does not exist (except as text) outside of the environment of the database in which it is being executed.

Nonetheless, if an application developer avoids relying on the procedural additions to SQL, there remains a significant amount of compatibility across vendors, allowing application developers to build their application with one database back-end and then switch to a different database back-end for deployment. SQL also provides client/server architecture access to relational databases in a hardware and system software independent fashion, allowing applications running on different operating systems to access the same database. SQL also provides for ad-hoc querying, namely the ability to interactively access the data in the database without having to write application programs.

To improve readability of SQL statements, the standard supports the use of optional "noise words" which make the statements look more like English sentences but which are ignored by the DBMS. For example, the phrases "INSERT INTO" and "DELETE FROM" can be used in place of simply "INSERT" and "DELETE", which are the only required parts of these phrases.

The SELECT Statement

I feel somewhat obligated, at this point, to introduce the reader to a basic SQL statement, rather than continuing to try to discuss the "language" in only vague terms. Although I will in no way attempt to teach SQL, something well beyond the scope of this book, there is sufficient consistency across all variations of SQL in how the single most important SQL command, SELECT, is implemented that it is worth briefly discussing this statement as an example.

The SELECT command is used to retrieve data from a relational database. The basic statement consists of three components, the list of attributes (columns) to be retrieved, the list of entities (tables) in which to find these attributes, and the criteria used to limit the data retrieved (Figure 5-18).

The attribute list consists of table/column name pairs, usually using the "dot" notation in which the table name is followed by a period and then the column name. If a column name occurs in only one of the tables specified in the FROM clause, only the column name needs to be listed in the attribute list (that is, the table name can be omitted). The tables containing the attributes are then listed in the "FROM" clause.

The most complex part of the SELECT statement is the WHERE clause. This clause includes a list of selection criteria expressed as conditional expressions, separated by the logical keywords AND or OR. The order of conditional expressions in the WHERE clause is irrelevant. There are two types of conditional expressions. The first type is referred to as a "join", and defines how the data in one of the tables is related to the data in another table. Basically, it matches the foreign key in one table with its corresponding column in the other table. In the example shown, the first line in the WHERE clause indicates that rows in the Person table are to be joined with rows in the Address table when the value in the add_id column of the Person table is equal to the value in the add_id column of the Address table. In general, if there are n tables listed in the FROM clause, there should be at

Person			
Last	First	p_id	add_id
Sinard	John	p1	a1
Mouse	Mickey	p2	a2
Potter	Harry	p3	a3
Torrance	Jack	p4	a4
Duck	Donald	p5	a2

Address				
add_id	Street	City	State	Zip
a1	310 Cedar St.	New Haven	CT	06510
a2	Disney World	Orlando	FL	32300
a3	4 Privet Drive	Little Whinging	Surrey	
a4	Overlook Hotel	Sidewinder	CO	80200

```
SELECT Person.Last, Person.First, Address.City, Address.State
  FROM Person, Address
 WHERE Person.add_id = Address.add_id
   AND Address.State = "FL"
```

Last	First	City	State
Mouse	Mickey	Orlando	FL
Duck	Donald	Orlando	FL

Figure 5-18: A sample SELECT statement in SQL. The select statement specifies what data elements (attributes) are to be retrieved, the tables in which that data is stored, how multiple tables included in the SELECT statement are related to each other, and the criteria to determine which subset of the data to return. The result is returned as a "table" and may contain data elements from multiple tables. Note that the SELECT statement does not specify how the data is to be retrieved, simply what data is to be retrieved. The "how" is up to the discretion of the optimizer built into the DBMS.

least n-1 joins in the WHERE clause, so that each table is joined to at least one other table.

The other type of conditional expression in a WHERE clause specifies value criteria which a row must meet in order to be included in the result set. In the example shown in Figure 5-18, the second line in the WHERE clause indicates that only rows in the Address table in which the State column has a value of "FL" are to be included in the result set. There can be as many of this type of conditional expression as needed to define the data desired.

SELECT statements return data in a tabular format. However, the columns in the "result table" can come from multiple different actual tables in the database. The result table can have one, many, or zero rows. Because of the potential one-to-many relationships in the database, result tables may have redundant data even though the database is properly normalized and does not have redundant data.

As mentioned above, there should be at least one join expression linking each table in the FROM clause to at least one other table in the FROM clause. Forgetting to do this is one of the most common mistakes made by novice SQL users. One might intuitively think that if one included a table in the FROM clause, but did not "link" it into the rest of the tables by providing a join expression for that table, the DBMS would simply ignore that table when building the result set. In fact, just the opposite happens. The WHERE clause should be thought of as always limiting the result set. In the absence of a WHERE clause, every row of every table listed in the FROM clause is paired with every row of every other table listed. Value criteria expressions limit which rows of each table participate in this pairing, and join expressions restrict which rows of each table are paired with each other. In the example shown, the Person table has five rows, and the Address table has four rows. If one were to execute the same SELECT statement shown but without the WHERE clause, the result set would contain 20 rows, where each row in the Person table is paired with each row in the Address table. This is known as a "cross-product", potentially disastrous if two of the tables included in the FROM clause were the patient table and the specimen table! If one were to include only the second conditional expression in the WHERE clause shown, the result set would contain five rows, with each row in the Person table being paired to the one row in the Address table which satisfied the "FL" criteria.

Note that no where in the SELECT statement is the DBMS given any instructions or clues as to how to fulfill the request, specifically which table to search first or how. That is the responsibility of the DMBS's optimizer.

The SELECT statement supports some additional keywords such as ORDER BY, GROUP BY, and HAVING, but these will not be discussed here.

Processing SQL Statements

Each SQL statement received by the DBMS is processed in a series of five steps. Each must finish successfully before processing can proceed to the next step.

- Parsing: The DMBS goes through the command, determining which words are command key words and which are arguments. The syntax of the command must be correct. If, for example, a SELECT statement is being parsed, and there is no column list or expression (a required part of the statement) or if there is an extra comma somewhere, the command will be aborted a syntactically incorrect. Note that the position of line breaks is NOT part of the syntax of an SQL command. They are often included to make the command more readable, placing the various clauses on separate lines, but this is not required. Line breaks are treated like a "space" when the SQL statement is parsed.

- Validation: Once the various arguments of the SQL statement are identified, they are validated against the database. This basically means checking to be sure that each of the tables specified actually exists, and that the columns indicated are present in the tables listed, and that there are no ambiguous column designations (as would occur if the same column was present in two of the tables, but only the column name was provided in one of the expressions). Validation also involves access privilege checking. If the person submitting the query does not have appropriate access to the tables and columns included in the query, the processing of the statement is aborted due to an "insufficient privilege" error.
- Optimization: As discussed above in the section entitled "Query Optimization" under "Database Management Systems", this is the process by which the DBMS determines how it is going to perform the command. Which table will be searched first? Will an index be used? Will it search first and then do the join, or join first and then search? These decisions are made based on internal algorithms, knowledge of what columns are indexed, and statistics about how the data in each table is, in general, distributed.
- Generation of an Application Plan: This is the DBMS equivalent of compiling the code. However, since true machine code is not produced, the term "binding" is often used rather than compiling. After deciding how it is going to execute the command (based on the results of the optimization process), the DBMS builds executable code, using internal pointers to the tables and columns involved in the query.
- Execution of the Application Plan: The application plan generated is executed. It is sometimes not possible to cleanly stop an execution once it has been initiated, short of administratively killing the database session performing the query.

SQL Access to Database from Computer Programs

Thus far, the discussion of SQL has been focused on what the database does when it gets an SQL command. This is fine for ad-hoc queries where one simply writes a command and submits it to the database for execution. However, since SQL is supposed to provide a mechanism by which computer programs can access databases, some consideration should be given to how computer programs integrate access to databases using SQL.

Embedded SQL

Some application development environments allow SQL commands to be directly embedded within the source code of the application. Then, at the time the application is compiled, the source code is first passed through a pre-compiler, which parses and processes the SQL statements. The pre-compiler inserts any needed code to connect to the database, pass the SQL commands, and retrieve the result set, and the code to disconnect from the database when the application quits. Embedded SQL requires an application development environment which not only supports a complete application language but also has the added features necessary to parse and validate SQL commands, as well as the ability to communicate with the database.

Two types of embedded SQL can be used. In static SQL, complete SQL statements are hard coded into the source code. During the pre-compile step, these statements are pre-processed through the parsing, validation, optimization, and application plan generation steps. The resulting application plan is stored either in the object code for the program or in the database itself. Then, at program execution time, the plan can be immediately executed, since the other four steps of the statement processing have already been completed. This results in much faster execution and better program performance. A potential disadvantage is that the optimization is done based on the database's information about the structure and distribution of the data in the database at compile time. If this structure changes, the application plan developed may no longer be the most optimum, and in fact the plan may become invalid (for example, if a column or an index is deleted). For this reason, the original SQL statements are often stored as well so that rebinding can occur at execution time if needed.

The other type of embedded SQL is dynamic SQL. This is used when the source code does not contain complete information about the query to be run, because it is built at runtime using information obtained either from the user or from the database. At program execution time, the SQL statement is built, usually in a host string variable, and then submitted to the database for parsing, validation, optimization, plan generation, and execution. Dynamic SQL is therefore slower than static SQL, because these steps cannot be performed in advance. Additionally, if the corresponding section of the computer program is executed repeatedly, the entire SQL statement processing procedure needs to be repeated each time. However, in return for this slower performance, there is much greater flexibility at runtime in building the query, and the optimization will be performed based on the state of the database at the time of execution, so there is no concern about using an outdated optimization.

SQL Module

Use of SQL modules is a highly variable process, dependent upon the database and programming language used, and therefore will be discussed only briefly here. It is very similar to embedded static SQL, except the SQL statements are separated from the rest of the source code (rather than being embedded), and are called by the application program via named routines. The collection of SQL statement are put through a pre-processor up through generation of an execution plan, building an SQL module or library. When the application source code is compiled, the SQL module is then linked to it for execution. One advantage this approach provides is that the development of the application source and the development of the SQL statements are separated, and can be performed by different individuals with different expertise. However, as there is great variation in how this solution is implemented (for example, whether the SQL module is embedded within the object code, stored as an external library on the client computer, or stored in the database), switching of the database or programming language may require extensive modifications.

API SQL and ODBC

Another common approach to allow application programs to access databases and perform database operations is through an Application Programming Interface or API (*ay-pee-eye*). This is sometimes referred to by the term Call-Level Interface, or CLI, but these terms are synonyms. With an API, the SQL code is not directly embedded within the source code, and no special pre-compiler or application development process is needed. Instead, the API consists of a library of function calls which communicate with the database management system. This library needs to be defined and linked to the application at compile time. Typically, within the application, the programmer will make a "call" to a library routine to establish a connection to the database. It will then build an SQL statement, dynamically, in a string variable, and then call another API library routine to pass this statement to the DBMS. Another API call is used to retrieve the result set, often one row at a time. At program termination, another API call is used to disconnect from the database. The capabilities of the database which are made available to the computer program are determined by the calls available in the API library. SQL APIs are frequently used by web server languages such as PHP and Perl to develop database driven web pages.

API libraries are specific for the database being accessed and the processor on which the application is running, and may even be specific for the programming language being used (although since the API library is pre-compiled, the language used to call that library should not be relevant). If an application developer wants to switch to a different database, a different API library will be needed, and the names of the routines in the library are likely to be different, so changes to the application code will be needed, even though essentially the same operations are being performed. In addition, if the application developer wants to access two or more different databases from the same application program, multiple libraries are needed, and the source code for access to each databases could be slightly different. To attempt to standardize this process somewhat, Microsoft developed and released, in the early 1990's, Open DataBase Connectivity, or ODBC.

ODBC is a generalized API implementation of database access from computer programs running in a client-server environment (Figure 5-19). It standardizes the front-end calls from the application, independent of what database is on the back-end of the deployment. Because of Microsoft's marketing position, most of the major database vendors have developed ODBC compatible drivers which recognize the standardized set of program calls made available to programmers through ODBC. Since the front-end seen by the application developer is the same, the back-end database can be changed simply by reconfiguring the ODBC manager and adding an appropriate driver.

Simultaneous access to different databases is also possible. The

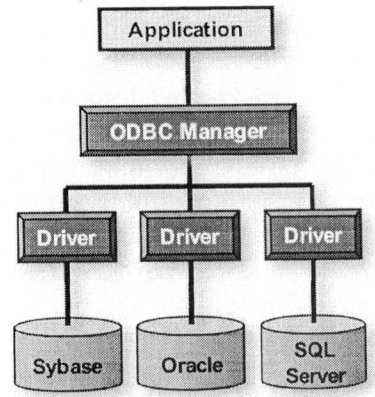

Figure 5-19: Open Database Connectivity. ODBC allows applications to access multiple databases through a common API. Each database to be used must have an ODBC compliant driver.

application routines submit a request to the ODBC manager, which is running as an operating system service. The ODBC manager determines which data source is to fulfill the request, and passes that on to the appropriate ODBC driver for that database. The driver then does whatever translation is necessary for the specific database. The results of the query are collected by the ODBC driver and passed back to the ODBC manager which in turn passes them on to the application.

Since not all databases support all the same operations, and since the ODBC API is intended to be largely database independent, not all database functions will be available through ODBC, and not all ODBC calls will work in all databases. However, the major data manipulation and retrieval commands are generally well supported.

World-Wide-Web-Based Access to Databases
One of the most popular methods for deploying databases has been to integrate access to them into web pages. This is what has made possible

such things as on-line shopping, banking, investing, bill-paying, etc. In fact, any web site where the user has to log-in with a user specific identifier and password must be using a database to store those usernames and passwords. Search engines and airline reservation systems are more examples of database driven web pages.

A general introduction to the world-wide-web and web servers was given near the end of Chapter 4 on Networking, and in particular Figure 4-13 diagramed a typical client browser accessing a static web page from a web server. The concept of server-side processing was also introduced, and will be elaborated upon a little here.

The whole point behind database driven web pages is to be able to deliver customized information to a user, based on information entered by that user. Information is returned to the user in the form of an HTML web page – that is the only thing which the user's web-browser can display. Clearly it would not be possible to "pre-make" every possible web page which a user might request and select from among them when the user's request is received. Instead, the web server has to build, in memory, a customized web page and return that to the user. The elements which are needed to make this system work include a way to get request information from the user, a template web page used to build a response page, a programming language which can use the information in the user request to access a database, retrieve requested data, and generate a "dynamic" web page containing the results, and then a server to deliver this newly created web page to the user.

Processing of user requests and generating dynamic web pages occurs on the server, and is an example of server-side processing. As discussed in Chapter 4, a number of programming/scripting languages can be used to achieve this, including CGI, ASP, PHP, JSP, and ASP.net. Each of these solutions provides similar functionality, but achieve it in different ways. CGI (Common Gateway Interface) was among the first server-side processing languages, but its use has largely been replaced by newer, more powerful languages. Microsoft's Active Server Pages (ASP) have become very popular, despite the limitation that they can only run on Microsoft's web servers, but this is now being replaced by a new Microsoft product ASP.net, a similarly named but completely different architecture solution which also can only run on a Microsoft web server. PHP (a recursive acronym which stands for PHP: Hypertext Preprocessor) is an open source solution which is very popular. It works with a variety of web servers, multiple operating systems, and can be customized to meet the particular needs of a developer. Java Server Pages (JSP) has some advantages over PHP in that the server-side programs, called servlets, are pre-complied, can support multi-threading, and provide better performance under heavy use.

JSP is more difficult to set up, but also provides better separation of the processing code from the visual HTML (hypertext markup language) code, and therefore may integrate better into team development groups.

To illustrate the process of delivering a dynamic database driven web page, I will describe a simplified example using PHP for server-side processing. Equivalent solutions based on one of the other server-side programming languages would follow a similar process, although some of the details will be slightly different.

The process begins with the user on the client computer being presented with an HTML form (Figure 5-20). This form is a method for gathering information from the user. That information could be as simple as a username and password or as complicated as multiple drop-down lists, radio buttons, and free response text fields. The user must provide enough input

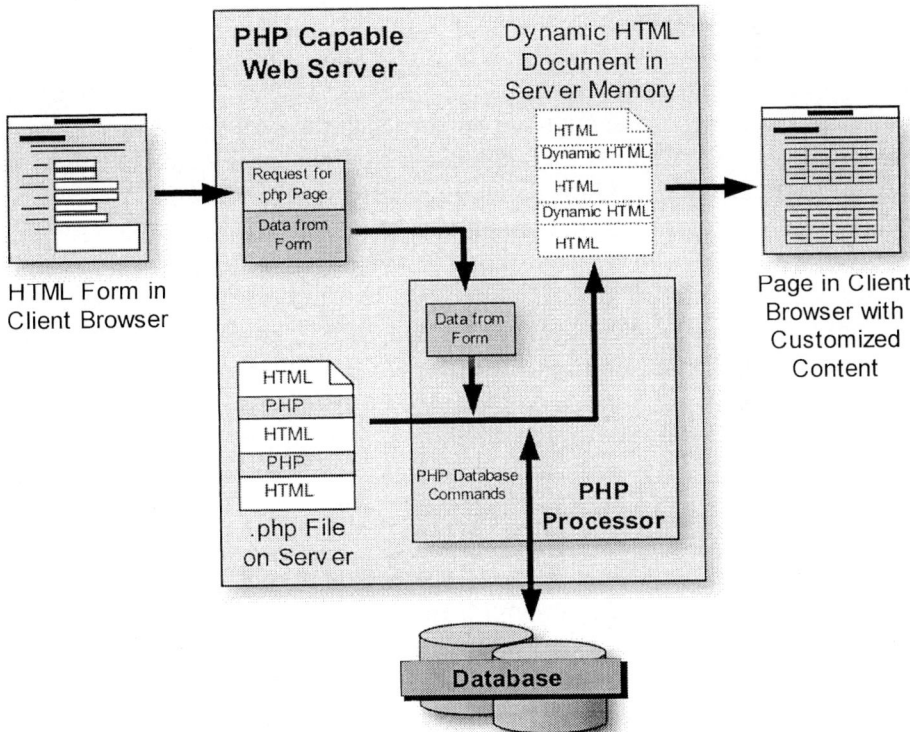

Figure 5-20: Using a server-side processing language (PHP) to generate a dynamic web page. The user submits a request to the server using an HTML form. The data from this form is used, in conjunction with the PHP code on the requested page, to access data from a database and then build, in memory, a dynamic HTML page containing the requested data. This process is discussed in more detail in the text.

so that the server will be able to determine what custom information is being requested. HTML forms themselves are often static pages pre-made by the developer of the solution, and although they frequently contain some JavaScript code to allow client-side processing and interaction (again, see Chapter 4), they usually do not contain PHP code (at least not when the user sees them). After the user completes the form, he/she presses the "Submit" button. This sends a request back over the internet to the web server. The request specifies a .php file on the web server, and attached to the request is all of the data entered by the user. The .php file requested will have a combination of PHP code and HTML code in it, with the HTML code generally representing the "static" portions of the page, including the formatting information, and the PHP code representing the dynamic portions. The web server recognizes the presence of PHP code in the requested web page and hands off that page and the data from the form to the PHP pre-processor which is running within the web server application. The pre-processor on the server executes the PHP code embedded within the .php file using the data from the form submitted by the user to retrieve specific information from a database (which may also be on the web server or, more commonly, on another server to which the web server has access). The PHP processor uses an API specific for the database being accessed to hand off SQL statements to the database's DBMS and additional API calls to retrieve the results of those data requests. The PHP processor then uses this retrieved information to build, in the memory of the web server, a dynamic HTML web page based on the .php file requested but in which the PHP portions of the file have been replaced with "custom" HTML code containing the information requested by the user. This dynamic web page, which exists only in the memory of the web server, is then delivered across the internet to the browser on the client computer of the user as if it were a regular, static, HTML web page, and the page is then rendered by the browser, displaying the requested data to the user.

If the dynamically generated web page also contains HTML form elements, one can begin to see how a series of user-initiated and request specific interactions can occur. With this approach, fully functional web-based applications with database access can be written. This type of application solution is becoming very popular because the code for the application resides in only one place, yet can be accessed from any networked computer, independent of the operating system on that computer.

Chapter 6

PATHOLOGY LIS: RELATIONSHIP TO INSTITUTIONAL SYSTEMS

Pathology laboratory information systems (LIS) form the core of most pathology practices. After the pathologists, in many places they represent the next most crucial asset, without which all practice operations soon screech to a halt. Additionally, the information contained in these systems, especially systems which have been around for a while, is invaluable for quality patient care.

Pathology practices are most commonly affiliated with health care institutions, and most health care institutions have other departments whose operations are also closely integrated with their information systems. Some of these computer systems may be institution-wide, whereas others are more limited with respect to the scope of the people they serve.

When multiple information systems are present within a single institution, issues of systems architecture, management, and integration invariably come into play. This chapter will try to begin to address some of those issues, including intranets, information system access delivery, management philosophies, systems integration, electronic medical records, and data warehousing.

Medical Intranets

An intranet is a network based on TCP/IP protocols (like the internet) which, although connected to the internet and providing access to the internet, is protected to varying degrees from computers and network traffic outside of the institution by a firewall. Intranets are "owned" by an organization or institution, and the full resources of the computers connected to the intranet are available only to other individuals within the institution. Information within the institution can be shared, but since the intranet is "behind" the firewall, it is protected from unauthorized external access.

An intranet is defined by the firewall which protects it, dividing the network into those devices which are inside or behind the firewall (on the protected site) and outside the firewall (on the internet side). A firewall is a combination of hardware and software, most commonly associated with a router computer (see Chapter 4 on Networking for more information about routers). Devices which are inside the firewall can freely communicate with each other over the network of the intranet. However, all network traffic leaving the intranet or entering the intranet from the internet must pass through the firewall. The firewall can thus protect the intranet in one of a few ways. One method is to examine each packet of data and block traffic which does not come from a pre-defined set of IP addresses or domain names. Another is to block traffic based on the socket (port) number, thereby allowing, for example, web traffic while blocking FTP traffic. Still another is to require a certain level of authentication at the time the connection is established, but once established freely allow all traffic for that connection. Usually, a variety of different methods are employed in different combinations. A firewall is only one way of protecting data on an intranet from the internet. Data encryption is another approach which can be used, usually in addition to a firewall.

Note that a similar level of security could be obtained simply by using a proprietary communication protocol on the segregated portion of the network. However, this requires a level of cooperation difficult to achieve in large institutions, as well as placing constraints on device selection and increasing deployment times, management issues, and costs. In contrast, creating intranets using the same communication standards and browser-based tools used by the internet markedly facilitates speed of solution development and minimizes the need for employing unique solutions. Any computer which can connect to the internet can be configured to participate in an intranet.

Because the most common protocol for both internet and intranet access is the hypertext transfer protocol used for the world-wide-web (see Chapter 4), many individuals restrict use of the term "intranet" to those instances in which browser-based tools are used to access information. However, here I use the term to refer to any network using any non-proprietary TCP/IP based protocol but to which access is restricted to members of an institution. While we are talking semantics, a third term, "extranet", should also be defined. Extranet is used when limited, authenticated access to an intranet is enabled, allowing individuals physically outside of the institution owning the intranet to access its resources as if the person were at the institution.

Medical intranets introduce a few unique elements of security not relevant for corporate networks or networks at most other institutions. An important difference is that the data we are protecting is not our own data per se but rather information about our patients. Inappropriate "leakage" of data is not simply an issue of loss of corporate secrets or even sensitive financial information: it can irrevocably change a person's life... forever. Whereas corporate secrets only have an inherent lifetime of a few years, medical histories are permanent. There are also federal regulations dictating security measures which must be employed when communicating protected health information. Poised against this need for security, however, is the desire to make the information about a particular patient as available as possible to the physicians treating that patient, since accurate and complete information forms the basis of high quality medical care. These conflicting goals of information sharing and patient privacy make for complicated technological, procedural and political issues. More information about patient privacy regulations is included in Chapter 12 on External Regulations.

A typical medical intranet is likely to include a variety of different types of hardware (Figure 6-1). In addition to the ones which most of the medical staff see every day, namely the desktop computers, printers, and perhaps

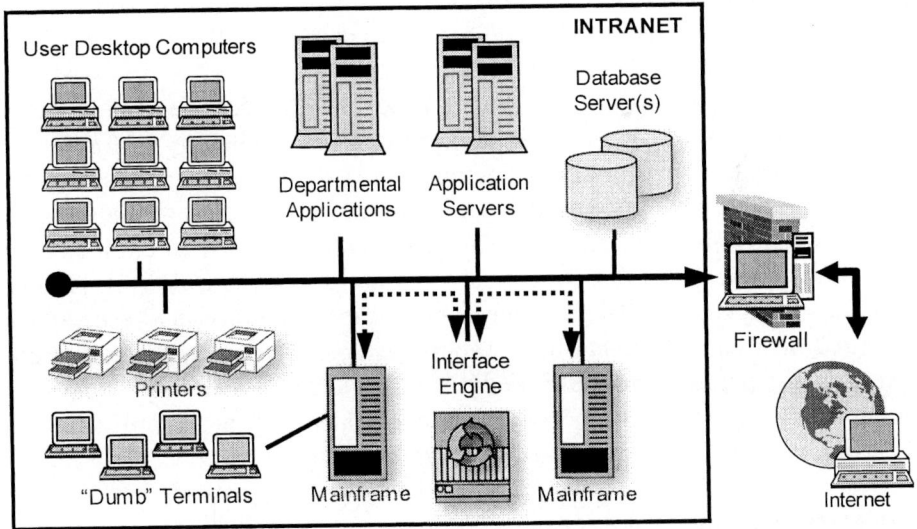

Figure 6-1: Medical Intranets. Medical intranets can be very complex. In addition to the desktop computers and printers which everyone sees, there are a number of higher-end computers behind the scenes, including large mainframe systems interconnected by one or more interface engines, application servers distributing core functionalities to various locations, and, of course, multiple database servers. A computer acting as a firewall protects these systems and their data from unauthorized access via the internet.

some additional terminals, the main machines which house the applications and data are traditionally sequestered away in a secure location, with appropriate environmental controls, backup power supplies, and limited access. These devices are actually responsible for most of the traffic on the intranet, since the vast majority of network traffic other than that between desktop computers and the internet is either heading for or coming from one of the main servers. Devices likely to be found include mainframe computers, interface engines, multiple database servers, computers housing departmental applications, and application servers. The heterogeneity reflects not only the varying needs of different departments but also the different models for distributing application functionality to the end users. These models for application connectivity, which define the mix of devices on an institution's intranet, will be the topic of the next section.

Distributing Application Functionality to Desktops

Few laboratory information systems reside totally on a desktop computer. While small, single user programs like word-processors and spreadsheets can simply be installed on a user's desktop computer, the need for multiple users to access the laboratory information system simultaneously and share a common data source, the "back-end" database, requires a different model for distributing the functionality of that application.

Although this discussion may seem a little out of place here, it is difficult to truly contemplate the relationship between a pathology information system and other institutional information systems without understanding the different models for connecting large information systems to their users within a health care environment. The last decade has seen an explosion in the features and capabilities of clinical information systems. Driven largely by the doors opened by faster processors, cheaper memory, and essentially unlimited disk space, clinical information systems have grown from simple menu driven operations to multi-media extravaganzas! With this increase in capabilities has come an increase in complexity. That complexity has necessitated changes in their distribution architecture.

Mainframe Systems

Early multi-user information systems were relatively simple with respect to the architecture of user access. The software and any associated databases and data resided on a large mainframe computer, sequestered away in some environmentally controlled room in a location which few people knew and even fewer ever visited. The user's interface to these mainframes was

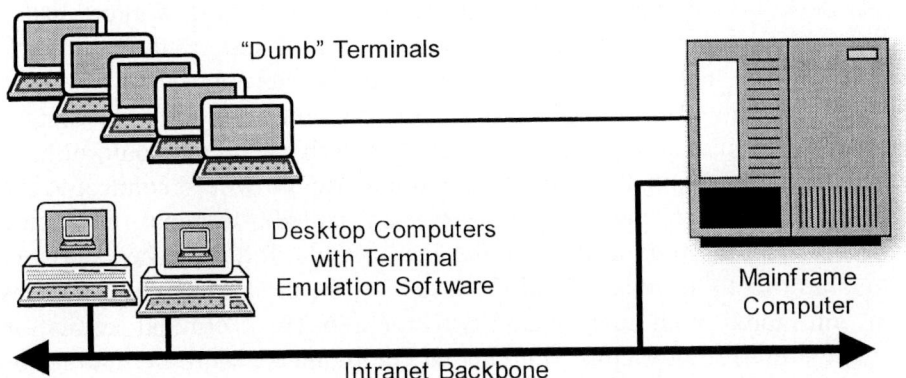

Figure 6-2: Early Mainframe Systems. With a mainframe computer, all of the computational capabilities are in the central computer. The terminals which connect to them have no central processor and are therefore commonly referred to as "dumb". Desktop computers can often connect to mainframe systems by simulating a "dumb" terminal via terminal emulation software.

usually a monochromatic "dumb terminal". (Some people use the term "black and white" to describe these displays, but in reality the characters were usually more yellowish and the background was generally dark-green to gray) (Figure 6-2). These terminals are referred to as "dumb" because although they have the cathode-ray-tube displays and keyboards of modern desktop computers, they have no internal processor (hence no internal intelligence), no random access memory, and no local data storage capabilities. They are simply windows into an operating system on a computer which is "somewhere else". Each terminal is equivalent to every other terminal, and each can be turned on and off at will. The connection to the mainframe computer is usually a "direct" connection via a serial interface, NOT through any network. Remember, since dumb terminals are not computers, they have no network interface cards and no networking capabilities. The wires for these connections are run as one would telephone wires, and in fact telephone wire is often used for this purpose. Because of the long distance, there is often some terminal serving hardware device between the wall plates and the actual mainframe, but this was invisible to the users.

All of the processing in such a system architecture takes place on the mainframe computer, which can support multiple simultaneous connections by different users. However, every connected user shares the processing power of the mainframe. If the main system goes down, everyone's screens lock up, or go blank, and no one can do anything.

As desktop computers became more popular, and most workers had a fully functioning networked computer on their desk to support their other job responsibilities, it was a waste of space to have to have a second CRT and keyboard on the desk simply to be able to connect to the laboratory information system (and that was the only thing that terminal could do). A program can be installed on a desktop computer to allow it to connect to the main information system.   This program, called "terminal emulation software", can communicate over the institution's TCP/IP based network using a protocol known as TELNET, assuming the mainframe computer has been configured with this capability (Figure 6-2).   Terminal emulation software allows the desktop computer to communicate with the mainframe computer as if it were a dumb terminal; what would normally appear on the display of the terminal now appears within a window on the monitor of the desktop computer.   When the terminal emulator program is active, all keyboard input is transmitted to the mainframe computer.   However, all of the processing still occurs on the mainframe computer. The processor in the desktop computer is largely an innocent bystander, merely sending keyboard input to the mainframe and receiving and displaying monitor output.

A new capability afforded by terminal emulation software is the ability to "capture" the output to the screen and save it in a local document which could be opened and edited with a word-processing application. While this allows doing new things with the output of the mainframe computer, it also means that sensitive protected health care information could now be stored locally, making it potentially available to other individuals who have access to the desktop computer but not login access to the laboratory information system. This represents a possible security/privacy breach issue which must be properly managed.

The mainframe system architecture has the advantage of being simple to understand and maintain. Since there is only one system, any modifications or upgrades to the system are seen immediately by all users. Also, any improvements in performance are also shared by all users. Dumb terminals are relatively inexpensive (compared to desktop computers). They are not capable of storing information locally, so as long as users remember to log out before wandering away there are no security or privacy concerns.

However, there are clearly disadvantages of the mainframe configuration. The main one is that all of the processing is done by a single computer. As more users are added to the system, the performance of the system decreases and all of the users suffer. In addition, because of the limited graphics capabilities of dumb terminals, as well as of the TELNET communication protocol, more advanced features such as digital imaging and even elements of a graphical user interface are not possible. These systems can also be difficult to install in a pre-existing building. Although installation of the mainframe itself is not problematic, distributing system access to dumb terminals scattered about the institution can involve a lot of wiring. In the modern environment, this simply would not be done, and terminal emulation software communicating along networks (undoubtedly needed and most likely already present in the building) would be the only reasonable solution.

Client-Server Systems (Distributed Processing)

With the proliferation of desktop computers within work environments, most users require a desktop computer for other purposes. Those desktop computers each contain their own processor. Rather than all users of the central information system sharing a single processor, it makes more sense to try to leverage the processing power that was in each desktop system. However, all of the users had to access the same data, so some degree of central processing was still important to preserve the integrity of that data and manage the access of multiple users to that data. Thus entered the era of client-server technology, otherwise known as distributed processing, because some of the processing is done on the desktop client, while some is done on the central server. In this configuration (Figure 6-3), the central server usually houses the database and the core of the database management system, and therefore is often referred to simply as the database server (see Chapter 5 for more information on database management systems). The bulk of the application software (the user interface by which the users access and manipulate the data) is installed locally on each desktop computer. The local processing is done by the CPU in the desktop computer. Data is then sent to the database server, over a network connection, and the processor in the database server then handles the storage of that data, as well as other database management tasks.

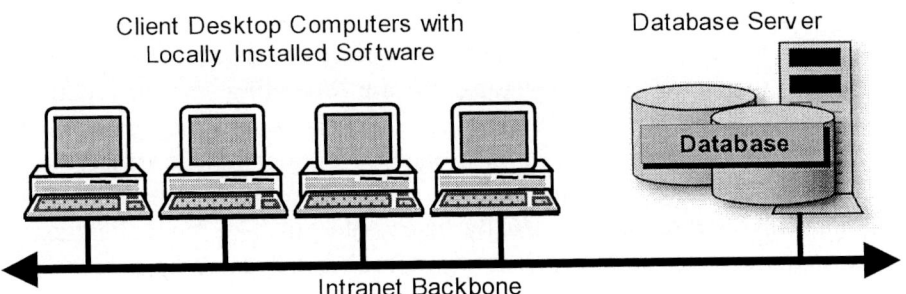

Figure 6-3: Client-Server Architecture. In a client-server system, computational tasks are split between a powerful database server and intelligent desktop computers. These systems communicate with each other via the institutional network, usually a protected intranet.

The advantage of a distributed processing configuration is that the user tasks related to the clinical information system are not handled by just one processor or just two processors but rather by the multiple processors present in all of the desktop computers accessing the system. Each user's own processor handles each user's own local tasks, thereby leveraging the processing power already present in their computer. However, the central processor in the database server still has to handle all of the database accessing.

In addition to the processing advantages, having the application software running on a computer with advanced graphics capabilities opens the door to new functionalities, graphical user interfaces with mouse controls, buttons, drop-down lists, etc. Technologies such as imaging and speech recognition are now also possible.

However, client/server architecture solutions are more complex to set up and maintain. Each user is required to have a desktop computer, and not just any desktop computer: it has to be one with the operating system specifications and hardware capabilities dictated by the vendor of the laboratory information system. If one is converting from a mainframe-based information system to one with a client/server architecture, purchasing the needed desktop computers is likely to constitute a significant added cost. Modifications and/or upgrades to the information system after the initial installation requires re-synchronization of the software among all of the workstations on which the application is installed, to assure that everyone is using compatible versions of the software. In practice, this often means visiting each client computer, which, for a large organization, can be hundreds. Depending upon the features added by an upgrade, the originally recommended desktop hardware may no longer be adequate to run the software efficiently, requiring not only upgrading of the software but also upgrading or even replacing the hardware. This has to be done for each workstation which accessing the clinical information system. Other issues which need to be considered include the potential effects of different desktop computers using different versions of the operating system, potential incompatibilities or conflicts with other software which may exist on the desktop computers, and the need for protection from computer viruses.

Just as the singular term "client" in client-server is inaccurate, the singular term "server" is also usually inaccurate. In fact, most client-server implementations use multiple servers, including the database server, print agents, fax agents, and synchronization agents, over which the business logic of the application is distributed. Each of these machines introduces new requirements for hardware and software, server administration skills, and backup procedures. Each also represents a potential site for system failure.

A final disadvantage of the client/server architecture is that operation of the information system now becomes dependent upon the institution's network. Unlike mainframe systems where the dumb terminal is connected to the main system essentially directly (along communication lines which were not shared by other users), clients generally connect to their database servers along the institution's intranet network. Insufficient networking resources resulting in transmission delays, poor network management, or failure of the network all can hinder or incapacitate the functioning of the clinical information system.

Thin-Client Technology

An alternative architecture exists for deployment of client-server based systems, referred to as "thin-client technology", which shares some similarity to terminal-emulation software. This architecture is even more complex, because it requires the presence of another high-end computer, referred to as the application server, which sits between the user's desktop workstation and the database server. The application server must contain special software which allows it to support multiple simultaneous sessions.

In this architecture (Figure 6-4), the "client software" is installed on the application server rather than on the individual user workstations, and it is the application server which communicates with the database server. The user desktop workstations run, instead, a small program called the thin-client. This program establishes a connection to the application server, which starts a new "headless session" and runs the client software for the clinical information system. (The session is referred to as headless because

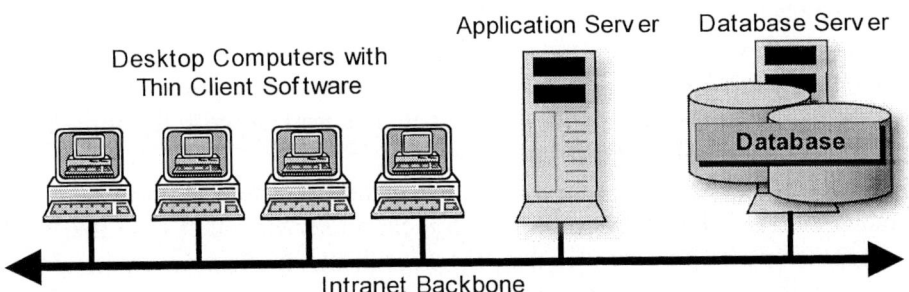

Figure 6-4: Thin-Client Architecture. Thin-client systems are based on the client-server model, except that the client software is installed on a central application server rather than the local desktop computers. To run the application, users at the desktop computers establish a connection to the application server, creating a "window" into a virtual desktop computer on the application server. This virtual session communicates with the database server. The application server can support multiple simultaneous virtual sessions.

you cannot see the output of the session from a monitor – the head - connected to the application server.)   Much like terminal-emulation software, the desktop workstation has a window into the session established on the application server.   However, whereas with terminal-emulation software the local computer is acting as if it were a dumb terminal, with thin-client software the local computer is emulating another desktop computer.   The workstation receives the screen output from the session running on the application server and sends keyboard and mouse input to that session, but all of the real processing occurs on the application server.

Thin-client software is available for a variety of different operating systems.   Therefore, regardless of what operating system the clinical information system has to run on, the desktop computers can be the same or a completely different operating system.   The actual client software is running on the application server, so the hardware and software requirements of the information system have to be met by the application server, constraining the choice of options for the server.   The desktop computers, however, only have to run a small thin-client program, and different versions of that software are available for different operating systems.   It is thus possible to have a Macintosh desktop computer, for example, with a "window" representing the clinical information system running in a Windows environment.

With the thin-client solution, the clinical information system software only needs to be installed in one location, the application server, eliminating issues of client synchronization.   If the software is upgraded, only the application server needs to be upgraded, and all of the thin-clients see the new version of the software.   If the new version of the clinical information system application requires a hardware upgrade, again only the application server needs to be upgraded.   The thin-client software requires only minimal computing power, so that it, in and of itself, will not drive the upgrade of the user desktop computers.   Operating system issues and potential conflicts with other desktop software are significantly minimized with the thin-client approach.

Since all of the users connected to the clinical information system are actually running the software on the application server rather than the local desktop computer (that is, it is the processor in the application server which is performing the tasks of the application, not the processor in the desktop computer), computing resources are largely centralized.   Although processing is still distributed between the application server and the database server, all of the users share the resources of the application server, and as more users are connected, everyone's performance will be degraded. However, increasing the power of the application server improves all user's performance. Therefore, application servers tend to be very powerful, multi-processor computers with a lot of main memory.

The centralization of processing tasks to the application server creates a single point for overall system failure – if the application server goes down or needs to be upgraded, all access to the system via this route is compromised. Much greater protection from server failure can be achieved by having two application servers which are load balanced: when a new user connects as a thin-client, the session established for them is created on whichever available application server has the greatest remaining capacity. If one application server goes down, all users simply connect to the other.

Although thin-client solutions are difficult to set up and administer, the advantages afforded are significant and generally worth the effort, especially for environments with a large number of occasional users. Much like traditional client-server solutions, thin-client solutions are also highly dependent upon institutional network performance.

An important issue which needs to be considered before deploying a thin-client architecture as the information system distribution solution is that software features which require direct interaction with hardware connected to the user's desktop computer will not work with this architecture. Some features such as image acquisition and speech recognition require the application software to communicate directly with hardware connected to the user's computer (such as a digital camera or a microphone). With a thin-client solution, the software is running on the application server, but the hardware in question is plugged into the user's desktop computer. This problem is, for most purposes, insurmountable, so if these features are important to your practice's workflow, then the thin-client solution may not be the right one for you.

Philosophical Spectra of Information System Management

Workflow in anatomic pathology laboratories is integrally tied to their information systems. Pathology practices, and (I would strongly argue) pathologists themselves, need to have a role in the information system decisions which are going to govern their practices. Occasionally, a pathology practice can function as an island, administratively isolated from external management forces. That is, however, the exception, and most pathology practices are affiliated with larger institutions. Within these institutions, the pathology laboratory may be a fully integrated department administratively falling within the hierarchical management structure of the hospital or medical school. Alternatively, the practice may be largely independent, sharing physical space but with little overlap in management.

Even in this latter situation, however, the housing institution can have significant influences on pathology practice decisions related to information systems, because, as illustrated in the previous section, most deployment options for large pathology information systems rely heavily on networking, and the owner of the building usually controls the network in much the same way that they control the electricity and telephone services.

Dozens of models exist for pathology information system management, and it is probably safe to say that no two institutions share the exact same relative mix of internal and external forces driving their information technology decision making processes. It is almost pointless to argue which model is better than another; not only does each have its own advantages and disadvantages, but the evolution of the model at any institution is so deeply rooted in the history and politics of that institution that it is often very difficult to change the rules under which any given practice is constrained, except perhaps in small steps. Nonetheless, for your particular practice, it is important to understand your particular rules, the philosophies underlying any constraints imposed, and how much flexibility you have within those constraints.

Philosophies are promulgated by decision making bodies. Knowing the mix of individuals who constitute the decision making body for information technology issues is crucial to understanding those philosophies. In some environments and situations, it can be easy to determine that mix. If your institution is currently undergoing or has recently undergone an information system selection process, simply looking at the membership of the selection committee can give you great insight into the forces with which the pathology practice will have to contend to assure that its issues are addressed. At some health care institutions, the decision making body is made up predominantly of physicians, and the relative capabilities of competing systems are most critically evaluated based on the impact they will have on patient care and care management workflow. Unfortunately, such a physician dominated decision making body is the exception rather than the rule. The other players are administration and information technology support. Administration is likely to be more influenced by the quality of the "back-office" solutions, such as billing, account management, scheduling, reporting, and record keeping. Representatives from information technology support will be more influenced by the underlying software upon which the system is built, such as operating system and database selection, because the quality of support they can provide will be affected by the overlap between the support needs of the system and the expertise of the support personnel. The relative input of these three groups, as well as the history of the institution, will determine the philosophies underlying the information system decision making process.

I have found it very helpful to consider three philosophical spectra which influence the decision making process for clinical information system selection and management, and for the adoption and integration of new technology. Regardless of the clinical information system chosen or the architecture used to deploy that system within an institution, someone locally has to be in charge of managing that system. In many instances, issues such as customization, upgrading, bug fixes, etc. are handled by the software vendor, but day-to-day management tasks such as controlling user access, maintaining dictionaries, monitoring interfaces, and performing back-ups need to be handled locally. Lots of options exist for this, and the power to choose from these often does not lie exclusively in the pathology department/practice. Nonetheless, understanding where your institution sits on each of these three philosophical spectra is important in determining your flexibility in the process.

Enterprise vs Specialty Solution

A fundamental underlying dichotomy exists between enterprise and specialty-based solutions. This decision was probably already made many years ago at your institution, and was most likely made at a high level. This is, therefore, one of the most difficult philosophies to attempt to change.

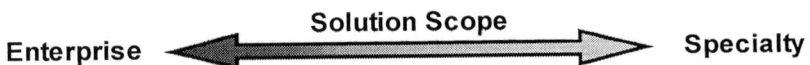

In an enterprise solution environment, a decision is made, usually at the institutional level, to go with a single vendor solution for all departments in the institution. Sometimes this decision is made by joint agreement amongst the departments; other times it is made by the administration and imposed upon the departments. This solution allegedly provides the advantage of built-in integration, although the level of integration actually varies quite a bit from vendor to vendor. When an enterprise solution is selected, the institution, rather than the individual departments, generally foots-the-bill for the system. The main disadvantages of this approach is that no enterprise solution is best for all departments. Thus, a particular vendor's solution may, for example, be very feature-rich in accounting and reporting and physician order-entry, but offer very few features for laboratory medicine, pharmacy, or radiology. The institutional decision will be biased in favor of a system which is stronger in the areas which the decision makers consider most important. In the grand scheme of hospital administration, anatomic pathology does not generally produce sufficient revenue to warrant a large say in the selection of the enterprise solution for the institution.

In a specialty solution environment, also known as "best-of-breed", each department individually selects the vendor(s) and product(s) which are best for their particular department. This freedom to choose can increase the efficiency and productivity of that department and allow for better attention by the vendor, since departments are not generally competing with each other for vendor services. This solution, however, places greater burdens on the department for selecting, maintaining, and perhaps purchasing the information system. The system also will need more sophisticated interface capabilities if communication with other institutional systems is required. A more detailed discussion of electronic interfaces in the health care environment will be provided in Chapter 10 on "Electronic Interfaces".

Not uncommonly, "discussions" will occur between a department preferring a specialty solution and their housing institution preferring the department accept the enterprise solution. It is generally best to approach these with good data contrasting the capabilities of the two solutions and the impacts the decision will have on the workflow. Feature analysis of clinical information systems can be a confusing task. The Chapter 7 provides an approach which can be used to facilitate this process.

Some would argue that the decision between an enterprise and specialty solution is not really a spectrum but rather two distinct points. Proponents of this belief have held that if even one department or practice within an institution has an independent information system, then by definition an enterprise solution does not exist. I am less interested in the semantics of the argument than the practical assessment of whether or not it is feasible for a single department to have an independent information system at an institution where all of the other departments share an enterprise solution. In fact, I have personal experience with such an institution, where the only department running on an information system different from the solution used by the remainder of the institution is anatomic pathology. Of course, in such a situation, the isolated department should anticipate taking on a much greater role managing their own system and not expect a great deal of support at the institutional level.

The choice between an enterprise solution and a specialty solution also occurs at a level within the pathology practice as well as at the institutional level. Anatomic pathology departments frequently consist of several units or divisions: surgical pathology, cytopathology, autopsy pathology, perhaps even molecular diagnosis, flow cytometry, and cytogenetics. Can each unit have its own information system solution, should they all be forced to use one system decided upon by the department as a whole, or is there a middle ground? All of the same arguments made above for institutional enterprise solutions apply to departmental ones (except perhaps the financial ones).

Off-the-Shelf Software vs Custom-Built Software

Another important philosophical decision to make is whether to develop one's own custom software/information system or simply buy a pre-packaged, commercially available system. This decision will be based, in a large point, on how closely the "off-the-shelf" system being considered meshes with the workflow of the department and on the availability of resources to develop a custom solution. A common mistake made when looking at information systems is to concentrate on the features it offers (see Chapter 7). Although clearly important in evaluating a system, features are an element of a system which can and will evolve over time. The workflow design, however, is far less likely to change. Does the workflow supported by the system match the workflow which your practice has developed over time? At some level, this analysis can be rephrased as a choice: "Is the information system supposed to help run our business the way we want to run it, or do we adjust our workflow to match what the information system can do?"

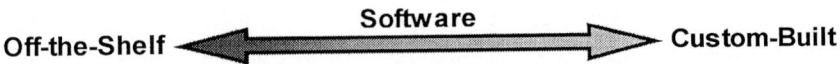

Off-the-Shelf ⟵——— **Software** ———⟶ **Custom-Built**

Some readers may take exception to my describing this philosophy as a spectrum, considering it rather a dichotomy: one either buys a system, or builds it. The increasing modularity of large applications allows for the integration of customized components with commercial solutions. Depending on the level of integration needed, many of these customizations may need to be developed by or at least in cooperation with the commercial vendor. However, remember that not all of the information system elements of a pathology practice need to be integrated. This concept is a bit of a mental obstacle for some, but consider the possibility that, for some needs, a stand-alone solution might be the best solution for that need. For example, at my home institution, our most used imaging solution, by far, is not the off-the-shelf one integrated into our clinical information system, but rather a stand-alone home-grown solution. Similarly, the best solution for a specialty laboratory might be one which is not integrated into the rest of the clinical information system. Of course, any home-grown elements require an appropriate level of expertise within the pathology department/practice to develop and maintain these solutions. Nonetheless, once one accepts the concept of "degree of customization", we have a spectrum.

Off-the-shelf solutions are faster to deploy. They have very predictable costs, and can generally be included in capital budget purchases. Commercial systems designed with input from multiple sites may have useful features which were developed and tested elsewhere, and may suggest workflow improvements in your own laboratory. Commercial solutions also carry more secure long-term service/support (the department is not at the mercy of the one or two programmers who develop a custom system), although that support can often be quite expensive.

Developing one's own system, or even just elements of a system, requires a lot of resources (money, personnel, expertise) and a lot of time. There is also a higher risk of bugs, since the system will not have been tested at multiple sites, and it can be difficult to budget just how much developing such a system will cost. Finally, long term management and maintenance issues must be considered as well. However, the pay-off is that it is theoretically possible for the system to function exactly as desired, and the system can be adapted as the workflow needs change.

Institutional vs Departmental Management

Regardless of the type of solution developed and/or deployed, it will have to involve some level of on-site management. This may be as simple as adding new users and new physicians to dictionaries, or more complex such as writing reports, or even small customizations. A final philosophical spectrum to consider is how the scope of on-site support will be distributed between the institution and your individual department/practice. This has to be considered on multiple levels, from as mundane as who gets called when a keyboard doesn't work, to something more complex such as the process for requesting a vendor customization.

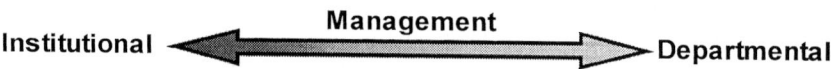

Institutional support allows consolidation and sharing of human resources. A larger support team can generally be maintained, and the level of expertise is often higher, although if your department has a specialty information system solution, the expertise present at the institutional level may not have a significant overlap with the expertise needed to maintain your particular system. When on-site support is centralized at the institutional level, different models for cost recovery exist, from a fully institutional cost center, to fee-for-service, to a fixed monthly fee. When human resources are limited, individual departments may have to compete for institutional support, and anatomic pathology may not be considered a high enough revenue generator to warrant top-level support – for example, a hospital is likely to prioritize fixing a computer in the operating suite area over fixing an anatomic pathology transcriptionist's terminal. Finally, when support is provided by the institution, departments are generally expected to conform with institutional practices and procedures, and there is not infrequently an element of "big-brother-knows-best" imposed on the departments.

In contrast, as each level of support is made more local to the department/practice, the responsiveness of the service is likely to be better, more attentive to the departmental needs, and more aligned with departmental priorities. However, it may be very expensive to maintain the level of expertise needed to provide this local support, and this expense will almost certainly need to be borne by the department. As a significant departmental support unit is built in an environment in which the institution charges departments for institutional level support, the institutional support group may view the departmental support unit as competition for potential revenue, and this can complicate resolution of issues which require institutional cooperation, such as network problems.

Electronic Medical Record Systems

Consider a scenario in which there are three databases containing clinical information on patients: an anatomic pathology system, a laboratory medicine system, and a diagnostic radiology system. Each of these databases contain information on a similar population of patients. Clinicians would rather not have to look up each of their patients three times (once in each system) to review recent clinical data. They would rather have one system in which they can look up the patients and obtain all the information available about each patient from all three primary databases. The advantages to patient care and to clinician efficiency are clear.

With rapidly increasing frequency, clinicians access laboratory data on their patient through a centralized system rather that the individual LIS's, which become feeder systems. In fact, the printed report is more and more being relegated to simply an instrument of documentation for the hard-copy medical record. This has direct implications for what data generators such as pathologists should view as our "product", because in many settings, that product is no longer the printed report. We should maintain some stewardship of our data, even when it is transferred to another information system. More on that later.

The centralization of clinical data from multiple information systems into one electronic location formed a nidus for the subsequent layering of additional information and functionality, and the concept of an electronic medical record was born. The dream of transforming, at some level, that often onerous, difficult to navigate collection of papers known as the patient chart, which is often incomplete and can only be in one place at a time, into a well structured, easily searchable, always complete, and diffusely available electronic form has now been around for some time, although it is still very much in its infancy. This goal goes by several names and abbreviations, among which the more common are electronic medical record (EMR), clinical data repository (CDR), and computerized patient record (CPR). Depending upon the environment, each of these terms not uncommonly carries a somewhat different connotation. EMR often implies a comprehensive system, involving all aspects of the clinical record, and sometimes even suggests a completely paperless system. EMR systems usually include added functionality beyond simple data aggregation such as physician order entry and decision logic. CDR is more commonly used when there is aggregation of data from multiple systems, but it is not necessarily comprehensive, and some functions within the health care environment still remain separate from the central system. CDR also suggests a particular architecture (warehouse) and possible use for research. CPR is perhaps the most generic of the three and therefore carries the fewest implied connotations. In this sense, it is, perhaps, the preferred term to refer to the broader topic of a centralized, electronic collection of patient information. Unfortunately, the computerized patient record shares an acronym with the more commonly understood cardiopulmonary resuscitation.

A Resurgence of Interest

Despite the fact that these terms have been around for so long, very few institutions have successfully managed to put together and routinely use what others would accept as a true computerized patient record. However, there has been a tremendous resurgence of interest in this area over the last few years, and essentially every large healthcare organization is reexamining the issue and developing plans to move toward an EMR of some sort. Why the recent interest? I feel a number of forces have converged to make the timing opportune for movement in this direction.

- Critical mass of computerized systems: Over the past decades, one by one, data storage and health care operations have been switching over to computerized information systems. Enough of these systems now exist for centralization to become feasible and even, perhaps, fiscally sound.
- Shared communication capabilities of these systems: Not only are most of the departments and services within health care organizations now computer based, but these computer systems often have, built in, standardized inter-system communication capabilities (eg HL7

interfaces), enabling automated background data aggregation. More and more standards for encoding, storing, and transmitting medical data are being developed and made available.

- Evolution of the workforce: Familiarity with computers among members of the health care workforce, and a certain level of comfort in using them, has reached a critical mass. Groups in the health care workforce who even ten years ago would never have considered looking up test results in a computer are now quite willing to order tests "on-line". This has come about as a result of slow, incremental steps as individual functions have been, one by one, computerized. This progression has been enabled by an influx of computer savvy individuals into these various health care groups, retraining of existing health care providers, and some degree of replacement/displacement of earlier generations.
- Wireless technology: One of the barriers touted to acceptance of an electronic medical record has been that charts could be moved anywhere, but electronic information could only be entered or accessed from a computer terminal. The increasing number and availability of computer terminals in medical environments, and the introduction of wireless access and data entry are removing these obstacles.
- Demands on health care workers: As health care organizations are increasingly required to provide care for more patients with a reduced workforce, the need for efficient management of these patients has become even more pressing. When properly designed and managed, centralized electronic records can facilitate more efficient patient care.
- Patient safety: Medical errors and patient safety have reached a heightened level of public awareness. Many of the "errors" reported to be threatening the lives of thousands of Americans each year relate to medications. Computerized provider order entry (CPOE) systems can greatly reduce misinterpretations of drug names and/or dosages, and can integrate dosing recommendations, formulary restrictions, and adverse drug interaction warnings.
- Professional society recommendations: Medical professional societies such as the American College of Physicians[1] and the American

---

[1] American College of Physicians. (2003) The paperless medical office: digital technology's potential for the internist. Philadelphia. "The purpose of this paper it to illuminate the great potential going paperless can have on quality of care, patient safety, administrative efficiency and overhead, physician productivity, practice revenue, and profitability." (p 2)

Academy of Family Physicians[2] have formally endorsed the adoption of electronic patient records.

• Greater utility of electronic information: Having information available electronically, especially when structured and coded in a standardized fashion, creates new opportunities for decision support, research, evidence-based treatment selections, and portability.

• External demands: There has been an almost continuous influx of government regulations and requirements being imposed upon the health care industry. Compliance with these regulations can be incredibly expensive. For many institutions, consolidation of information systems is the only financially feasible solution to achieving any level of compliance. In addition, it is likely that the government is not too far away from issuing "recommendations" aimed specifically at moving institutions toward electronic patient records.

Some Issues of Data Centralization Unique to Health Care

Health care data is very unlike any other scientific, commercial, financial, or industrial data collection. The data elements are so individualized, the value and potential impact of inaccuracy is enormous, and the longevity of the usefulness of the data often exceeds that of even the patient. If my credit card number is compromised, or the results of my experiment are accidentally lost, or the accounting records for my business are inaccurate, the consequences can range from inconvenient to life altering, but in each of these cases I can conceive of a remedy to the situation. I cannot, however, get a new medical history.

The nature of medical data introduces some unique issues to be considered when planning or evaluating any data centralization solution. Many of these issues are obvious – the data must be accurate and must be protected from unauthorized access or usage. I do not mean to trivialize these issues, but it doesn't require much insight to realize they are issues. Here, I will try to focus on a couple of less obvious issues which might

---

2 Task force 1 writing group, Graham R, Bagley B, Kilo CM, Spann SJ, Bogdewic SP. (2004) Report of the task force on patient expectations, core values, reintegration, and the new model of family medicine. Annals of Family Medicine 2: S33-S50. "Family physicians will rely increasingly on information systems and electronic health records to provide assessments, checklists, protocols, and access to patient education and clinical support.... Electronic health records with a relational database design and meeting national technical standards are essential." (p S42).

otherwise be overlooked but would compromise the value and perhaps usability of any proposed data centralization solution.

With all of the recent emphasis on patient privacy and protecting health care information from unauthorized access or leakage, an arguably insufficient emphasis has been placed on making this information available to those who appropriately do need to access it. An important element of any security solution is making sure that the information is readily available to those who need it. It is relatively easy to lock information away in a fashion in which it so incredibly protected that it is available to no one, but even the most complete and comprehensive electronic medical record is useless if your physicians cannot get to it when they need to treat you.

In most circumstances, constant availability to the correct people requires knowing, in advance, who will need access to an individual patient's data. In the modern world of multi-physician teams, specialty consultation, and patient mobility, that is no small task. For non-emergent situations, one can require each physician to go through the proper procedures of securing patient permission, submitting forms, and having information access granted, but that is not only time consuming and inefficient but also, in practical terms, poses such a burden that the physician is far more likely to do the best he/she can with limited information. On the other end of the spectrum, an institution may elect to grant all physicians access to information on all patients, but log each access and audit that access, either routinely or at least in the event of suspected inappropriate use or disclosure of the information. Finally, the middle road approach is to restrict access to physicians known in advance to need access, but then offer all other physicians a "break-glass" entry, a metaphor from manual fire alarms. With this functionality, a physician who attempts to access information on a patient for which that physician has not been previously granted access is presented with a warning, but then allowed to proceed. These "break-glass" accesses should routinely be closely monitored for inappropriate activity. However, busy consultative services are likely to have so many "hits" that meaningful auditing may not be practical.

Constant availability of clinical data also has implications for repairing and upgrading a clinical information system. This can be somewhat akin to attempting to repair a ship while at sea. While it would, in general, be a lot easier to dry-dock the ship, do the repair, and then re-launch it, all health care environments in general, including pathology departments, cannot simply close down for more than an hour or two while they repair their systems. Regulatory agencies require that every clinical laboratory have backup contingency plans on how their operations can continue even in the event of a complete information system failure, but few would argue that this is at best a short term solution with compromises to overall quality.

In the typical electronic medical record solution, data from individual departmental system is collected and made available to users through a common interface. The centralized data solutions must be flexible enough to accommodate the broad spectrum of data types which need to be stored. This includes not only numeric results with normal ranges and free-text reports as in anatomic pathology and radiology, but also more complicated results as with electrocardiographic tracings, flow cytometry data, and genetic studies. The system must also be able to respond to the increasing demands for accommodating the diverse data types being produced by new molecular studies, which often generate enormous datasets and require special tools for data display.

Data display is a very important and often overlooked issue in electronic medical records. Individual departments are very familiar with how the data is made available to them and displayed in their own information system, but frequently have no clue how the same data will be displayed once electronically exported to a centralized data solution and then presented to authorized users. The information which physicians derive from clinical data is determined not only by the content of that information by also by how the information is presented and displayed. Factors such as font selection, screen size, data field size, and sometimes even color can limit the amount of "information" which a clinician can obtain, even if the content is

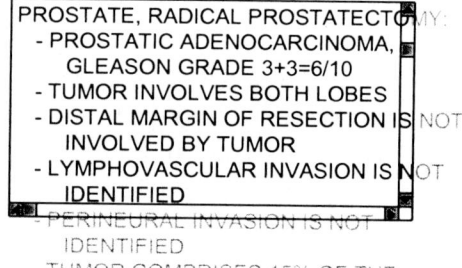

FINAL DIAGNOSIS:

1) PROSTATE, LEFT APEX, BIOPSY:
  - NEGATIVE FOR MALIGNANCY

2) PROSTATE, LEFT MID, BIOPSY:
  - NEGATIVE FOR MALIGNANCY

3) PROSTATE, LEFT BASE, BIOPSY:
  - NEGATIVE FOR MALIGNANCY

4) PROSTATE, RIGHT APEX, BIOPSY:
  - NEGATIVE FOR MALIGNANCY

5) PROSTATE, RIGHT MID, BIOPSY:
  - PROSTATIC ADENOCARCINOMA,
  GLEASON GRADE 3+3=6/10

6) PROSTATE, RIGHT BASE, BIOPSY:
  - NEGATIVE FOR MALIGNANCY

FINAL DIAGNOSIS:

PROSTATE, RADICAL PROSTATECTOMY:
  - PROSTATIC ADENOCARCINOMA,
  GLEASON GRADE 3+3=6/10
  - TUMOR INVOLVES BOTH LOBES
  - DISTAL MARGIN OF RESECTION IS NOT
  INVOLVED BY TUMOR
  - LYMPHOVASCULAR INVASION IS NOT
  IDENTIFIED
  - PERINEURAL INVASION IS NOT
  IDENTIFIED
  - TUMOR COMPRISES 15% OF THE
  PROSTATE

Figure 6-5: The size of the display field for anatomic pathology data can affect how that data is interpreted. Electronic medical record systems often allocate limited screen space to the display of test results. For anatomic pathology reports, this can result in key diagnostic information lying outside of the display area. Clinicians who do not scroll vertically (left example) or horizontally (right example) can misread and misinterpret the results reported.

fully present. Particular attention needs to be paid to the location of comments or addenda which might significantly alter the interpretation of the data. Anatomic pathology reports are generally free text, and therefore simply stored and displayed as text, but even this can be problematic if the display field size is small and the user has to scroll to see all of the text (Figure 6-5). Vertical scrolling is not as problematic, since most users are likely to be used to that from having visited a number of web pages, but horizontal scrolling can be very problematic, both because not all users will think of that, and because key words like "not" can easily "disappear" off the right side of the display margin.

Another issue which should be considered early in the design process is the tremendous potential value of the information stored in electronic medical record systems for clinical research and the advancement of medicine. Although this may not be part of the initial intent of the system, and some have even been deployed specifically with the thought that the system would not be made available for research purposes, the incredible value of the information will not long escape the notice of members of the institution at all levels, and forces will mount to find some mechanism to tap into and leverage that value.

Models for "Centralized" Data Storage and Access

Whether one calls it an electronic medical record system, a computerized patient record, or a clinical data repository, the practical need for some centralized data storage solution is easy to understand. Two basic architectures exist for satisfying this need (Figure 6-6).

In the first, the data is actually aggregated into one physical location or database. This is known as the true "data repository", or "data warehouse" model. I should mention here that, for some individuals, the term "warehouse" carries a more specific meaning. In addition to implying a higher degree of comprehensiveness, the term "warehouse" may suggest specific rules for data management. In some contexts, its use is restricted to instances in which all transactions are catalogued into a centralized storage, from which no data is ever erased or removed. Any modification of the data involves flagging the old data as obsolete and adding the new data, usually with a link to the data it is "replacing". All data changes and entries are logged based on when they occurred and who did the modification. Because of the extensive audit trails included in this very specific use of the term "warehouse", it is possible to "return" the warehouse to the state it was in at any point in time. This warehouse model is often too cumbersome for health care environments, in which there is usually no need to return to a particular point in the past. When I use the term "warehouse", I am not using the term

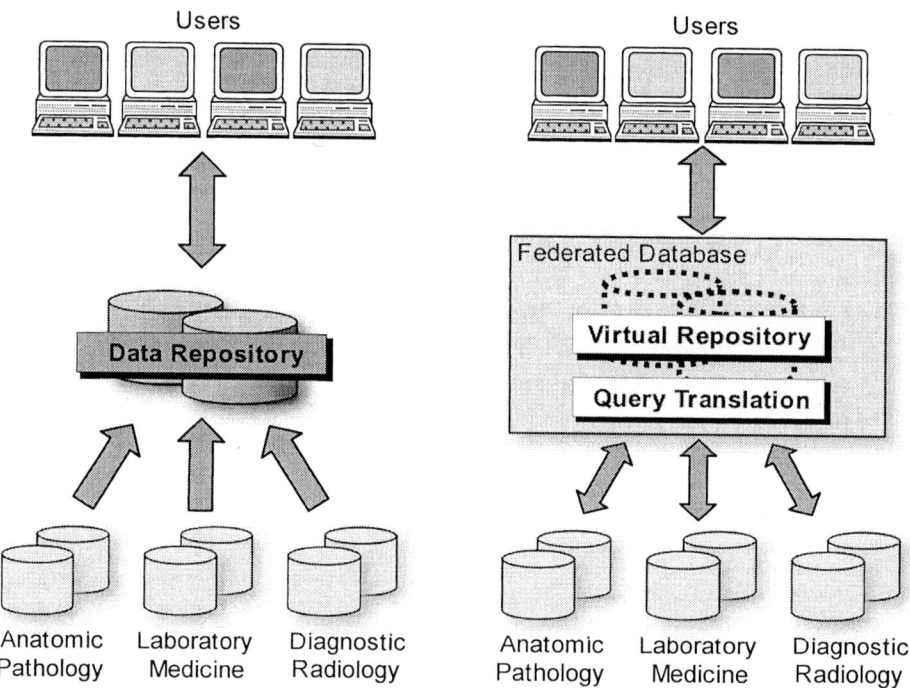

Users   Users

Federated Database

Virtual Repository

Query Translation

Data Repository

Anatomic   Laboratory   Diagnostic   Anatomic   Laboratory   Diagnostic
Pathology   Medicine   Radiology   Pathology   Medicine   Radiology

Figure 6-6: Data Repositories and Federations. In the data repository model, data is collected from multiple primary systems into one central database. Users access information from this central repository. In the data federation model, a virtual repository is created. The data remains only in the primary systems, but because of the virtual repository, the data appears to the user to have been aggregated into a single system. Requests for information are actually executed against the primary systems.

so restrictively in this discussion, but simply refer to a single database into which data from multiple other databases is "deposited". This can be done "real time", in which additions to the source databases are almost immediately reflected in the repository, or on a regularly scheduled basis, like once or twice a day, but most commonly occur on a "triggered" basis, in which an event in the source application, such as the signout of a surgical pathology specimen, triggers the transfer of the data to the repository. Modifications of the data in the source database eventually also result in modifications to the repository copy.

With a central data repository, the structure of the data storage does not need to be the same as in the source database. This allows optimization of the storage for data mining (as opposed to transactional) uses. Frequently, data repositories will have more indices than the source system, in order to better support dynamic queries.

The second model for "centralized" data storage is known as a "data federation." In this model, the data is not collected into a central database, but rather remains only in the source databases. A "virtual" data repository is created, in which the federation engine knows the data models for each of the source databases, including the scope of the data stored, the names for each of the entities and their attributes, and the organizational structure within the database. When the user submits a query to the "virtual database", the federation engine determines which source database actually contains the data being sought. It then translates the query into an appropriate structure for the source database, retrieves the data from that database's database-management-system, and then returns it to the user. If the submitted query requires data from multiple source databases, the federation engine submits appropriate queries to each, collects the results from each, and then performs whatever additional processing is needed to produce the final result set, which is then returned to the user.

Federated databases offer some definite advantages over the traditional repository approach. All of the data obtained is "up-to-the-minute", since there is no transfer of the data at discrete points in time to the central repository. Therefore, there is no risk of a user getting an "old" copy of the data. Each source database maintains the data in a "native" environment, so there are no issues related to data conversion errors or component data loss resulting from trying to store data in a structure not specifically designed to hold that data. For example, a surgical pathology report typically consists of a clinical history, a gross description, a final diagnosis, and perhaps a microscopic description. In the anatomic pathology information system, these fields will be stored separately and are separately identifiable and searchable. When the report is transferred into a central repository, will it be stored as individual fields, one large report, or even as simply a picture of the report which is no longer searchable at all? Data federations allow access to the greatest level of data granularity represented in the source systems. Finally, political issues associated with data ownership are less of a concern with a federated database model, since there is no copy of the data created in another location. The "owners" of the source databases retain ownership of their data, and they can "remove" their data from the federation at any time simply by disconnecting their system from the query translation engine.

Of course, federated databases have some disadvantages as well. In addition to the obvious technical complexity of setting up the query translation, requiring special capabilities not only in the federation engine but also in each of the source database systems, there are some practical concerns as well. The "up-to-the-minute" access to data is not necessarily a good thing, because the source database may hold data which its owners do not want released for general viewing. For example, the anatomic pathology database may hold the "working" version of the diagnosis of a case which is still being evaluated, but as the pathologist for that case, I would not want the diagnosis released outside of the pathology department until I had signed out the case. This logic might exist in the anatomic pathology information system application, but would have to be reproduced in either the application used to access to data federation or in the query translation used to get the data from the anatomic pathology system in order to prevent the data from being prematurely released.

The data federation model dictates that when users perform a search for data, they are not accessing a copy of the data in a secondary database but rather the primary copy in each production source database. Each query to the virtual repository will draw upon database management resources in each of the source databases, and thereby degrade the performance of the clinical information systems in each of the source departments. An inappropriate search run at an inopportune time could potentially cripple multiple institutional production systems.

One of the greatest problems encountered with respect to data aggregations by either model is how to handle inconsistencies between data in different source databases. Every user of any clinical information system has had the experience of stumbling across data which is not accurate. After all, at some point, the data was entered by a person at a keyboard, and no person is infallible (some less-so than others). For example, consider an instance in which the same patient (correctly identified by medical record number) has a date of birth of "Jan 1, 1960" in the anatomic pathology database, but a date of birth of "Jan 1, 1961" in the diagnostic radiology database. In the data federation model, a query arrives to obtain the date of birth for that patient. How does the query translation engine address this? Because it knows the data model for all the connected databases, it knows that that information is available in all three data sources. Does it always get the data from the sources in a particular order? If so, that would draw unfairly upon the resources of one of the connected databases. Does it randomly choose which data source it will use? If so, the same query run two successive times might return different results. Does it poll all three sources and use the value which occurs the most frequently? The issue of data inconsistency has to be addressed whether one is using the federated database model or the data repository model. The only difference is that the repository model allows the centralized database to detect the inconsistency in advance, flag it for resolution, and allow the intervention of a person (database curator) to investigate and resolve the conflict. In the federated database model, the inconsistency needs to be dealt with on-the-fly, and the inconsistency is unlikely to ever be corrected because the individuals in charge of the federation are unlikely to have authorization to edit/change the data in the source systems.

With both "centralized" database models, a special application allows the users to access the data in the repository (real or virtual). The user list does not have to bear any particular relationship with the users able to directly access any of the source systems. Therefore, transcriptionists in the anatomic pathology department have access to the data in the anatomic pathology database via the pathology clinical information system application, but do not need access to all of the data made available through the "electronic medical record". In contrast, treating clinicians can have access to all of the information on the patients through the centralized repository, without requiring individual access to the source databases. The centralization of access to all of the clinical data creates an opportunity for centralization of access control and auditing of user access. Rather than each department having to keep track of who is allowed to access data on which patients, and to log all of those accesses, a centralized data storage allows all of those accesses to be controlled/monitored at one entry point.

Most of the access to a centralized data repository will be "read-only", and all of the issues discussed in the previous section with respect to data display apply to either data storage model. However, the models differ dramatically with respect to the implications of allowing data edits. In the true repository model, data edits affect only the copy seen by users of the repository, but do not affect the data in the source systems. This creates an opportunity to manually curate the data, resolving any inconsistencies, but those manual edits can at any point be overwritten by incoming data from the source system, which presumably would still have the bad data. With a data federation, any modifications to the data could directly affect a source database, correcting the bad data at the source and eliminating concern for subsequent overwriting of the corrected data. However, this is generally not allowed in a data federation model, since the administrators of the source databases are unlikely to release update control of their source data to a centralized group who may not fully appreciate the implications of such data alterations. In addition, for data present in multiple source systems, the virtual repository model is supposed to present this data as a single data element, and therefore it is unclear how any modifications to redundant data should be distributed to the source databases.

Obstacles to the Adoption of an Electronic Medical Record System

Some form of centralized data storage and access within an institution has obvious advantages. These advantages would be even greater if that centralized electronic version of the patient's chart could be transportable from institution to institution, or even available globally, creating the concept of a "Universal Electronic Medical Record". Yet, despite the advantages this could have for patient care, and the almost universal agreement among clinicians that this would be a good thing, few institutions have been successful at deploying an effective solution even within their own doors, and inter-institutional solutions have, for the most part, been experimental and limited. What are the obstacles? Many are unique to individual institutions, and are beyond the scope of this discussion. However, I would like to briefly mention a few issues which seem to come up at multiple institutions. This is not intended to represent a complete coverage of the topic, and indeed several consulting firms derive the bulk of their livelihood exploring and discussing this dilemma.

Economics

It is largely touted that computerized patient records will yield vast savings in total health care expenditures. This is based on the fact that it has been estimated that between 20 and 50% of diagnostic laboratory tests and procedures are performed needlessly simply because the results of previous test or a complete medical history is not available to the treating physician at the time the new tests are ordered.

I do not pretend to be an economist or a financial analyst. Nonetheless, I am familiar with the concept of supply-and-demand upon which most business are based, and I know enough about the health care environment to realize that it operates under a completely different set of rules. In the standard supply-and-demand model, providers of a product or service price their service based on how many consumers want it, and how many other places they can get it. If I charge too much, consumers will get it elsewhere, and I will go out of business. If I don't charge enough, I can't make enough income to pay all my expenses, and I will go out of business. A good business plan involves balancing these forces, and the consumers ultimately dictate whether or not I have the right balance. Health care doesn't work that way. In addition to providing a service which everyone wants and hopes they will never need, the entities which provide the services are so disconnected from the entities which set the fees for those services. The individuals receiving the services, the patients, generally have little to no say over whom they can receive those services from, since these decisions are often pre-made based on the health care plan which happens to be provided by the individual's employer.

So what is the point of my meanderings on the economics of health care? Well, there is a similar disconnect with respect to the funding for electronic medical records. To develop and deploy any sort of electronic medical record system is expensive, both in terms of up front capitalization costs as well as ongoing support and maintenance costs. As there is no external funding source for this activity, and since it cannot be charged back to patients, health care institutions, specifically their administrations, are being asked to foot this bill. However, the primary benefits of an EMR will be realized by the patients and those paying for their care, and not only do the health care providers not see any short term benefits, there are also likely to be short term losses, beyond the cost of the EMR systems themselves. Sure, there are likely to be some long term improvements in patient care, and a long term greater convenience for the medical staff (once the new system is in place and everyone learns how to use it), but an EMR will not attract new patients, will not increase payments to hospitals, and is unlikely to shorten patient stays. Having a patient's medical record electronic and consolidated in one location will make it easier to transfer that information to another institution, should that patient decide to seek care elsewhere, but that is not something hospitals are particularly eager to make easier until they can be on the receiving end of this information transfer. In short, there is little incentive for administrations of health care providing institutions to make this information system investment. In addition, this possible expenditure is being proposed in the wake of two other large, recent, expensive, un-funded electronic information systems projects, namely the "Y2K" hype and more recently HIPAA (Health Insurance Portability and Accountability Act) compliance. The latter of these is mandated by law, and is costing larger health care institutions literally millions of dollars in real money and manpower allocations.

For completeness, I should point out that there are some health care delivery systems in which this separation of payers and providers does not exist. With the Veterans Health Administration system, for example, the Federal government funds the hospitals providing health care as well as pays for the care delivered. In such a closed system, the increased provider costs of implementing a computerized patient record can be offset by savings in the cost for the care provided. A similar closed system exists for large health maintenance organizations like Kaiser Permanente. In fact, in both of those cases, deployment and adoption of EMR systems is already well underway.

Vendor Choice

There are literally only a handful of players on the vendor list for institutional level electronic medical record systems. Most of these vendors market enterprise solutions for health care organizations, and for those institutions who have already committed their future to the longevity of a particular vendor by adopting an institution-wide enterprise solution, the next step to a clinical data repository or electronic medical record is a relatively small one. For others, however, especially those who have held to the "best-of-breed" approach to meeting their information system needs, there is tremendous uncertainty about which vendors to consider in selection of an electronic medical record system. Recent years has seen the rise and fall of many "IT" organizations, including some in health care, and bankruptcy, buyouts, and mergers are all too common in this marketplace. One of the greatest barriers to moving toward an electronic medical record solution, in addition to the cost, is the concern about choosing the wrong vendor, which, millions of dollars later might not even be around long enough to see the system go live. As medical records are so critical to the operation of any health care provider, the concern over resting the future prosperity of the entire organization on the success of a largely untested information system solution is certainly not trivial. This market is also very resistant to new players entering the field, since hospitals are even more reluctant to go with a new kid on the block.

Adding to the uncertainty over vendor selection is uncertainty about the future role of the government in this process. HIPAA has clearly demonstrated that the government is quite willing to impose rather specific constraints, formats, and coding system choices on health care organizations for the storage and exchange of electronic patient information. Their justification, all along, has been to improve the portability of that information. The only way to truly assure that portability is to dictate specific standards for the electronic storage of all patient data. Will these standards be simply at the level of data storage, or will the government dictate a particular application which compliant health care organizations will be expected to use? Uncertainty over what "next-step" the government might make has caused health care administrations to pause, waiting for all the rules to come into play before prematurely going with a solution which may not be as compatible with new regulations as an alternative vendor's solution.

Universal Patient Identifier

In August of 1996, congress passed the Health Insurance Portability and Accountability Act, otherwise known as HIPAA. More information on this act is included in Chapter 12 on External Regulations. However, among the components listed in the section entitled "Administrative Simplification" was a requirement to create a universal patient identifier system, also known as the unique patient identifier and the National Health Identifier for Individuals (NHII). While the other components of HIPAA have moved forward, no progress has been made toward establishing a system for identifying the same patient across health care institutions and health care insurance companies. In fact, in September, 1997, the National Committee on Vital and Health Statistics formally recommended to the Department of Health and Human Services that "we believe it would be unwise and premature to proceed to select and implement such an identifier in the absence of legislation to assure the confidentiality of individually identifiable health information and to preserve an individual's right to privacy"[3]

It is generally believed that an unique, universal identifier for patients is an essential element in achieving the administrative simplification "promised" by HIPAA. In addition to reducing administrative costs across the entire health care system, it would improve patient care, since accurately identifying an individual and their medical history at the time of provision of care is essential to the quality of the care. Especially in the growing environment of patient mobility throughout the health care systems of the country, and the involvement of numerous specialty consultants, there are significant costs and risks associated with lost data, repeat testing, and incomplete treatment histories. The advantages are clear to anyone in the health care field, and in recognition of this, Great Britain has recently adopted a nationwide universal patient identifier system.

However, the culture in the United States is different. Privacy is of utmost concern to the American culture, and many believe that any unique identifier for individuals represents a threat to that privacy. For some, that privacy threat outweighs any benefits which might be derived from the identifier, such as improved health care and decreased administrative costs. In the absence of a universal identifier, only the patient would have access to all of their identifiers across institutions, and therefore elements of the patient's medical history could only be linked together with involvement of the patient in the process. For those acknowledging the advantages of a universal identifier within the health care system, controversy exists as to whether or not use/linkage of this identifier outside of health care should be allowed. Proponents argue that the greatest public benefit would be derived if health care records could, for example, be linked to police accident reports, allowing investigation of the costs and benefits of passive restraints and airbags, or to environmental exposure records. Opponents fear that even if a universal patient identifier exists and is kept secure, linkage to less secure identifiers would compromise patient privacy.

For the time being, the lack of a universal patient identifier represents a barrier to integration of health information across institutions. However, it

---

[3] Letter to Donna Shalala, Secretary of the Department of Health and Human Services, from Don Detmer, MD, Chair of the National Committee on Vital and Health Statistics, dated September 9, 1997.

also represents a barrier within an institution. Although we would like the believe that a patient's institutional medical record number (MRN) is sufficient to serve the purpose of a unique identifier within the institution, the fidelity of management of these numbers varies significantly from institution to institution. Many patients have two or more medical record numbers, even within the same institution, either because their initial MRN could not be identified when the second was assigned, or because the institution represents a fusion of two formerly independent organizations who could not agree on a unifying mechanism for patient identification. There is no way to reliably link data from prior to the assignment of an institutional medical record number (as is seen with referrals from other treatment environments), and even after assignment of an MRN, data obtained during outpatient visits is not always reliably linked to the patient's record. A universal patient identifier system would externalize identifier assignments to a centralized, hopefully well run agency. Duplicate identifier assignments would be less common, since fewer people will be empowered to do the assigning, and since identifiers will have been pre-assigned to all patients prior to any encounter with the health care system (except, of course, new births).

Mention should be made of the proposal to use the social security number (SSN) as the universal patient identifier. When originally established in 1935, the SSN identified an account number, not an individual. However, in 1943, an executive order from President Roosevelt required Federal agencies to use the SSN for any new record systems, and it was subsequently adopted for military identification, federal employee identification, and taxpayer identification. Although the Privacy Act of 1974 placed some requirements for the protection of SSNs when used for Federal purposes, there are few restrictions on the use of this number by private organizations, other than the individual's right to refuse to provide their SSN as an identifier except for government related activities.

Arguments in favor of using the social security number as the universal patient identifier include the fact that, for many health care institutions, it is already the patient identifier, making it a *de facto* standard. Most individuals already have a SSN, and a system already exists to administer the assignment of this number, greatly reducing the time and cost needed to adopts this number as the patient identifier.

However, not all individuals have SSNs, and a system would have to be established to provide SSNs for newborns and non-citizens receiving health care in the United States. Medicare's use of the SSN was done in an unfortunate way, since the Medicare identifier consists of the SSN of the wage earner on whom the benefits are based, with an appended letter designating the relationship of the patient to that individual. As a result, many couples essentially share the same SSN, and similar sharing occurs within immigrant families to which only one SSN was assigned.

An important privacy concern about using the social security number as the universal patient identifier is that many record keeping systems which already use the SSN are not sufficiently secure to protect this number, and it is "too late" to retrospectively secure these systems. Using the SSN would also promote linkage of patient health information with non-health information, further compromising patient privacy.

The future of the universal patient identifier is still very much unclear. The progressive merging of health maintenance organizations into large health care provider conglomerates with their own unique patient identifier may make many of the arguments against a universal identifier moot.

Anatomic Pathology Outreach Services: A unique EMR Problem

The preceding discussion has been somewhat generic and although applicable to anatomic pathology information systems, is not unique to them. However, many anatomic pathology practices evaluate material not only from their housing institution but also from private physician offices and referral material from other institutions. This "outreach" practice has been made possible by the fact that specimens can travel more readily and further distances than patients are likely to be willing to travel. In addition, with increasing specialization within anatomic pathology, a greater catchment area is needed to provide a sufficient specimen volume to support the increasing number of specialists required to provide the highest level of service. Finally, the income generated from outreach practices has been directly responsible for the continued solvency of a number of pathology departments and groups.

In the absence of a universal patient identifier, most health care institutions developing a centralized data repository have based patient identification on their institutional medical record number. Unfortunately, the very nature of an outreach practice means that many of the patients from whom the pathology department receives specimens will not have an institutional medical record number, or at least it will not be known to the pathology department. This means pathology clinical information systems must use their own identifiers for patients, as well as being able to store the institutional medical record numbers for these same patients should specimens be later received from their hosting institution.

The storage of non-institutional patients in a pathology information system creates unique problems in an environment where an electronic medical record system or clinical data repository exists and therefore data is being exchanged electronically. Although not insurmountable, these problems need to be addressed. Does the pathology information system have the ability to filter which results it sends to the institutional data repository? If not, what will the repository do when it receives a specimen on a patient without a medical record number? What should happen if the pathology information system has an institutional medical record number for the patient, but receives a specimen as outreach material rather than through an encounter with that institution? Should that result be provided to the institution with the goal of a more complete medical record, or does this constitute a privacy violation? Many of these issues relate to electronic interfaces between a pathology information system and institutional record systems, and will be discussed in more detail in Chapter 10 on electronic interfaces.

Chapter 7

EVALUATING ANATOMIC PATHOLOGY INFORMATION SYSTEMS

Whether your department/practice has decided to buy a new clinical information system, or you already have one and you are considering activating some new features, or you are trying to defend your selection of a system against your institution's attempt to "persuade" you into adopting their enterprise solution, you need to approach evaluation of your information system in an organized and methodical way.

This chapter will present a useful framework for evaluating features of a clinical information system, and then apply this framework to a number of common and some state-of-the-art features of anatomic pathology information systems. Before embarking on this journey, however, I would like to put forth a couple of underlying, guiding principles.

General Principles

Workflow

Workflow. Workflow. The single most important element to consider when evaluating a clinical information system for your practice is, you guessed it, workflow. Unfortunately, this can be one of the most easily overlooked, and sometimes even difficult to evaluate characteristic of any information system. One can get so absorbed in what the system can and can't do (the features) that it can be easy to forget to pay much attention to how the system does things – not at a technical level, but at an operational level. Features will come and go (mostly come), but the underlying workflow of the system is so fundamental to the system design that it is unlikely to change significantly over time.

Your practice already has a particular workflow. That probably did not arise by accident, nor as a random selection. Although it may have started out with a somewhat arbitrary choice, years of operation in your particular environment, with your particular staff, have resulted in subtle modifications and fine tuning to a workflow which meshes best with your practice environment. An information system with a different concept of workflow can really muck things up.

So what types of things do I mean by workflow? If your practice handles consult specimens differently than routine surgical specimens, does the information system allow you to do that? Does the system require you to enter certain information at the time of accessioning which you do not have available to you at that time? Does the information system require each specimen to be associated with an encounter, and if so, are all of your specimens really associated with encounters? Do the slides come out of the histology lab in numerical accession order, or grouped by pathologist, or by resident, or by priority? Does your histology lab handle special stains on a rolling basis or in batches, and how does that compare to what the information system does? How and where do you print your final reports? Do you send just one copy of the report to the primary ordering clinician, or a copy to each clinician? Do you send an extra copy to the physician's practice, or perhaps only the extra copy with no copy going directly to the clinician(s)?

The best way to get a sense of the workflow of the system is, during a demonstration, take a couple of real specimens (for privacy reasons, change the name, etc.), and put them through the system, start to finish, to see how the system assists you or hinders you at each step in your process. Although this is a far cry from putting a hundred or more specimens a day through the same mock processing, it will be a start, and should uncover any major inconsistencies.

Finally, don't immediately assume that if the computer system does something in a different way than you have always done it, that your way is necessarily better and the system's way is necessarily worse. Assuming you are evaluating a commercially available system which is in use in other pathology practices, the "system-way" may represent an aggregation of workflow analyses from a number of different practices, and there may be definite merit to considering that alternative. However, the choice should be yours, not forced upon you. Any concerns you have about the workflow should be taken up not only with the vendor (who, surprisingly, will assure you that their system will work well in your environment) but with other pathology practices who are using that vendor's system. Ideally, you should contact references which have a similar volume and specimen mix to your own. If they report having had problems initially with a particular element of the workflow, discuss how they have solved the problem, and consider whether or not that solution is viable in your environment.

One last comment: vendors may offer to "work with you" to develop a software solution to whatever particular concerns you might have about their product's capabilities. This is a great opportunity, and one which will not appear again once the contract is signed, so consider it, but ONLY if there are individuals in your department/practice with the time, inclination, and skills necessary to develop a reasonable collaboration.

Traps and Pitfalls

Every journey has obstacles, and they are easier to avoid if you know about them ahead of time. Many of them might be unique to your particular practice environment, and you are likely to be already familiar with these. However, as a general rule, it is important to remain practical and realistic when evaluating a clinical information system's capabilities and in predicting what impact it will have on your practice.

Understand and distinguish between what is not possible, what is possible but not practical, what is practical but not appropriate, and what is actually a good idea. This is probably best be defined as managing expectations. I have observed that one of the best ways of detecting unrealistic expectations is to pay attention for certain key phrases which often foretell impending disappointment, either for your implementation team or for the planners and/or users of the information system. A few examples of these are presented here.

"This is really cool! We must be able to use this for something."

Technology can be quite enticing, and even clinical information system developers, the presumed "experts" in the field, can be lured into integrating technology which not only adds no real value to the system but also increases its complexity and cost. Just because a technology exists doesn't mean it has to be used. (For example, I would put whole slide imaging into this category, at least for the present time.) Incorporation of new technology should be driven by need and by the ability of the technology to meet that need in a way which is not currently being done as effectively. Sometimes, my attempts to counter the "really cool" position by requiring a definition of need results in "this fulfills a need which we didn't even know we had." First of all, if you didn't know you had the need, it wasn't a very significant need. Rather, it is usually a case of "I've invented a need to justify purchasing a technology which I want to have". Adopting a technology which is not needed is a good way to spend a lot of money and resources on something that few people will ever use.

"It only takes a few seconds to capture a digital image. We should be doing this for every case."

This is one of those top-down extrapolations generally made by someone who lacks a solid grasp on what actually occurs on the "front lines" of a pathology practice day after day. This would fall into the "just because something is possible doesn't necessarily mean it is practical" category. Unlike the previous category which I might paraphrase as "we don't even want to go there", this category would be more along the lines of "we want to be able to go there, but only when warranted." Technology must fit will into the workflow, meaning it must be integrated in such a way as to not disrupt that workflow, or users will resist it and become surprisingly incapable of learning how to use it. However, having advanced capabilities available for appropriate "special cases" can be a source of moral inspiration and genuine support for the information system.

"Special stains are ordered through the computer system. The fact that they aren't out until 4PM is an IT problem."

There is a fine line between enabling the workflow and determining the workflow. Left unchecked, information technology groups can rapidly become a dumping ground for every workflow or administrative problem in the department. This is especially true if your practice happens to have a particularly competent IT group. Nearly everything an anatomic pathology practice does with specimens involves the information system. That does not mean that every solution, especially workflow solutions, should be driven by the IT group. Certainly IT groups should be part of the team involved in the solution development, especially in offering assessments as to what the computer system is capable and incapable of doing, but workflow decisions should be made by directors and managers of the appropriate units within the department, and then IT can be involved in helping to deliver those decisions.

I know I typed 88304, but I meant 88305. 88304 is never used for a GI biopsy. Why can't the computer catch that?

First of all, information systems, even the most advanced ones, cannot read the mind of the user. Although they can be made to recognize valid from invalid entries (for example, the computer can prevent you from entering an ICD-9 code where it expects a CPT code), it cannot easily recognize right from wrong when both are valid entries. Data entry constraints are logic which is applied to entries to try to determine if they can't possibly be right (e.g., "date of autopsy" prior to "date of death"). Some computer systems allow a degree of flexibility in defining such constraints, although their definition often requires a more sophisticated IT group. These entry constrains may be institution specific. It is important to remember that if created, these constraints will function all of the time, not just when you want them to. They can also be very labor intensive to maintain, especially if they are buried deep within the system. Good documentation is necessary as these constraints can be forgotten with time, and may become the hidden cause for "unusual system behavior" later when the needs of the institution change. Although data entry constraints can be very helpful in improving the integrity and accuracy of the data in the clinical information system, care should be taken in deciding when to use them and when to simply try to employ better trained data entry personnel.

Evaluating Informatics Activities in Anatomic Pathology

Categories of Information Technology Impact

It is easy to be overwhelmed by features of clinical information systems. In fact, their appeal to users, or potential users, is exactly what vendors use to sell their products. However, it is important to look past the glamour of high technology features and make a realistic assessment of whether or not any particular feature actually solves a problem or whether incorporating it into your workflow will create more problems than it solves.

To assist in this evaluation, it is useful to have a framework to assess how your practice of pathology is impacted by a particular information system feature or other technology component. I refer to this framework as "Categories of Information Technology Impact", the components of which are shown in Table 7-1. This system is by no means the only such system, but it is generic enough as to serve at least as a starting point for developing an evaluation framework more customized to your practice.

Using the impact categories defined in Table 7-1 as a framework, a number of features which have been integrated into anatomic pathology information systems or otherwise incorporated into the practice of anatomic pathology as non-integrated entities will be discussed. The list is not intended to be exhaustive but rather representative. Some straight-forward examples will be provided first, followed by more controversial discussions. Each feature or functionality will be "graded" in each of the framework categories. If that category is felt to be significantly impacted by the feature, its icon will be shown as a solid square. If a feature has only minor or indirect impact on a particular category, that category's icon will be shown hollow. Remember, the details of the analysis may vary based on your particular practice environment, and are provided here to raise some of the more important issues and to serve as a sample analysis.

Table 7-1: Categories of Information Technology Impact.

PM	***Practice Management:*** These are functionalities which expedite the day-to-day processing of specimens. They are internal to the pathology department/practice, and their benefits only indirectly extend beyond the pathology department.
PC	***Patient care:*** These are functionalities which directly improve the quality of care delivered to patients, either by improving the accuracy of the diagnoses themselves or by improving how those diagnoses are communicated to the clinicians.
E	***Education:*** These features advance the education of pathologists, other physicians, students, residents, patients, and/or the general public.
R	***Research:*** These functionalities assist in the advancement of our understanding of diseases by making material from and/or information about patients available in an appropriate way for medical and/or outcomes research.
M	***Marketing:*** Perhaps the most controversial category in this list, information technology is being increasingly drawn upon to market pathology services. The fascination of the general public with technology has led to the sometimes inaccurate perception that "high tech" means "better." In an increasingly competitive market where, unfortunately, the accuracy of the diagnosis is taken for granted and therefore not a marketable commodity, flashy presentation, even when devoid of any true added value, does have perceived value and therefore becomes important for any pathology practice hoping to remain in business.

Traditional Features of Anatomic Pathology Information Systems

Specimen Tracking   **PM** **PC**

The use of information systems to track the status of specimens from accession through signout, reporting, and billing, has greatly facilitated the workflow in pathology departments, has decreased the amount of paper used, and helps prevent the loss of specimen reports. This concept is fundamental to the design of essentially every anatomic pathology clinical information system. However, other than by increasing the efficiency of specimen processing, this has had no direct impact outside of pathology departments. Its impact has been primarily on Practice Management, with some secondary benefits to patient care from improved efficiency.

Histology Block/Stain Ordering/Tracking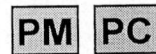

A number of histology related procedures have been greatly facilitated by computerized information systems. The ability to categorize blocks, compile logs, and print slide labels improves the efficiency and throughput in the histology lab. Additionally, electronic stain ordering allows this to be done from any computer terminal in the department, and the system can automatically batch these to accommodate the workflow in the laboratory. The primary impact here, again, is on Practice Management.

Identification of Previous Specimens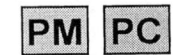

When a specimen is received for evaluation, it is not uncommonly accompanied by an all too brief clinical history. Knowing the clinical history of the patient can be crucial to the appropriate interpretation. Much of that clinical history can be deduced from the previous material received from that patient, and thus it is important to know what previous material from that patient was processed in the department, and where the corresponding slides are located. Computerized information systems which contain historical information facilitate this process by eliminating the need for pathology personnel to manually index and record each case, and manually search that index (often in the form of a card file) as each new specimen arrives. However, more importantly, the automatic identification of previous material from a patient can redirect the pathologist's interpretation of the case and as such directly improves patient care. Electronic identification of previous specimens also allows that material to be more easily retrieved for direct comparison with the current case.

Computer Assisted Report Distribution   **PM PC**

Patients often have multiple physicians involved in their care, each of which may wish to receive a copy of the report, in addition to the chart copy, which should go either to the patient's floor or to medical records. Information systems can easily generate the additional needed physician copies, addressed to those physicians. The "chart" copies can be batched and printed sorted by the inpatient unit for delivery to the patient floors, or by medical record number for delivery to medical records. If there is an active admission-discharge-transfer interface feeding the pathology information system, that interface will update the patient location as the patient moves from unit to unit in the hospital. This allows the inpatient chart copy to be sent to the floor the patient is currently on, not the floor the patient was on when the specimen was received. Computer assisted report distribution is primarily a practice management issue, but the greater efficiency of communication with all the appropriate physicians can yield some direct benefits to patient care.

Automated Reporting (Faxing, Web Access)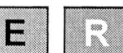

This functionality has similar benefits to those described above for computer assisted report distribution, but allow even more rapid communication of results. In theory, faster should be better, especially for outreach material where the clients are off-site. In a very real sense, however, these theoretical benefits are often not realized. High volume clients often do not want their fax machines tied up during the day and prefer to have the faxes arrive at night. This dilutes the benefits of "rapid communication". In addition, faxing at night carries the risks associated with machines running out of paper or jamming. Web reporting, if done well, can be an effective solution, but requires that the submitting physician look up the results, an "active" process which, if not done, raises issues about who is responsible for the failed communication of the diagnosis. Web interfaces are also not easy to maintain. The increased internal costs and management issues associated with keeping either a web or a fax delivery systems functional, as well as appropriately addressing security concerns, often offset any benefits otherwise realized. Nonetheless, the "high technology" nature of automated faxing and web based reporting can be leveraged as a marketing strategy.

Case Identification by Diagnosis

One of the greatest advantages of electronic data is the ability to rapidly search that data in ways which would not be practical to conduct manually. This is a "new" capability, made possible by electronic information systems. Case identification by any number of criteria other than patient name is routinely used to select cases for research projects, for teaching conferences, and quality control issues. Both the educational and research benefits of this capability have been tremendous, but this functionality has had little effect on practice management or patient care. Various approaches to case identification by diagnosis, including coding systems and natural language searching, are discussed in greater detail in Chapter 11.

Electronic Signout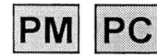

Traditional signout of reports includes multiple iterations of the pathologist making changes on written reports which are then returned to the transcriptionist for retyping. This can delay the signout of some reports for days. Electronic signout (ESO) allows the pathologists to make minor changes themselves, and immediately release the report to clinicians, avoiding at the least the last printing/manual signing cycle. ESO also allows the pathologist to have the "last word" with respect to other data elements such as fee codes and ICD-9 codes. The disadvantage is that the pathologist takes on some editing responsibilities in the computer system, but the advantages to both practice management and patient care generally outweigh these disadvantages.

Management Reporting Tools   PM   E R

In addition to patient reports, most clinical information systems can also produce management reports, addressing such things as counts of specimens received, turnaround times, staff workloads, etc.   These reporting capabilities often require special skills to customize reports, and additional administration to regulate who can run what reports.   Since some of these reports may draw significantly on system resources, slowing down the performance of the overall system, inappropriate use of management reports during busy work times can hinder overall productivity.   This can be particularly problematic because the individuals running the reports may have minimal knowledge or appreciation for the effect they are having on overall system performance.   It would be important to investigate whether or not the system has the capability of scheduling reports to be run at off-hours or at a lower priority.   It is also important to know if all of the data in the system is available for reports, or only some pre-selected fields.   However, when the necessary skills to write good reports are available within the department, and management reporting is appropriately managed, the data generated can be used to improve elements of practice management, as well as being useful for education and research.

Newer "High Technology" Features

Electronic Interfaces: Input (ADT Streams)   PM PC

Clinical information systems which support incoming electronic data transfer from other hospital systems, in particular admission/discharge/ transfer (ADT) data from the patient management system, can save entry time and improve the accuracy of patient information in the pathology information system.   It can also facilitate billing for services.   Updates with new patient locations allow reports to be sent to where the patient is at the time the report is signed out rather than where the patient was at the time the specimen was received.   The main disadvantage of input interfaces is the risk of introduction of duplicate patients or even erroneous information into the pathology information system.   This can be a real problem, since the relatively large number of people manually manipulating the data in hospital patient management systems can lead to significant quality control concerns.   Management and correction of these duplicates and errors within the pathology information system can be very time consuming.   Nonetheless, input interfaces can improve practice management and affect patient care by increasing the accuracy of information and report delivery. ADT interfaces are discussed in more detail in Chapter 10.

Electronic Interfaces: Output (Results; Billing) PM PC   M

At most institutions, not all clinicians have direct access to the anatomic pathology information system. Results interfaces allow reports to appear, essentially instantaneously, in other information systems to which the clinicians do have access. This improves patient care, but also assists in practice management. Limiting access to the pathology information system to individuals within the pathology department is also a way of off-loading some of the HIPAA privacy issues to the administrators of a different information system. If any of those other systems are available to clinicians outside the institution, this capability can be used to market anatomic pathology services to community physicians. Automated electronic billing is also an essential element of any modern pathology practice. It is difficult to imagine any manual billing process being as rapid and accurate as electronic billing. With billing interfaces, billing batch files can be created and sent to contracted billing services either within or outside of the institutions. Billing routes can be different for different patient types (inpatients vs outreach), and most information systems will allow separate handling of the technical and professional components of the billing.

Gross Photographs: PM PC E

Digital Image Acquisition   Photomicrographs: E

Most pathology practices routinely photograph complex specimens for documentation. Emulsion-based photographs need to be developed, labeled, sorted, and stored. With the increasing availability of digital imaging hardware, many practices are beginning to capture digital images as an alternative to traditional "silver photography". When used for gross photography, the advantages of digital imaging are numerous. (A more detailed discussion of the advantages of digital imaging can be found in Chapter 8.) Digital images are more difficult to lose, can be immediately viewed, and can be directly labeled with the case number, facilitating accurate cataloguing. These features, plus the elimination of film developing, slide storage and photograph duplication services, enhance practice management. The greater availability of these images, potentially allowing attending pathologists to routinely see, during signout, what specimens grossed in by others looked like, can improve patient care. Finally, the pool of images combined with a searchable clinical database can provide an incredibly valuable teaching resource.

The advantages of digital imaging for microscopic image acquisition are less impressive. This is mainly due to the fact that most pathology practices do not routinely take photomicrographs of all cases, and thus doing so digitally represents additional work. It is quite disruptive to try to do this during routine signouts. Nonetheless, if this is done, and if the microscopic images captured are stored in a retrievable way, this can add to the value of an educational resource. The faster turn-around time on digital images (essentially zero for digital presentations) can facilitate preparation of educational conferences, increasing their value.

Incorporating Digital Images   Gross Photographs: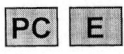
      into Reports   Photomicrographs:

Digital image acquisition can be done as a stand alone solution, or as an integrated component of the clinical information system. When integrated into the information system, digital imaging may offer the ability to incorporate images into patient reports. There is an increased workload associated with identifying the images to include, but these images do improve the appearance of the reports, which serves a marketing role. Including gross images in reports can allow clinicians to correlate the gross pathology with their clinical assessments, serving an educational role. The advantages to patient care are less obvious, but can be real. Consider the scenario of a patient who notices blood in his urine. He has no other symptoms. His physician performs an imaging study identifying a mass in the kidney. The patient is referred to a surgeon, and undergoes a nephrectomy. The pathology shows a renal cell carcinoma, with renal vein extension. From the patient's point of view, the fact that he has cancer can be difficult to accept. After all, he has never felt sick. Having a gross photograph of his kidney in the pathology report can be a useful tool for clinician interaction with this patient, and in helping him accept the possible need for further therapy.

I am far less enthusiastic about the value of incorporating digital photomicrographs into patient reports. Few clinicians, and even fewer patients are likely to be able to interpret such images. Those clinicians who feel they can interpret these images may attempt to second guess the pathologist's interpretation. This can be very problematic. The pathologist makes his/her diagnosis based on evaluation of the entire specimen. In general, the diagnosis cannot be captured in one or two images. Including one or two images in the report suggests that perhaps it can, and that the images should be able to stand by themselves as justification of the diagnosis. This is clearly not practical, and may introduce issues of trust between the pathologist and the treating clinician. Therefore, I feel that including photomicrographs in reports, except under special circumstances, can have a negative effect. Nonetheless, this practice definitely can have a marketing impact.

Checklist-based/Itemized/Synoptic Reporting   PM PC E R

Traditionally, final diagnoses have been entered into anatomic pathology information systems simply as text, using tools comparable to a word processor.   Depending upon the capabilities of the system, but more importantly on conventions adopted by the department, that text can be entered with or without structure, such as a bulleted list of elements of the diagnosis. Nonetheless, this text, from the computer's perspective, is simply text, and although the formatting may make the text easier for the clinician to read and digest, it does not, in general, make the information more searchable or otherwise analyzable.

For specific types of cases, most notably malignant neoplasms, it is important to be sure that the report contains certain information about the specimen to allow for proper staging and planning of subsequent therapy. This includes things like tumor size, extent, involvement of other structures, status of margins, lymph node involvement, etc.   Recently, the results of some molecular studies have been added to this list. The details needed for any given specimen are determined by the site and the diagnosis.

Many pathologists simply include the relevant information in their free text report, knowing from experience what key pieces of data need to be included. In some practice settings, written "checklists" are used with pre-determined text phrases – essentially multiple choice questions (for example, "The left ovary is involved" or "The left ovary is not involved") from which the pathologist selects the appropriate choice. A transcriptionist then enters this information into the final diagnosis field as text, either by typing the text from the checklist or, if the computer system has the capabilities, entering a code phrase which is translated into the corresponding text and inserted into the final diagnosis field. These checklists can both assure the completeness of the report, and can have the added advantage of creating reports with a consistent structure and terminology so that the clinicians learn where to look for particular data elements. In practice settings where a number of pathologists may be signing out these cases, checklist-based reporting can promote a consistent look and terminology across pathologists. A variety of terms have been used to describe this practice: checklist-based reporting, structured reporting, itemized reporting, and synoptic reporting are just a few of the terms used.

Anatomic pathology information systems are beginning to incorporate the ability to load these checklists into the information system, and then allow users to select from the elements of the list "on-line" via checkboxes, radio buttons, and drop-down lists. Different vendors have implemented "checklists" in different ways. The ability to customize the language, alter the options available, and define new categories are important features to investigate when evaluating these systems. Also, the ability to edit the text which is generated as a result of the checklist selections is another important variable to explore. However, the various implementations of this feature break down into two fundamentally different categories, based on whether or not the details of the elements chosen are preserved beyond their use to generate the text. In the "transient data" model, the choices are used to generate a structured final diagnosis text, and once the text is generated the individual choices are discarded. With this type of solution, the generated text is usually editable, allowing the pathologist to fine tune the language for the particulars of the case at hand. However, there is no way to return to the checklist which originally generated the text, with the original choices selected. If one wants to go back to the checklist, one has to start over, re-enter the choices, and regenerate the resulting text. In the other model, or "data persistent" model, the individual choices are stored, and one can return to the checklist for the case with the original choices all pre-selected. In this model, the resulting text is often not editable, because changing the text would break the link to the underlying synoptic data elements, introducing potential inconsistencies between the stored data elements and the associated text. The storage of the individual choices, however, does potentially enable searching based on these granular criteria and also makes possible the generation of aggregate analyses.

Checklist-based reporting is an understandably controversial issue in pathology, and there are many arguments for both positive and negative effects on patient care. No one would argue with the fact that pathology reports should contain all of the diagnostic and prognostic information about the specimen needed to enable subsequent clinical care. In settings in which this is not being done, the greater completeness of the report which can be promoted by checklist-based reporting can improve clinical care. There is also probably some gain in the ease with which clinicians can obtain data from a consistently structured report. Why the resistance then? Unfortunately, some of the resistance may be political. Use of checklist-based reporting, or at least deciding which data elements "must be included" in reports, is not being driven by pathologists, and in some instances is not being driven by sound data that each of the elements is an independent predictor of prognosis. Rather, many of the required elements seem to be driven by a desire to accumulate data which may prove to be useful at some point in the future, thereby relegating pathologists to the role of data collection technicians for someone else's possible future research study. Some of the elements even seem to be driven by a lack of trust: the need to include all three dimensions of all tumor sizes when there is not a single staging system which uses anything more than the single largest dimension suggests that pathologists might not be able to determine which is the largest dimension. These issues aside, however, purely checklist-based reporting limits the language selection options available to pathologists, and I consider this a bad thing. Pathologists do not simply put names on tissue. We recognize that many lesions do not fit nicely into pre-determined, well-defined bins, but rather represent points on a spectrum, or more accurately points on multiple spectra, and we choose our language to communicate the subtle differences expressed by an individual case. Although standardization of categories and language may yield better understanding of these diseases in the long term by facilitating data aggregation across institutions, there may be short term harm to individual patients from an inability to tailor a diagnosis specifically to that patient's lesion. Also eroded by standardized checklists is the role of the pathologist as a clinical consultant rather than simply a data gatherer.

Another argument which has been raised about checklist-based reporting, or any form of reporting in which the diagnosis text represents pre-written text chosen from some bank of phrases, is the risk of accidentally selecting the wrong item from the list due to an aberrant click or a typographical error in entering a code number. When actually typing text, typographical errors are detected because the text typed is misspelled or simply does not make sense. With pre-formulated text, the text will always make sense and be correctly spelled, even if the wrong text is accidentally chosen. Therefore, this type of error can be very difficult to detect.

There are also philosophical issues related to template based documentation in medicine in general. Templates are certainly not unique to pathology, and in fact are routinely used for operative notes, procedure notes, and sometimes even admission notes. The documentation requirements in medicine have become so onerous that a physician can easily spend half of their professional time dealing with paperwork and documentation rather than providing direct clinical care. Pre-formed templates for "routine" procedures can greatly facilitate this process, providing fully detailed descriptions with all of the necessary elements documented. However, when the templates become very long and include details such as volume of blood loss and number of surgical ties, one has to begin to question the degree to which they reflect what really happened. Among my other responsibilities, I also head the autopsy service. Many have expressed surprise at the fact that I have not "computerized" the gross descriptions for the autopsies. Granted, a template does exist which is used by the residents, but this template is printed and is used as a dictation guide. All of our gross descriptions are still dictated. When a resident dictates what they found at autopsy, it is "just as easy" for them to dictate what they really saw as opposed to what the template says. However, if the template were preloaded into the computer system, it then becomes much more work to edit this to reflect reality rather than simply accept the default descriptions.

One can argue that it is not the responsibility of the programmer or informaticist to worry about how technology is used. After all, templates have facilitated the documentation process. However, they have also enabled bad behavior, and this trade-off needs to always be kept in mind when any type of templates are used.

Nonetheless, templates have already worked their way into anatomic pathology. A good example of this is microscopic descriptions included in reports for high volume biopsy services such as dermatopathology. I have seen many instances where the paragraph-long microscopic description of one patient's basal cell carcinoma is identical, word for word, to that of another patient. We all know that no two basal cell carcinomas look exactly alike. Nonetheless, the microscopic descriptions provided are generic enough that they remain accurate, despite differences in the histologic appearance of the actual slides. This then raises the question about the value of the microscopic description at all, especially since it is generic and really has no relationship to the specific case. After all, I can look up a generic description of a basal cell carcinoma in any pathology text book.

Most of the current electronic implementations of checklist-based reporting for the final diagnosis in anatomic pathology are far more granular than is being used in other fields of medicine, and the pathologist must make multiple selections, each corresponding to only one line in the diagnosis, to build the entire final diagnosis. Therefore, at least for now, many of the philosophical issues mentioned above do not pertain to the current discussion of checklist-based reporting. However, when evaluating a checklist-based reporting solution, be sure to consider the flexibility of the system and the ability to avoid the inclusion of inappropriate pre-canned phrases in the resulting reports.

Implementing a checklist-based reporting system will clearly impact practice management, and the specifics of the system selected as well as the workflow in the environment in which it is implemented will determine whether this impact is positive or negative. Issues to consider include maintenance of the checklists, ability to merge elements from more than one checklist for complex specimens, and determining who will select the choices from the checklist. Educational benefits may be gleaned for junior pathologists in that a checklist will guide them in generating more complete reports. Finally, if the solution chosen employs a data persistent model, the research capabilities of the information system will be greatly enhanced by being able to identify cases based on more specific criteria in the diagnosis. For example, if properly set up, it could be possible to identify not simply "all breast cancer cases", but rather "all node-negative breast tumors greater than 2 cm in greatest diameter."

Outreach Support   **PM** **PC**   **M**

Many pathology practices, in addition to meeting the pathology needs of the institution in which they are housed, also receive, process, and diagnose specimens from outside sources such as physician offices or independent surgical centers. This is not a particularly high technology feature, but it is relatively new in the anatomic pathology information system world. Pathology information systems vary in their ability to accommodate the processing of specimens received from physicians outside of the main institution served by the pathology practice. At the very least, needed capabilities would include specifying the client from which the specimen was received, the ability to enter patients who may not have a medical record number, and whatever control is needing over the reporting routes to meet the needs of the clients. Other features might include separate number wheels, distinct report formats, customizable interfaces, or even secure web-based reporting for the referring physicians. If billing is done from the pathology information system, attention needs to be paid not only to billing routes but also where patient insurance information is stored. For example, some information systems store insurance information linked not directly to the patient or specimen but rather to the encounter with the healthcare system. Outreach specimens are not likely to have an associated encounter in the pathology information system. If one wants to enter patient insurance information and this has to be linked to an encounter, then an encounter will have to be "invented" in order to have a place to put the insurance information.

In addition to the above practice-management issues, patient care can be improved by including outreach material in the same pathology information system used to store inpatient information. Since the majority of the outreach material usually comes from the same local vicinity, many of these patients eventually may be seen, for definitive therapy, at your primary institution. Having the initial biopsy material, or the old resection material, available at the time a new specimen is evaluated can improve patient care. If it is the initial biopsy which is seen as an outreach specimen, this may obviate the need to review that material when the patient is referred to the primary institution. The possibility of making information about outreach material available to other hospital systems, thereby enhancing the institution's electronic record for the patient, can also be explored, although appropriate privacy issues need to be considered. Finally if the pathology information system has a web-based reporting module, results can be more rapidly delivered to the submitting physicians, accelerating subsequent follow-up. Any of these capabilities, especially a web-portal, can be used to market the pathology practice to potential outreach clients.

Multi-Site/Lab Support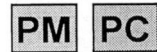

Not only are some pathology operations providing support for multiple clinical environments, but with increasing frequency the same pathology information system is being used to support multiple pathology laboratories, such as at affiliated institutions. As with outreach support, this can promote better patient care by making available to the pathologists the diagnoses and perhaps even glass slides from prior specimens seen at either institution and processed by either laboratory. If some of the same faculty staff both institutions, it may not be necessary to review material on patients who are treated at both locations. However, effectively managing two laboratories within the same pathology information system requires special capabilities of that system, and few commercially available pathology information systems offer all those capabilities. At the least, different specimen number wheels are needed, as are multiple medical record numbers, and multiple histology laboratories, with the ability to direct workflow to specific laboratories. Less commonly seen is the ability to filter staff based on practice location (some pathologists may practice at both institutions, but most will practice at only one or the other, and should be filtered from selection lists at inappropriate institutions). Laboratory tests should be filtered by laboratory, since not all tests (for example, some immunostains or molecular testing) will be offered by all of the laboratories. These more advanced capabilities can certainly improve practice management.

Bar Code Technology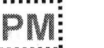

So many people have purported the remarkable, almost magical solutions which bar-coding is supposed to provide that I have become convinced that very few people actually know how bar codes work. Contrary to popular belief, scanning a bar code does not "make the computer do something" unless the computer is set up, in advance, to respond to a particular bar code at a particular point in the application in a particular way. ALL of the functionality related to bar code solutions is in the application which reads the bar codes; none of the functionality is in the bar code itself.

One dimensional bar codes are relatively easy to implement and use. Two options exist for creating them. Some dedicated label printers have bar-code character sets built into them. With the appropriately installed drivers and configuration, one simply send the text-string one wants expressed as a bar code, and then the printer does the rest. This limits the choices of printers significantly. Alternatively, one can use special bar-code fonts, installed on the system just like any other font. Since there is generally not a one-to-one relationship of characters in the string to bar-code representation (due to the presence of start and stop characters and interlacing), one generally has to "process" the text-string first with a string manipulation function. The string to be expressed as a bar code is processed by this function (so some programming capability is required) and then the result is printed with a bar-code font. For reading of bar codes, a variety of scanners (both wands and guns) can be used. "Keyboard wedges" in the form of either software or hardware allow bar codes to be used with any application by transmitting the scanned information as if it were simply typed on the keyboard, only fast and accurately. The application, however, has to be in the proper state, with the focus on the correct field, for the bar-code reading to have the desired effect. To use barcodes in this way, the bar code itself cannot contain any special characters needing further interpretation beyond what one would type on a keyboard.

Popular one dimensional bar codes include Code 25I, which is purely numeric, Codabar (used for UPC symbols), Code 39 (numbers, symbols, and upper case letters) and Code 128 (all 128 standard ASCII characters). However, one dimensional barcodes cannot store a lot of information in a small amount of space (Figure 7-1). In anatomic pathology, the most common use is to store the specimen accession number. This requires both letters and numbers, so Code 39 or Code 128 would be required. Since all bar codes require a "quiet-space" flanking the barcode of at least an eighth of an inch, and start and stop characters, Code 39 can accommodate only 3 coded characters on a one inch wide label when printed at 300 dpi, or 6-8 characters when printed at 600 dpi. This is not enough for an accession number. Code 128 is higher density, and can support 4 characters on a one inch wide label at 300 dpi or 8-10 characters at 600 dpi, so the latter scenario is just enough to be useful. Shrinking the bar code to try to fit more characters increases the frequency of unreadable bar codes.

Two dimensional bar codes can store much more data. The DataMatrix

Figure 7-1: One dimensional vs two dimensional bar codes. Two of the more popular bar code formats are shown. The one dimensional code is Code 128, which can accommodate all of the lower 128 standard ASCII characters, but anything more than a few characters takes up a significant amount of space. PDF417 is a more compact two dimensional bar code format which can store more data in a small amount of space, and do so with internal redundancy, but requires more complex programming both to make and to use.

code can store 20 ASCII characters in a square inch, and the PDF417 code can store up to 1000 characters in a square inch (Figure 7-1). However, these bar codes are more difficult to produce, requiring more sophisticated programming and more expensive printers and readers. Also, when reading two dimensional bar codes, the data needs to be manipulated before being sent to the application, so more advanced "keyboard wedges" are required. One advantage that some two dimensional bar codes offer is the ability to encode the information with internal redundancy, so that they remain readable even if part of the code is damaged.

With the right application, and the correct workflow, bar codes can improve practice management. Unfortunately, this is not typically the case. The greatest impact can be achieved if specimens arrive pre-bar-coded, and the pathology information system can interpret the information encoded, but this is also an uncommon situation except in environments with enterprise information system solutions. It is unlikely that bar codes, in anatomic pathology, improve patient care, since there are multiple other mechanisms available to confirm the identity of a specimen, block, or slide. There are no educational or research impacts of bar coding. Use of bar codes could be used to suggest increased workflow sophistication and therefore have minor marketing benefits.

Speech Recognition Technology　　　　　PM　　　　　　　　　M

Very few technologies have received as much "Oh, we must be able to benefit by using this" than speech recognition. (Note that many inaccurately refer to this technology as "voice recognition". Voice recognition software determines who is talking, based on the tonal characteristics of the voice. Speech recognition software attempts to determine what you are saying.) In reality, however, except in specific limited applications, speech recognition has not yet come of age in pathology.

Two basic types of speech recognition technology exists. In the first, speech is used to select an item from a relatively limited list of possible phrases. Since the software only has to figure out which of the items is the closest to what you said, accuracy is pretty good, even without any pre-training of the system to your particular voice. This type of system is used in many automated telephone trees such as those used by airlines to provide automated flight status information. To use this type of speech recognition in an anatomic pathology information system, the software has to be specifically redesigned to continually present the user with a list of choices. Much of the benefits gained come from building and implementing the lists of choices, and the speech recognition part can even be replaced with pointing and clicking with similar yields in productivity.

The second type of speech recognition is known as "free speech" recognition, in which the user can say anything, and it is typed. This technology usually requires pre-training the system to your voice, and requires a pre-loaded vocabulary. The choice of the vocabulary is very important in determining the accuracy with which the software will be able to figure out what you are saying. The software needs to know the words you are likely to use, and in what context you are likely to use them. As you speak each word, the software ranks its possible choices for what word you have said based on comparisons between what you have said, your voice profile, and its internal vocabulary. It then adjusts that ranking based on what word came before what you said, and what word comes next. This contextual editing allows the software to distinguish between homonyms like "to", "too", and "two".

Unless restricted to a specific subset of specimens, and therefore to a more limited vocabulary, the accuracy of speech recognition is not truly sufficient to facilitate workflow. Even 95% accuracy means that one out of every twenty words will be wrong and someone will have to fix it. If your transcriptionists are responsible for the editing, consider that editing is a very different skill set than typing, and some of the fastest transcriptionists can make very slow editors: it may be more time consuming to edit an existing document than to simply type a new version. Alternatively, the burden of editing can be placed on the resident or attending pathologist, further increasing their workload. In general, if a practice implements speech recognition with the aim of decreasing the number of employees doing transcription, and is successful at achieving a decrease, it is often because other employees are now doing that work. You may also have to hire a new information technology person to keep the speech recognition system running. Finally, consider that the transcriptionists are likely to be doing more than just typing. To the extent that they are responsible for other tasks like tracking down missing information, resolving discrepancies, creating procedures to store the diagnostic text, or managing workflow, someone else will have to perform these tasks if transcriptionist positions are eliminated.

Speech recognition software is operating system specific, and usually requires specific hardware in the computer to process the audio input. Therefore, it generally will not work with the thin-client solutions discussed in Chapter 6. Also, speech recognition is very processor intensive, so up-to-date hardware is required to use it effectively.

For these reasons, speech recognition functionality, as it exists today, provides no significant advancements in any of the categories being evaluated. Yes, it is "high-tech", and anything perceived as high-tech can be used as a marketing tool. With improved accuracy and the newer background recognition engines, more significant benefits may be realized in the future.

Customizability

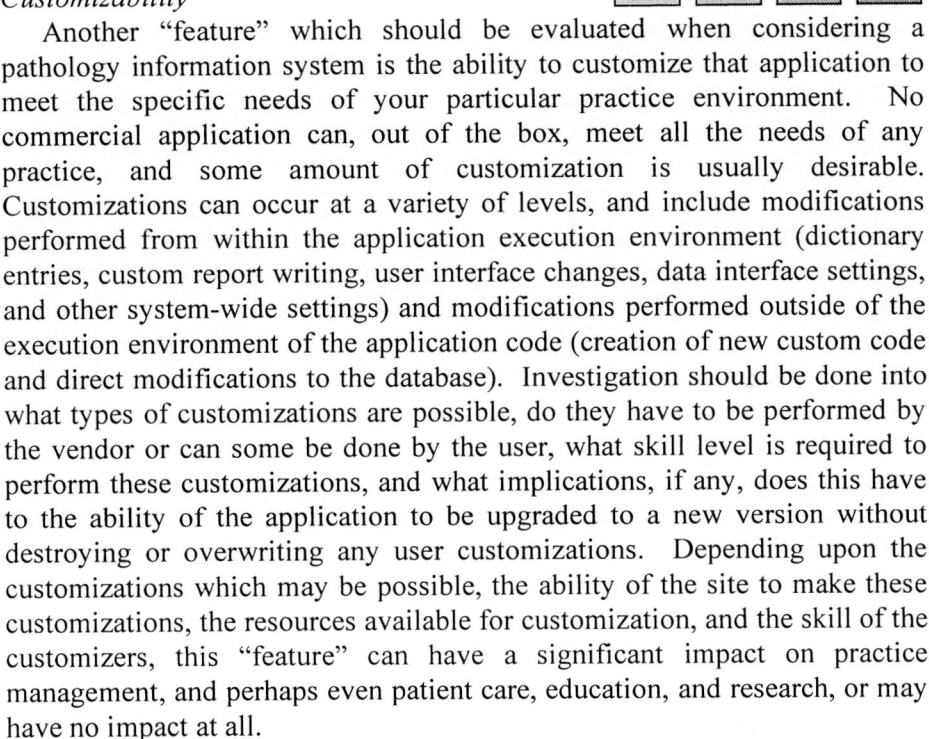

Another "feature" which should be evaluated when considering a pathology information system is the ability to customize that application to meet the specific needs of your particular practice environment. No commercial application can, out of the box, meet all the needs of any practice, and some amount of customization is usually desirable. Customizations can occur at a variety of levels, and include modifications performed from within the application execution environment (dictionary entries, custom report writing, user interface changes, data interface settings, and other system-wide settings) and modifications performed outside of the execution environment of the application code (creation of new custom code and direct modifications to the database). Investigation should be done into what types of customizations are possible, do they have to be performed by the vendor or can some be done by the user, what skill level is required to perform these customizations, and what implications, if any, does this have to the ability of the application to be upgraded to a new version without destroying or overwriting any user customizations. Depending upon the customizations which may be possible, the ability of the site to make these customizations, the resources available for customization, and the skill of the customizers, this "feature" can have a significant impact on practice management, and perhaps even patient care, education, and research, or may have no impact at all.

Informatics Activities Not Integrated into LISs

I include here a couple of informatics activities which are not routinely integrated into commercial anatomic pathology information systems. In many cases, non-integrated informatics solutions can be the best solution for a particular need.

Access to Online Literature Databases

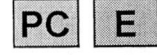

Recent advances in the molecular understanding of diseases and the effect this is having on classification systems is only one of the many diagnostically relevant areas of intense research and publication. Pathologist access to literature databases such as MEDLINE during signout allows quick an easy lookup of relevant recent articles, enabling review of the most recent diagnostic and prognostic criteria which can be specifically evaluated and addressed in the final diagnosis. Relevant references can be sited in the reports, improving their educational value to other clinicians. As such, this functionality serves both an educational function and can improve patient care.

Providing the capability of literature access during signout requires simply having an internet connected computer with a web browser application at the signout location. For some institutions or practices not currently equipped, this can represent a significant initial investment, but is probably well worth the expense, not only for providing this activity, but also because having computers at each signout station enables a number of other informatics activities during signout.

Pathology Web Sites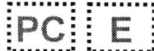

Nearly every major academic pathology department, most commercial pathology labs, and many private pathology practices have web sites. Serving primarily an advertising role, some of these sites also offer educational content, aimed mostly at patients but also at physicians. Initially, having a web-site was a sign of a "high-tech" laboratory, and had great marketing value. Now, however, this has become an expectation, and not having a web-site is often perceived as not being up-to-date, resulting in a negative marketing impact. Informational web sites are relatively easy to create, especially since there is usually initial excitement for the project, and any number of companies will host a web site on their hardware for only a few dollars a month. However, once completed, interest in updating the site fades, and maintenance of the site becomes an issue. A "static" site which is not updated becomes "stale".

Web-based reporting is beginning to surface as an alternative method of report distribution. The potential exists for either physicians or the patients themselves to access test results. This level of functionality is far more difficult to maintain, generally requires in-house hardware and more sophisticated information technology skills, especially with proper attention to security. Many of the security issues associated have not yet been addressed by the legal system. In addition, the psychological costs of having a patient discover, by themselves, perhaps in the middle of the night, that they have a malignancy, when there is no medical personnel available to discuss this with, are difficult to estimate.

Data Recovery from Legacy Information Systems

Much of the historical data at many institutions is trapped in older, legacy information systems, which for any of a number of reasons have fallen into disuse or at least disfavor. As new production systems replace older ones, and since gigabytes of storage can be bought for mere dollars, there remains a desire to keep all the old data "on-line" for continued use, and this almost invariably requires data conversion. Medical data is particularly valuable, not only for the potential treatment value it may still hold, but also for its tremendous research value. As new large scale parallel analysis tools like microarrays become more popular, there is a tremendous need for clean, mineable historical patient information to correlate with tissue analyses and outcomes data. To achieve this effectively, the data needs to be exported from legacy systems and moved into newer architecture databases. Recent more stringent security requirements for the storage of heath-related data, driven by the Health Insurance Portability and Accountability Act (HIPAA) has added increased urgency to moving this data into more sophisticated database systems.

Data conversion from any legacy information systems is a crucial element to investigate when evaluating any new clinical information system. Most pathology information system vendors include a budget in the contract to address data conversion. Make sure it is enough. The cost of this process has a bad habit of growing well beyond initial expectations.

The process of converting the data from legacy systems can be quite problematic. The reasons for this are many fold, but are based predominantly on the fact that data entry constraints are likely to have been relatively loose over the long lifetime of the legacy system. Examples of this would include changing data entry conventions over time (full capital letters vs title case; date only vs date/time), the same field being used for different purposes at different points in time (eg "Source" field initially indicating the clinical unit; then, as an outreach program is implemented, the same field is used to indicate the client), and a change in data types (e.g., switching from a free response field to a dictionary driven field). It is also common to see the appearance of new data fields over time, and the retirement of old fields. Finally, the new information system may require data which was not required on the old system.

The discussion which follows presents some of the issues which should be considered when exploring and budgeting the data conversion process.

Custom Conversion Programming

The vendor for the new information system has undoubtedly dealt with data conversions before, and almost certainly already has programs which will import old data into the new system. That data, however, will have to be in a specific format, and it is generally the responsibility of the pathology practice to get their old data into the correct format. This requires custom conversion software to export the data from the legacy system. It is generally necessary to "massage" the data being exported from the old system so that it can be successfully imported into the new system. There may be sufficient in-house expertise to write export routines from the legacy system, especially if it has been developed and maintained in-house. If not, you may get some assistance from the vendor who sold you the legacy system, if they still exist, but don't expect this to come cheap, since it is not in their best interests to assist you in abandoning their system for a competitor's. Hopefully, they will have some generic routines which will dump the data from the old system in some predetermined format. You will then have to resort to custom programmers to write applications which will convert that data into the format needed for import into the new system. This has to be done with close supervision. The programmers will know how to write programs, but are likely to be unfamiliar with the meaning or significance of the data they are manipulating. A lot of decisions will need to be made by someone with the proper domain knowledge, including such things as appropriate values to use for blank fields, what is the equivalent value in the new system for each data value in the old system, what rules should be used to determine how data needs to be modified or reformatted for the new system, etc. The longer the time frame covered by the legacy system, the more "special cases" will be identified and the greater the needed complexity of the conversion software.

The Conversion Process is Iterative

The data conversion software is never complete until all of the data has been successfully brought into the new system. It is unreasonable to expect a clean separation between the writing of the data conversion software and its use. Therefore, the custom conversion programmer(s) will have to be present during the entire conversion process.

Deficiencies in the conversion software often do not become apparent until the import of the exported data fails. When incomplete or inappropriately formatted data from the legacy system is "stuffed" into the new information system, one of two things can happen. Most commonly, the particular record (usually at the specimen level) is simply rejected. This requires identifying the problem and adjusting the data export/conversion routines to properly reformat the data for import. This reworking of the code can "fix" the problem for one record while simultaneously "breaking" it for others. Numerous iterations are likely to be needed. Alternatively, the incoming record may be accepted and filed into the new information system, but as soon as it is accessed, the new system behaves "unpredictably" because an expected data element is missing or an invalid value is present in one of the fields. "Unpredictable" behavior can, unfortunately, include system failure. If discovered, the solution is to remove the imported record, correct the conversion software, and re-import that record. Unfortunately, these "hidden bombs" within the new system can be difficult to ferret out, and may pop up intermittently for years after the data conversion. Therefore, the "best" errors are the ones that fail up-front. The "worst" errors are the ones that remain silent and hidden.

Accuracy is Paramount

This seems like a silly thing to have to actually state. No pathologist would sleep well at night knowing that some of the converted specimens may have been inappropriately linked to the wrong patients. Even less obvious problems like associating the wrong staff with the specimen can have potential legal implications. Unfortunately, impressing this need on for-hire programmers can be remarkably difficult. Whether it is due to the fact that programmers likely to be available for such a short term project are not particularly good ones, or that programmers are so accustomed to the concept of small "bugs" in programs producing unwanted results, exacting a high level of quality control from programmers should not be taken as a given. Extensive checking of imported records and comparisons against the same specimens in the legacy system is crucial.

Custom Conversion Programming is Expensive

Since conversion programming is very specific to the particular details of the source system, the destination system, and the choices made by the institution over the years as to how to use the source system, very little in the way of pre-written routines can be drawn upon. Most of the conversion programs will have to be written from scratch. This simply takes many hours and lots of testing. Custom programmers can charge anywhere from $80 - $300 per hour, depending upon the skill level required. This cost will be in addition to any contracted expenses with the vendor of the new software system. Adding insult to injury is the knowledge that the programs being produced will likely be used only this one time and then discarded.

An Alternative Approach

For relatively small conversions, on the order of a few thousand records, much of the data conversion might be doable with commercially available desktop database software. These packages are very user friendly, and can allow even the novice computer user to build an effective database. These desktop database applications often have extensive data import tools, which will allow you to import the data extracted from the legacy system. The data can then be directly viewed within the database software by someone familiar with the meaning of the data. Any of a number of views can be created, focusing on a limited set of data elements, to allow scanning for accuracy or needed modifications. Sorting the records by various fields can help identify invalid or missing data values. Calculated fields can be used to check the consistency of data elements. For example, a calculated field could be used to set a flag if the date of signout for a specimen is before the date of accession (which can occur if these are free entry fields in the legacy system). Then, selecting records by that flag can allow examination and correction of these records. Calculated fields can also be used to convert values from the old system into corresponding values for the new system. After all the manipulation has been done, the data can then be exported into a format appropriate for importing into the new information system.

In the pathology department at Yale, we used this approach to successfully convert approximately six thousand morgue records from our legacy system into a custom module in our new pathology information system. The data conversion was accomplished using FileMaker Pro on a Macintosh operating system.

Chapter 8

DIGITAL IMAGING IN ANATOMIC PATHOLOGY

Traditional 35mm photography has been used for decades by anatomic pathologists to document the appearance of specimens and lesions. Whether used primarily for medical legal, educational, or purely archival purposes, a camera and copy stand can be found in essentially every anatomic pathology gross room in the world. Digital imaging has made this documentation process faster, easier, and cheaper. Few pathology practices have not at least begun to consider the transition to digital imaging.

Digital imaging technology has become so much less expensive, compared to when it was first introduced, that even the initial setup costs are comparable to that of traditional photography. The veritable explosion in the availability and affordability of high quality, portable digital cameras has, in part, driven this revolution. Most digital cameras are easy to use, and even individuals who seem to have trouble programming a VCR can take high quality digital images. What can be the greatest barrier, however, to adopting this technology in the clinical setting is understanding the terminology and the features available, and then determining which features are actually desirable. To the uninitiated, understanding the technology, terminology, and elements needed for a viable solution can seem somewhat overwhelming. Much as one should have a framework for evaluating the features of an information system (see Chapter 7), one must be similarly critical in looking at the features of a digital camera, clearly separating what is needed and useful from what is just cool. Also, as will be discussed, the success or failure of a digital imaging solution deployment will depend on a large number of factors other than simply choosing the correct camera. This chapter will introduce digital images, discuss the elements needed for a complete digital imaging solution as well as many of the options available, and then present some very practical suggestions for successful deployment.

Digital Imaging vs. Traditional Photography

As with any new venture, one must have an understanding of what one hopes to attain from embarking on a new technology, as well as realistic expectations formed by an understanding of the limitations of that technology. In the clinical setting, digital imaging has both advantages and disadvantages over traditional photography (Table 8-1).

With digital images, the quality of the image can be immediately assessed at the time the image is "captured". One of the greatest shortcomings of traditional photography is that feeling one is often left with just after taking the picture of "I hope this comes out". We have all had the experience of taking a picture which we feel will be spectacular, and then are disappointed when, a few days later, either for technical reasons (the film didn't load properly or was scratched, the roll of film was lost) or artistic ones (unexpected highlights were present in the image, the background was dirtier than appreciated) the image turns out to be not quite as good as we had hoped. Sometimes, as insurance against this possible disappointment, we take the picture in several different ways, trying different lens apertures

Table 8-1: Digital imaging vs. traditional photography.

Advantages of Digital Imaging	Disadvantages of Digital Imaging
Quality and content of images can be assessed at capture time; no developing delays	Resolution of "usable" images is generally poorer than 35mm photographs; cannot rely on subsequent magnification
Images are immediately available for review by attending pathologist and clinical teams	Acquisition software and procedures vary from manufacturer to manufacturer; can be more difficult to learn
Presentations for clinical conferences can be prepared with much shorter notice	Need to develop an electronic storage system and cataloguing procedures to assure the preservation and availability of the images
Digital images are easily duplicated with 100% fidelity; don't have to take multiple copies	
No film costs; no developing costs	Presentation in non-digitally equipped conference rooms requires converting the digital images to 35mm slides
Images can't be lost (easily); can be directed into long term storage at acquisition, decreasing the risk of misfiling	
Eliminates need for physical storage space for slides, slide tracking procedures, slide developing procedures, slide labeling procedures, and slide retrieval/re-filing procedures	
Images can be accessed from any image capable terminal in the department; no need to request retrieval from storage	

and zoom positions, hoping to decrease the chance of being disappointed. This takes time – often valuable time. With digital imaging, you can view the image immediately. If it is not as anticipated, it is trivial to discard it and try again, or to shoot several and select the one or two best. This rapid availability also has advantages outside of quality assessment. If it is a resident or assistant taking the pictures, the resulting photographs can be immediately available for review by the attending pathologist or members of the clinical team (who invariably show up about an hour after the specimen has been already dissected). Clinical conferences can also be prepared with much shorter notice.

A number of administrative benefits can be achieved by switching to the routine use of digital images. They can't easily be lost, assuming you have a well designed and maintained storage system. Images can be directed into long term storage at the time they are acquired, decreasing the risk of misfiling. They can be duplicated in seconds with 100% fidelity, so there is no longer a need to take multiple copies of each picture (e.g., one for the main file, one for teaching, one for a personal collection). There are no ongoing costs of film or developing, and no costs associated with filing the images, retrieving the images, tracking the slides as they are borrowed, and/or re-filing them. Physical space does not need to be allocated to store them. One of the greatest advantages of digital images is that one can create a storage solution which makes the images far more accessible to everyone in the department/practice. They can be retrievable from anywhere in the department without having to formally request that they be retrieved from storage.

Digital images also have some disadvantages over traditional photography (Table 8-1). The most important of these is that the image quality is not as good as 35mm photography. This is not to say that it is impossible to take a digital image of comparable quality to a traditional photograph, it is simply not practical to do so routinely. This will become more understandable later when image resolution and file size is discussed. However, for the time being, suffice it to say that with digital images, one cannot rely on subsequent magnification to create a close-up view of a particular area. It is important that individuals taking digital photographs realize that they need to take both low magnification and high magnification (zoomed-in) pictures of lesions.

The image quality argument can be taken too far, however. Do not be overly critical. When Yale Pathology first switched to using digital imaging (for the Autopsy service), some of the attendings thought the images were not of sufficient quality since they could not make primary diagnoses just by looking at the images. Although often true, this is not the fault of the technology. The traditional photography which was being replaced was never held to this standard of "diagnosability", and in retrospect these same attendings found they could not make primary diagnoses from just the traditional photographs either.

Each manufacturer's digital cameras work a little bit differently, and as such learning to use digital cameras can be a little more difficult that traditional 35mm cameras. These cameras all come with corresponding software which can be installed on the computer to which images are downloaded, and that software will vary from manufacturer to manufacturer.

Developing an effective storage solution for digital images is essential, and will be discussed in greater detail later. This storage needs to be maintained and backed up on a regular basis. Although it is difficult to "lose" a single digital image, if one is not careful, one can "lose" ALL of the digital images.

One final disadvantage of digital imaging is that, in order to present a case at a conference, the images may have to be converted to a traditional 35mm slides. This takes time, and in the end is far more expensive than simply shooting the 35mm slide in the first place. However, only a small percentage of the images taken have to be converted, and with digital projectors and digital presentations becoming far more common in conference rooms, even this number is dropping essentially to zero.

Basic Digital Imaging Concepts and Terminology

Most technology carries with it a unique terminology. Digital imaging is no exception. When one starts to work with digital images, one needs to understand the terminology. The most important terms are pixel, image resolution, pixel density, and color depth.

In Chapter 3, two different types of digital images were introduced: vector images and pixel-based or bitmapped images. The former is used for diagrams and simple icons. Photograph-like digital images are all pixel-based, and that is the type of image dealt with in this chapter.

Digital Image Specifications

Pixel
The idea that life-like images can be created by placing different colored dots very close together was popularized in the nineteenth century by the impressionistic painter Georges Seurat. (Even traditional 35mm photographs are made up of dots, although for film the dots are very small.) Digital images are simply the electronic extension of a Seurat painting. All digital pictures are made up of "dots". These dots are called pixels (*pik-*

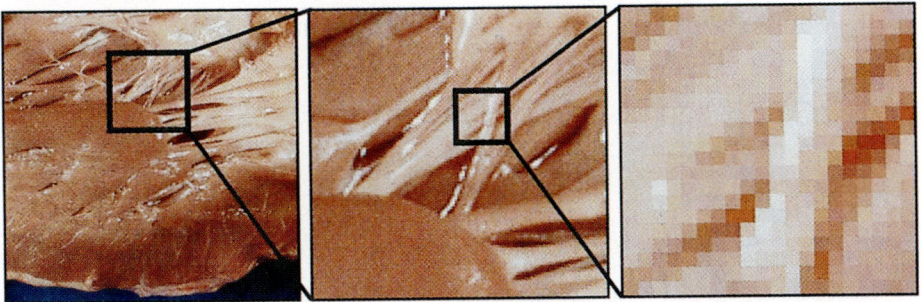

Figure 8-1: Pixels. Digital images are made up of pixels, a collection of square "dots", each of a single color, arranged in a rectangular array.

sells), which is short for "picture element". However, with digital images, unlike a Seurat painting, each dot is exactly the same size, and the dots are arranged in a perfectly rectangular array. The pixels are generally small enough that it is not readily appreciated that the image is composed of dots. However, repeated magnification (Figure 8-1) reveals the "pixilated" nature of these images. The number of pixels comprising an image determines the "resolution" of that image. Each dot (pixel) can be one, and only one color. The range of possible colors is determined by the "color depth" of the image.

Image Resolution (Pixel Resolution)

The term "resolution" is perhaps the most confusing term in digital imaging, not because it is a difficult concept but rather because different people use it to mean different things. Properly speaking, it should be used only to refer to the number of pixels in each dimension (width and height) of the image (Figure 8-2). Thus, typical image resolutions would be 640 x 480 or 1024 x 768. By convention, the horizontal dimension is usually listed first, but this convention is not always followed.

Pixel Density (Image Density; "dots-per-inch")

A digital image, in and of itself, has no actual physical size until it is printed or displayed. Once output, each specific instance of the printed or displayed image has a pixel density (Figure 8-2). This refers to the number of pixels per inch (dots per inch = dpi) AT WHICH A DIGITAL IMAGE IS PRINTED OR DISPLAYED. The value is meaningless unless one is referring to a specific output of the image (either displayed on a screen or printed on paper). Usually, the pixel density is the same in both the horizontal and vertical dimension.

Some people refer to the pixel density as the image resolution. This is unfortunate, since by itself it is a useless term. If someone asks me for a

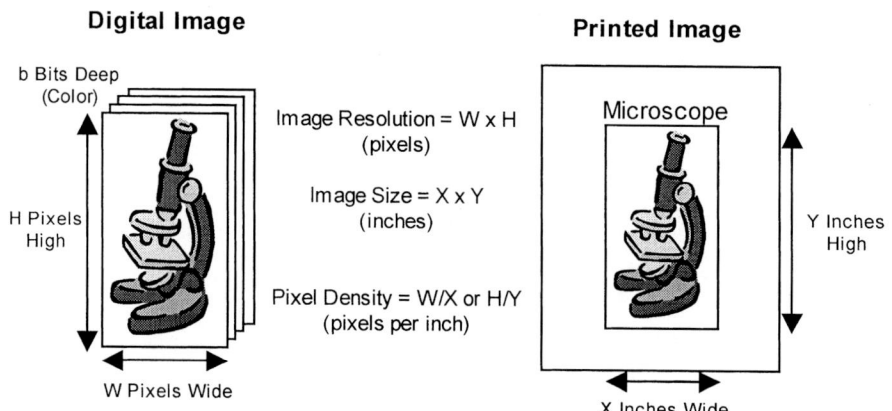

Digital Image   **Printed Image**

b Bits Deep
(Color)

H Pixels
High

Image Resolution = W x H
(pixels)

Image Size = X x Y
(inches)

Pixel Density = W/X or H/Y
(pixels per inch)

Microscope

Y Inches
High

W Pixels Wide

X Inches Wide

Figure 8-2: Pixel resolution and density. Pixel resolution is a property of the digital image itself. In contrast, pixel density is a property of each instance of a printed or displayed image, and is directly (inversely) dependent upon the physical size of the output.

digital image of something, and I ask what resolution they want, they often reply "300 dpi". I still have no idea how many pixels there should be in the image. This is equivalent to asking someone how far they live from where they work, and having them answer "30 miles per hour". If you happen to already know how long it takes them to get to work, then you can figure out the answer to your question, but otherwise you are not really much closer to an answer than you started. Likewise, "300 dpi" does not tell me how many d's I need unless I already know how many i's I have.

This confusion probably comes as a carryover from film photography. 35mm film has a grain density, and it is well known to most photographers that lower ASA film (e.g. 100) has a higher usable grain density than higher ASA film (e.g. 400). Thus, if you are planning to make a large blow-up of the image, you are better off starting with lower ASA film, because the image will be of a higher "resolution". For 35mm film, however, the film size is a constant. Since the usable silver grains in lower ASA film are at a higher density, lower ASA film provides a higher resolution because there are more silver grains devoted to the image. Equating the grain density to resolution works for 35mm film because the film size is a constant. That is not the case for digital images, which have no intrinsic size.

Color Depth (Pixel Depth, "Bit-planes of color")

Each "pixel" in a digital image can have one and only one color. The range of possible colors is determined by how much digital storage space is used to store the color for each pixel. Remember that all digital information is stored as collections of binary data elements called "bits". If an image is stored in "8-bit" color, that means that 8-bits are devoted to store the color information for each pixel. Therefore, 16-bit color allows for a greater range of colors, and 24-bit color for even more.

Digital color information is usually stored using what is referred to as "RGB Color Space" (Figure 8-3). This is based on the principle that all colors can be expressed by a combination of different intensities of Red, Green, and Blue

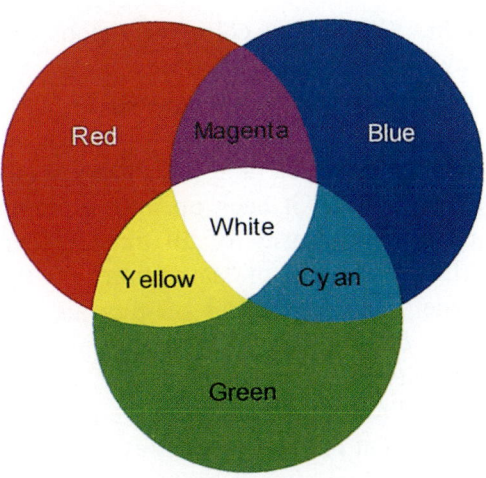

Figure 8-3: RGB color space. All colors can be expressed by combining red, green, and blue light in varying proportions.

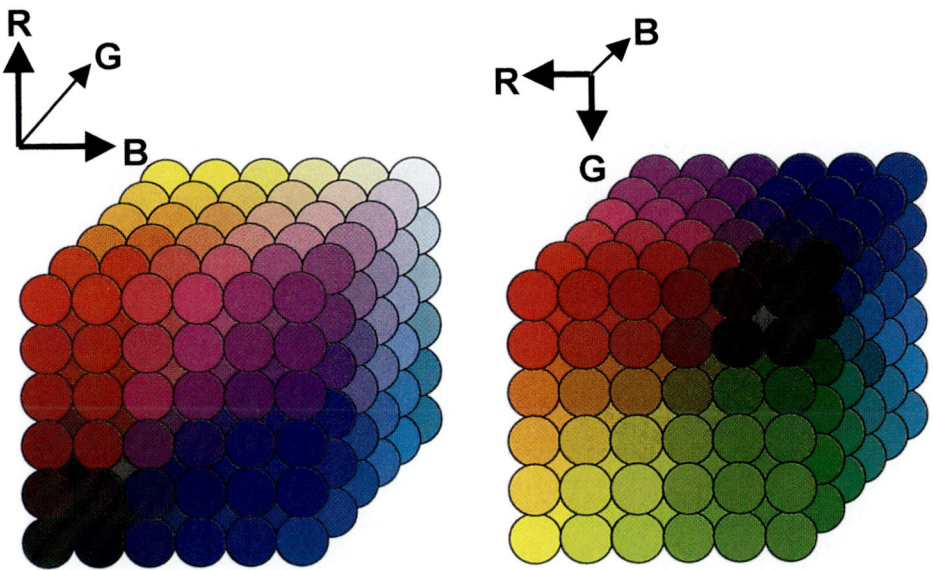

Figure 8-4: All colors can be expressed by mixing different intensities of red, green, and blue light. The cubes shown are the same, simply viewed from a different perspective. The front face of the cube on the left is the same as the top face of the cube on the right. The vector diagrams are drawn such that the intersection of the three arrows represents black (0% of each color), and increasing saturation of each of the three component colors is in the direction indicated.

light. (Projection color televisions operate under this same principle, and have red, green, and blue "guns" aligned to create the projected color image). Bright red is created by using full intensity of red light, and no green or blue light. White is created by using full intensity of red, full intensity of green, and full intensity of blue. (A prism is able to take white light and split it back up into its component colors.) Black is created by using 0% intensity of all three colors. By mixing these three colors at different degrees of "saturation" (0-100% intensity), all other colors can be made. Various shades of gray are created by using equal amounts of all three colors, but at different intensities (e.g., light gray could be 75% intensity of red, green, and blue, whereas dark gray would be 25% intensity of all three colors). Colors are created by mixing red, green, and blue light at different relative intensities (e.g. bright yellow is 100% red, 100% green, and 0% blue; pink is 100% red, 50% green and 50% blue). This mixing of colors is demonstrated in the color cubes shown in Figure 8-4.

In digital images, the color of each pixel is expressed by indicating how much red, how much green, and how much blue it contains. With 24-bit color, 24 bits (three bytes of 8 bits each) is used to determine the color of each pixel. That allow 8 bits (one byte) to be used for each "channel" (red, green, and blue). Since each bit can only be a 0 or a 1, 8 bits of information allow for 2^8=256 possible intensities of red (from 0 to 255 = 100%). 256 possible intensities of red, combined with 256 possible intensities of green and 256 possible intensities of blue create a spectrum of 256 x 256 x 256 = 16,777,216 possible colors, or "millions of colors" (Figure 8-5).

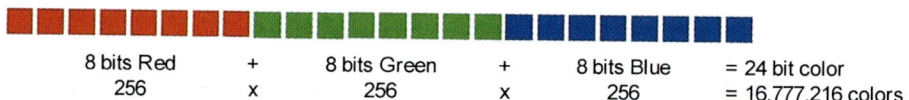

| 8 bits Red | + | 8 bits Green | + | 8 bits Blue | = 24 bit color |
| 256 | x | 256 | x | 256 | = 16,777,216 colors |

Figure 8-5: 24-bit color. This is the most popular color encoding scheme used for digital images and allows for more colors than can be discerned by the human eye.

With sixteen-bit color, two bytes of data is used to store the color information for each pixel. However, 16 doesn't divide evenly by three. Therefore, 5 bits are used each for the red, green, and blue channels, and one bit is wasted. One might argue that only 15 bits should be used rather than wasting one bit. However, computers are designed to work with and address data in 8-bit units (bytes), and splitting information across byte boundaries would significantly degrade performance and complicate the data retrieval. Therefore, it turns out to be far more efficient to simply waste one bit per pixel. 5 bits of data allows for 2^5=32 possible intensities for each color

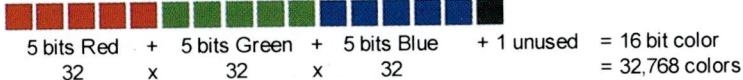

5 bits Red + 5 bits Green + 5 bits Blue + 1 unused = 16 bit color
    32   x   32   x   32   = 32,768 colors

Figure 8-6: 16-bit color. Only a highly trained eye can distinguish 16-bit from 24-bit color.

channel, for a total of 32 x 32 x 32 = 32,768 colors, or "thousands of colors" (Figure 8-6).

Eight-bit color works completely differently. If the same model were used, one would have only 2 bits each for red, green, and blue, with 2 bits being wasted. That would allow for only 4 x 4 x 4 = 64 colors. What is done, instead, is that a "color lookup table" is created, containing 256 different colors (Figure 8-7). Each position in the color table stores one color. Then, for each pixel in the digital image, rather than storing a color, an 8-bit index number is stored. That index number points to the particular position in the color table where the desired color is stored. This color model, referred to as "indexed color", allows 256 different colors in the image (as opposed to only 64). Early computer systems did not let you choose which 256 colors were available. The operating system pre-selected which colors would be in the "system color palette", and that

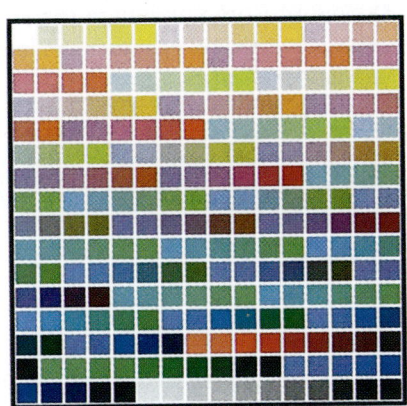

Figure 8-7: Color lookup table.

was that. What's more, the system palette used by the Macintosh operating system was different from that used by the Windows operating system, and only 216 of the colors were the same in both. This was fine for icons and simple drawings, but not sufficient for photographs. Later, images could create their own custom palettes. It turns out that most images can be very well drawn with only 256 different colors, if you got to pick which 256 colors you needed. Since each image has a custom color lookup table, that table has to be stored in the image file.

Is 24-bit color enough, or do I need more? It is estimated that the trained human eye can distinguish approximately 100,000 different colors. Therefore, 24-bit color is certainly enough, and 16-bit color is probably enough. Higher color resolutions still have a role in image analysis applications.

Image Size

Why not always use the most pixels you can get at the greatest color depth possible? Because that takes up space – often a lot of space. More space means not only more space on disk and more space in memory, but perhaps more importantly, bigger means more time – time processing, time on the network, etc.

So how much space? The total size of the image is determined by the total number of pixels (width x height) multiplied by the number of bytes used for each pixel. Table 8-2 shows a pixel count and total image size, in memory, for some of the more commonly used image resolutions. Careful consideration must be given to your choice of image resolution. It can become incredibly inefficient to use images which are larger than needed for a particular purpose.

Table 8-2: Common image resolutions and the corresponding image sizes.

Image Resolution	"MegaPixels"	Color Depth	Image Size
640 x 480	0.31	8-bit	300 Kbytes
640 x 480	0.31	24-bit	900 Kbytes
1024 x 768	0.79	24-bit	2.25 Mbytes
1200 x 900	1.08	24-bit	3.09 Mbytes
1600 x 1200	1.92	24-bit	5.49 Mbytes
3072 x 2048 (PhotoCD)	6.29	24-bit	18.00 Mbytes
2550 x 3300 (8.5x11" @ 300 dpi)	8.42	24-bit	24.08 Mbytes

Note: 1 byte is 8 bits. 1 Kbyte is 1024 bytes. 1 Mbyte is 1024 Kbytes.

Storing Images in Files

While in memory in a displayable format, the structure of any pixel-based digital image is essentially the same. It is a two-dimensional array of pixels, each with a color represented by one (indexed) to three (full-color) numbers. To be displayed, printed, or manipulated, every image needs to be converted to this structure. For storing the image on disk, however, a large number of options are available. The details of how images are stored in a file determine the image file format, many varieties of which were introduced in Chapter 3. Of the image file formats commonly used today, most use either 16-bit or 24-bit color storage (e.g. JPEG, BMP, TIFF). Some image formats (e.g. GIF) use 8-bits. In this case, the color table has to be stored in the image file. Other image file formats (PICT, PNG) can support either type of color mapping scheme.

All of the image file formats contain a "header" followed by the actual image data. The header can be as short as a few bytes, but more commonly consists of several hundred bytes. The header contains information about the format of the data stored in the rest of the file. This includes information like resolution, color depth, perhaps a color table, perhaps data about how and when the image file was originally created, and information about any image compression algorithms used to store the image. The format of the header is different for each image file format. Image files themselves are not directly displayable as they are stored on disk. They have to be read into memory, and then converted into the two-dimensional array representation discussed earlier in order to be displayed.

Image Compression

To facilitate the storage and transport of large images, a number of compression algorithms have been developed to decrease the size of the image file. Initially, these were developed so that the files took up less space on disk. At a few megabytes per image, even a collection of a few dozen images starts to use up a lot of disk space. With the decreasing cost of disk storage, conserving disk space has become less of a motivating factor. However, images still need to be moved around, and the larger the image file, the more time it takes to transmit that image on a network. This became especially important with the increasing popularity of the world wide web, since most web "surfers" will not patiently wait two or three minutes for a web page to load.

Image compression algorithms have been developed to decrease the amount of space needed to store an image in an image file without significantly degrading the appearance of that image when converted to a displayable format. Compression algorithms take advantage of the fact that many images have a number of zones or regions where all of the pixels are the same color. Compression algorithms are generally classified as either "lossless" or "lossy", based on whether or not the EXACT original image can be reconstituted from the compressed image.

The most popular compression algorithm is JPEG compression. It is supported on all computer platforms and by almost all imaging software, and remains the most common image format used on the web. JPEG stands for "Joint Photographic Experts Group", and is a lossy compression algorithm developed by a group of imaging specialists to significantly decrease the size of the image file while only minimally altering the visual image quality. Crudely described, this algorithm breaks up the image into 8 x 8 pixel matrices. Rather than separately storing the color for each pixel in the

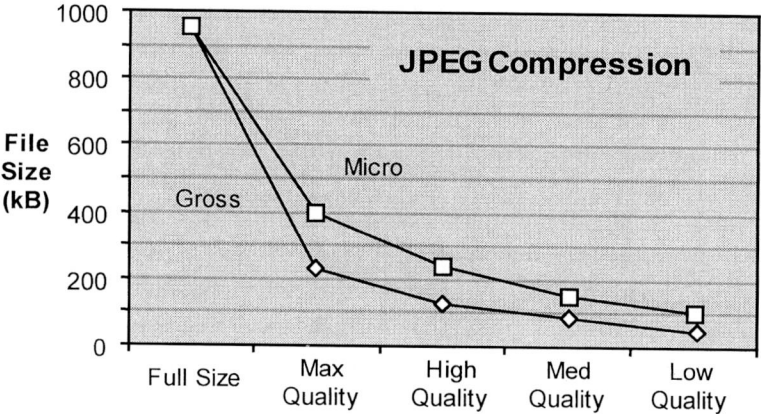

Figure 8-8: Effect of JPEG compression on image size. Depending upon the degree of compression requested (image quality), the size of the image file can be routinely reduced by 80-90%.

matrix, the algorithm stores a single color for the whole matrix, and then additional information about how that color changes over the matrix. The amount of "additional information" determines the level or degree of compression or quality. Highest quality images (minimal compression) store lots of information about how the color changes over the matrix; lowest quality images store the least amount of information. Using this approach, one can typically achieve compression ratios of 5:1 to 20:1 (Figure 8-8), with very little effect on the viewed image quality. Examples of the same image with different levels of compression are shown later in this chapter. Digital images of gross specimens tend to compress to a greater degree than digital photomicrographs because images of gross specimens tend to be taken on a background, and that background is usually one color.

Lossy image compression algorithms introduce subtle artifacts into images. Therefore, they should not be used for any applications in which one plans to do image processing such as densitometry. Also, it is generally not a good idea to manipulate images by cropping or adjusting color balance or contrast once they have been JPEG compressed. Ideally, all image manipulations should be done on an uncompressed image, and then compress it when done. This, however, is not always practical.

Remember that no matter what compression algorithm is used, or what degree of compression is obtained, image data is only compressed when stored in a file on disk or transmitted over a network. The image still needs to be unpacked in memory back to its full size in order to be displayed. Therefore, using compressed images may decrease the amount of disk space you need, but will not decrease the amount of RAM you need in your computer.

Elements of a Digital Imaging System

What is needed to implement a digital imaging solution depends upon what types of images will be taken, who will be acquiring the images, and what will they be used for. Less than a decade ago it was important to consider specific hardware requirements which one's desktop computer would have to have in order to be able to view and create digital images. Now, however, essentially every desktop computer sold has sufficient hardware capabilities to accomplish these tasks. Therefore, this is really no longer a significant concern.

This section will serve as a brief overview, introducing the elements of a digital imaging solution. The following section will specifically address more practical aspects as they apply to anatomic pathology.

Basically, three steps need to be addressed for any digital imaging solution: image acquisition, image storage, and image utilization (Figure 8-9). All three should be considered before beginning any implementation of a digital imaging solution because no solution will be successful unless appropriate solutions are identified for all three steps.

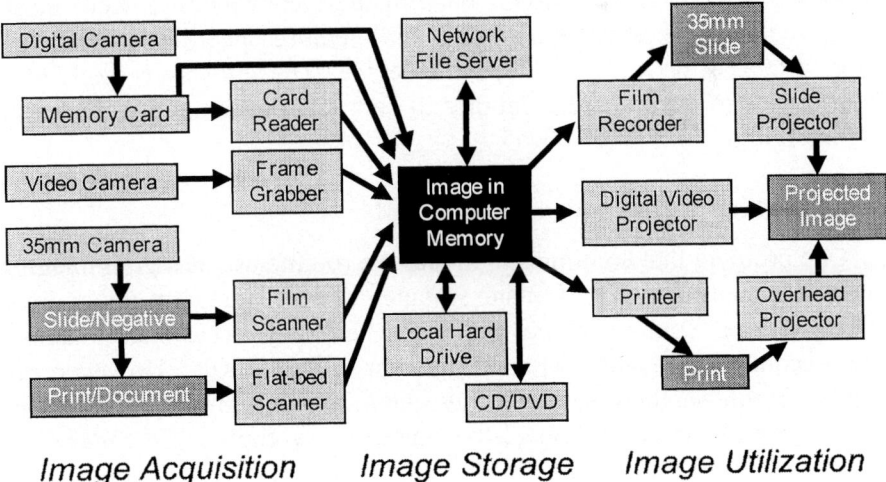

Image Acquisition   _Image Storage_   _Image Utilization_

Figure 8-9: Elements of a digital imaging system. A complete digital imaging solution includes hardware to acquire the images, store the images, and use the images. Not all of the components listed are required, but at least one in each of the three steps is needed.

Image Acquisition

Eventually, we want to end up with a digital image in a computer. The choices are to acquire a digital image directly, or to acquire a non-digital image and then convert it to a digital image.

Direct acquisition of a digital image requires a digital camera. Some digital cameras can be directly connected to the computer, perhaps even controlled from the computer, and the images are acquired directly into the computer. Other digital cameras temporarily store the image internally (in memory or on a removable card). These can later be connected to a computer and the images downloaded, or the removable card can be put into a card reader connected to the computer and the images downloaded from there. When selecting a camera, one must consider such issues as range of focus (many off-the-shelf digital cameras cannot focus on objects closer than 5 feet, and therefore would not be practical for gross specimen photography) and, for photomicroscopy, the availability of hardware to mount the camera to a microscope.

The process of converting a non-digital image to a digital one is dependent upon what kind of non-digital image one has. If the image is a static video signal from an analog video camera, one needs a frame grabber device, either a circuit board installed in the computer or an external video capture device, to do the conversion (see Chapter 9 for more details). If the starting image is a 35mm slide or a negative, a film scanner can scan the image at high resolution. If the starting image is a print or a document, a flat-bed scanner is usually used. Each of these conversion devices must be connected to the computer and each will require specific software (often referred to as a "driver") to operate the device. The software is likely to vary from device to device and computer to computer, although some standards are emerging.

Image Storage

One problem that continues to hinder the routine use of digital imaging in the clinical setting is that of image storage. Simple storage of image files on office desktop computers may suffice when only occasional images are being acquired by a single or small number of individuals. However, as the number of images increases, or if multiple individuals are involved, the issue of storage and retrieval of images becomes more complex. To engage in this activity at a departmental level requires a more substantial solution. Radiology departments routinely rely on commercial picture archive and communication systems (PACS) to manage their images. These often require the images to be in a DICOM (Digital Imaging and Communication in Medicine) compatible format. This solution has worked well for radiology since there are generally a limited number of image acquisition stations, operated by specifically trained individuals. However, complete enterprise solutions are often quite expensive, and although appropriate for radiology departments in which the primary data set is the image, this solution is not generally the best solution for smaller imaging endeavors, even at a departmental level.

Options for where to store digital images depend on how many images one plans to acquire, and how accessible they need to be. Local storage on the hard disk of the computer used to acquire the images is the easiest solution, but least likely to provide adequate accessibility to other users. Images can be burned onto CDs relatively inexpensively by most computers. Finally, departmental file servers allow access to the images by others through a network.

Unfortunately, simply determining where the images will be stored is not sufficient. One has to decide how the images will be stored. How includes not only the image file format and the file names, but also how those image files will be organized. These decisions have implications for the ease with which images can be retrieved, and how much effort is required to manage the storage and back-up of these images. A number of commercial image archiving applications are available which may assist in this process, or you may elect to develop your own solution. If you are using an imaging solution integrated into your pathology clinical information system, that is likely to have a built-in storage solution.

Image Utilization

The only real reason for capturing an image of any sort is because you want to be able to use it later. Viewing digital images on the computer monitor simply requires being able to access them from the storage solution chosen. Projecting these images so that others in, for example, a conference room can also view them requires one of three steps, diagrammed in Figure 8-9. If a digital video projector is available, and the images can be accessed from a computer connected to the digital projector, then this is the simplest and best solution. If there is no digital video projector available, or the images cannot be brought to the projector, then one has to convert the digital images into a more traditional format. This means either printing them on paper (color printers of varying qualities and speeds are available) or using a film recorder to convert the images to 35mm slides. Many institutions as well as commercial photography stores offer this service.

A digital video projector is an important part of a complete digital imaging system, because many of the benefits of digital imaging (with respect to presentation preparation time and cost) are minimized if one has to convert the presentations to traditional 35mm slides. Digital projectors are often sold based on the maximum resolution they can accommodate. Be careful about distinguishing what inputs the projector can accept from what output it displays; many projectors can down-size or up-size a video input, allowing them to accept multiple input resolutions, but only project at a single output resolution. Acronyms like "VGA" and "XGA" are often used to define digital projector resolutions, in just the same way that they are used for video monitors and other video display devices. A table defining the various resolutions is included in Chapter 2 on Desktop Computer Hardware, under the section describing the Video Display Controller.

Practical Aspects of Clinical Imaging for Pathology

The previous sections have introduced/discussed many of the technical aspects of digital imaging. However, the success or failure of any venture into this realm will depend on how much attention is paid to the practical considerations more so than the technical ones. These practical consider-ations are extremely dependent upon the problem which needs to be solved and the specific workflow issues of the environment in which it is solved.

Anyone can take a digital image. Even people who cannot program their VCRs can operate a digital camera. Additionally, most pathologists would agree that digital images offer a number of advantages over 35mm photography. Why, then, are not ALL pathology departments routinely using digital photography rather than traditional photography? The answer is because of the lack of availability of, and often attention to, practical solutions to the workflow and environmental constraints of the problem. Using the same 3-step framework as above for the technical aspects of a complete imaging solution, let's now address some of the practical issues.

Image Utilization

Although using the images is the last step in the imaging process, it is actually the one which needs to be considered first, because it will drive the other steps in the process. What will the images be used for? The range of possibilities includes documentation, viewing at signout, embedding in patient reports, projection at conferences, incorporation into lectures or other presentations, quantitative image analysis, and building an educational resource. Deciding what the images will be used for will determine what image resolution is needed, how many images are likely to be acquired, how much storage space will be needed, what image file format should be used, and how the images need to be made available to users. It is tempting to take the approach of "I want the highest quality images, at a high resolution, in a lossless format, since I'm not sure what all of my needs will be and I want to be able to adapt to any future need." This is simply not practical. It is true that large uncompressed images are more likely to be usable for a greater number of purposes, but the overhead associated with accommodating rare uses is more likely to hinder an imaging effort that help it. Inability to reach a decision on these issues will seriously compromise the success of any imaging solution developed. Pick an approach which meets your initial or current needs. The decision can always be changed later if and when your needs change.

Other utilization issues which need to be considered are how the images will be made available to the various members of the department/practice, and whether or not the level of access needs to be restricted or otherwise controlled.

With the above discussion as a disclaimer, I do have some recommendations about image resolution for two of the most common uses, projection as part of a digital presentation, and routine printing.

Images for Digital Projection

Digital images are frequently used with digital presentation software such as PowerPoint or Keynote. Most digital video projectors project at a full-screen resolution of 1024 x 768 pixels. Therefore, even if the image being projected uses the full screen-width, it makes no sense to have more pixels than the projector resolution, because those extra pixels cannot be displayed. Therefore, more than 1000 pixels in the greatest image dimension makes no theoretical sense.

In general, fewer total number of pixels is needed for gross photographs than for photomicrographs. The more rapidly the detail of the image changes across the image, the more pixels are needed to represent that detail. Gross photographs do not tend to contain a lot of detail which changes rapidly. Therefore, fewer pixels are needed. Photomicrographs on the other hand, especially low magnification micrographs, contain a lot of detail, and benefit from a higher image resolution (more pixels).

Texture information is expressed by subtle changes in color. Gross photographs contain important texture information, and therefore having an adequate color palette is important. Sixteen-bit or 24-bit color is recommended for gross photographs. For photomicrographs, neither color fidelity nor texture information is crucial, so shallower color depths are adequate.

In practice, I have found that 500 pixels in the greatest dimension is usually more than adequate for a full-screen image. If one is preparing a composite slide with multiple images, the needed image resolution is proportionately less. Therefore, for a composite of 4 images (2 rows of 2 images), a resolution of 250 x 150 pixels for each image is usually quite adequate.

All images included in digital presentations of any length should be JPEG compressed. If this is not done, the size of the presentation file on disk rapidly becomes enormous, and the digital presentation software is more likely to fail. It is also crucial to consider how the images are incorporated into the presentation. In general, one should first edit the image as desired, including cropping or resampling to a smaller image size, in your image editing program of choice (e.g., Photoshop, GraphicConverter, etc.). Then, save the image using JPEG compression into a file. Finally, from your presentation program, use the "insert picture from file" procedure to insert the image. It can then be resized as needed in the presentation software. It is very tempting to try to skip the "saving to a file" step, and simply copy the image from the image editing software and paste it into the presentation software. THIS IS A MISTAKE. Remember that image compression is a method of storing images on disk, and all images must be un-compressed in order to be viewed. Therefore, even if you started with a JPEG compressed image in your image editing software, what you are copying to the clipboard is the un-compressed image being viewed, and that is what gets pasted into the presentation software, resulting in a MUCH larger file. On most operating systems, dragging an image from one application to another (if the application supports drag-and-drop) is equivalent to copying and pasting, so this should also be avoided.

Images for Printing

The key consideration when preparing a digital image for printing is knowing how large the printed image will be, and to a lesser extent the quality of the printer being used. In general, approximately 150 pixels per inch provides sufficient quality. This is illustrated in Figure 8-10. Minimal difference is apparent between the two versions shown at 200 dpi and 150 dpi. At 150 dpi, 1024 x 768 pixel images still allow nearly 5"x7" prints, which is usually adequate for most applications. However, the image quality is significantly degraded at 50 pixels per inch.

The level of the JPEG compression used will also significantly affect the final file size. Various programs use different terminology to set the JPEG compression level. For example, some use a 100 point scale with higher numbers meaning more compression. Others, like Photoshop, use a 10 or 12 point scale (depending upon the software version), with higher numbers meaning higher quality and thus less compression. Higher levels of compression are better tolerated (have less of an effect on image quality) when the image has more pixels in it. In the examples shown in Figure 8-11,

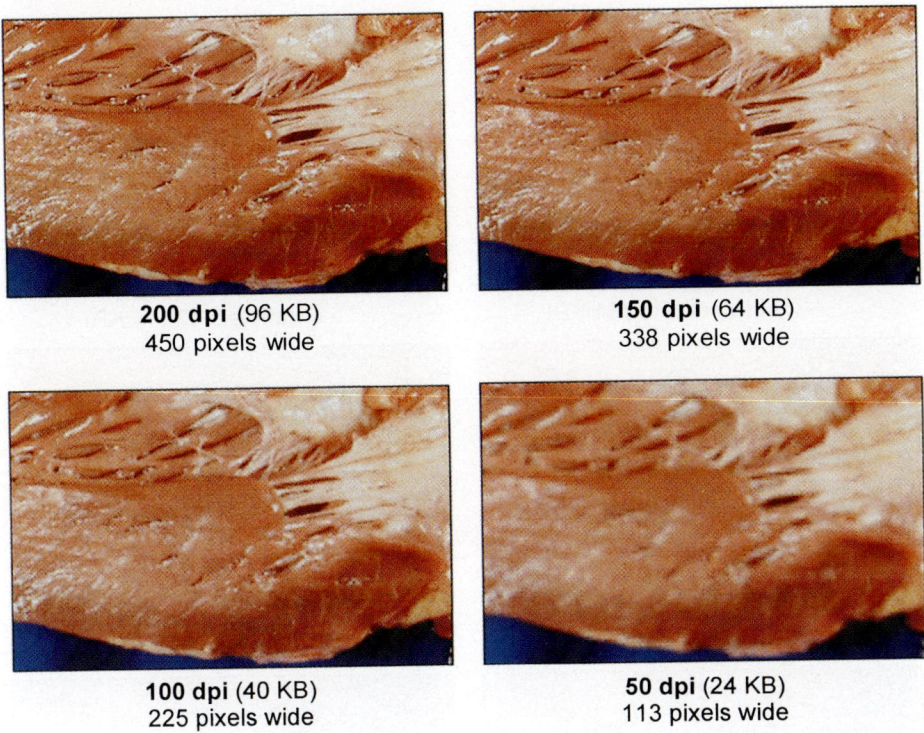

200 dpi (96 KB)
450 pixels wide

150 dpi (64 KB)
338 pixels wide

100 dpi (40 KB)
225 pixels wide

50 dpi (24 KB)
113 pixels wide

Figure 8-10: Effect of pixel density on image quality. Each of these images represents a different resolution digital image of the same subject. The pixel density of each is adjusted so that all of the images are printed at the same size. In all cases, the images are JPEG compressed (Photoshop JPEG Quality = 10/12). The pixel density, image file size, and horizontal resolution are shown for each image.

the images are all printed at 150 dpi, with varying levels of quality/compression (actual file sizes will vary with the software used).

As illustrated in the examples in Figure 8-11, even the 4/12 quality image is nearly indistinguishable from the 10/12 quality image, even though the file size is about one third that of the higher quality image. The uncompressed image would be 215KB. This illustrates the power of the JPEG compression algorithm to preserve image quality while significantly decreasing the size of the file on disk.

In the digital imaging solution we have deployed at Yale Pathology, we routinely use 1024 x 768 resolution images with JPEG compression at the 8/12 level for all of our clinical gross imaging. We do not yet have a standard for microscopic images, but I personally tend to go a little higher, usually 1280 x 1024, also with the same level of JPEG compression.

Some individuals have argued that JPEG compression should not be used for clinical images, because it is a lossy compression, and the legal

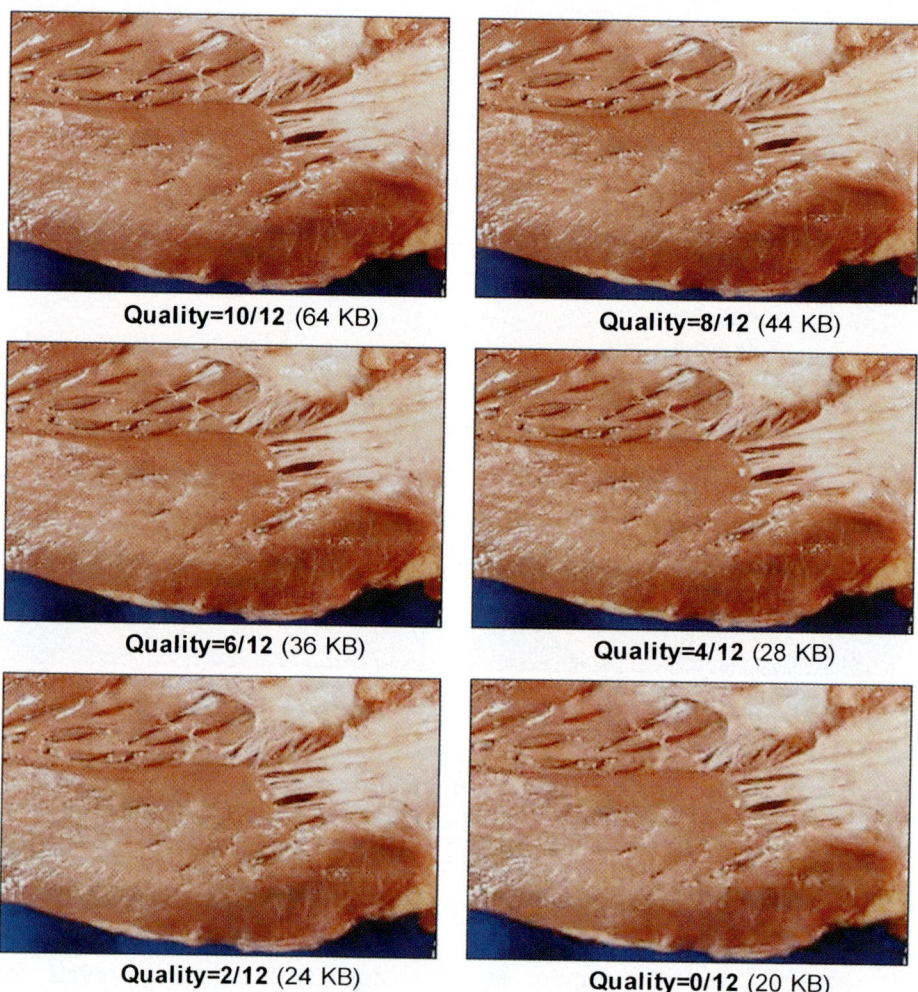

Quality=10/12 (64 KB)   Quality=8/12 (44 KB)

Quality=6/12 (36 KB)   Quality=4/12 (28 KB)

Quality=2/12 (24 KB)   Quality=0/12 (20 KB)

Figure 8-11: Effect of JPEG compression on image quality. Each of these images are shown at the same resolution (same number of pixels, 150 dpi), but at different levels of JPEG compression, from the least compressed (upper left) to the most compressed (lower right). Note the decrease in image file size with increasing levels of JPEG compression.

implications of "discarding" image information have not yet been tested in the courts. I don't consider this a valid argument. Pathology departments have been taking traditional 35mm photographs for years to document specimens. I am not aware of any legal standards for film speed, aperture, focus, or any other aspect of image quality. Perusing the archives of 35mm photographs taken by the department, I have seen some pretty awful images, and although in many cases I consider it a crime to have lost the opportunity to get a really great teaching photograph, to the best of my knowledge no one has ever been arrested for the quality (or lack thereof) of their photographs. It would be unreasonable to require more of digital photographs.

Perhaps the least demanding use for the digital images acquired in a clinical setting is the embedding of those images in patient reports. Essentially any digital image with at least 300 pixels in the widest dimension will be adequate for this, unless you plan to include full page color images in patient reports, in which case I would recommend at least 600 pixels. This is because the quality of the printer used to print these images will limit the overall final quality of the images, and having a greater number of pixels will not help. If you print your patient reports in color, you will most likely do this on a color laser printer. These produce very reasonable prints, and are appropriate for this purpose. It is unlikely that you will be using a color sublimation printer (at a cost of approximately $5 per page, or more) to print routine patient reports.

One issue which does come up is publication of the images and publication quality photographs. Can these be done digitally? The answer is certainly. In fact, some major advantages that digital images provide over traditional is the ease with which one can construct composite photographs with multiple panels, the ease with which one can add annotations, the ability to produce prints at precisely the size they will appear in the journal, and the reproducibility of getting multiple copies which have exactly the same color balance and color saturation, even if printed weeks apart (assuming you use the same printer for all the copies). You will most likely need a high level color sublimation printer to produce the prints which you ultimately submit, since the output from a color laser printer may not be adequate for the journal. These are expensive printers, but this service can be provided by a centralized institutional resource or by commercial photography studios.

Some journals allow direct submission of electronic digital images, without having to print them out at publication quality yourself. What minimum specifications are required for submitting digital images for publication? With traditional photography, photographs were not held to any measurable quality standard: if they looked good, they were good enough. With digital images, one can get numerical specifications such as pixel resolutions and compression levels, and many journals have created standards like "the images must be TIFF files (no compression) and must be at 300 dpi resolution". This is an example of someone inventing a standard simply because one can, and in my humble opinion is absurd. I have seen some very high resolution digital images which are out of focus and just plain bad. I have taken many myself. The concept that these would be acceptable because of the resolution and the file format makes no sense to me. I still think that the old standard of "if it looks good, it is good enough" is the best standard, and I think we will get back there eventually. Unfortunately, the rest of the world is not currently so reasonable. I have this "friend" (not me, of course, but a friend) who once submitted to a journal for publication some images that he thought looked pretty good, but they were JPEG images. The journal gatekeeper sent them back because they did not meet their submission requirements for digital images, which was a certain number of pixels and a TIFF file format. So I, I mean my friend, took the JPEG images he had submitted, opened them in an image editing software package, up-sampled the images to increase the number of pixels, and saved them as TIFF files. Now, since he started with the JPEG images, there is no way that the final TIFF images could have any more information than was in the original JPEG images. On resubmission to the same journal gatekeeper, however, he was informed that the new images were "much better". I'm not sure why I told this story, since I certainly would not recommend such behavior, not even to meet an unreasonable, arbitrary standard.

Image Acquisition

"I'm still using the same 35mm camera I bought 20 years ago and it works great. If I'm going to switch to digital images, I want to buy a camera which will meet all of my needs for the next 20 years, remain compatible with my current and future computers and software, and always be supported by the vendor in case I need to get it fixed." Be real. Many pathology practices are unable to break into digital imaging simply because they are so concerned about making the perfect camera purchase that they end up never getting anything. In reality, for most solutions, the digital camera will be the most "disposable" component in the overall imaging solution. Nonetheless, with so many camera options from which to choose, one needs somewhere to start.

If you plan to use an integrated imaging solution (see below) as provided by your pathology information system software vendor, you may have a limited selection of cameras which have been approved for use with their system. If that is the case, the discussion which follows here may not be relevant to you. However, if your software vendor's solution is more open with respect to camera choice, this information may be useful.

Digital cameras offer a myriad of features, and sifting through them can be such a daunting task that many people simply give up at this step. When evaluating a camera, try to separate its features into one of three categories: those which affect image quality, those which will determine or limit what you can use the camera for, and those which are "cute but probably useless." In the image quality category, you could take the approach of "is this a one chip or a three chip camera?"; "what is the chip size?"; "is it a CCD or a CMOS chip?"; "what is the native pixel resolution?" (some of the details of "chips" are discussed in Chapter 9). Alternatively, simply try to camera out, preferably in your own environment. If you like the pictures you get, the quality is probably good enough for your purposes, regardless of the specifications of the camera. Of course, be sure to try several pictures of several specimens, and try using the picture for the various purposes for which you would acquire a digital image.

In the "cute but probably useless" category, I would put such things as digital zoom, date/time stamping, and voice annotation. These features are designed to appeal to the mass consumer marked, but are really not relevant to an anatomic pathology setting. Digital zoom makes objects appear bigger without increasing their resolution. You will probably not want dates and times in the images themselves, and I have no idea where one might use voice annotation.

The most important group of features to deal with are those which will determine, or perhaps limit, the usability of the camera in different settings. Therefore, the correct mix of features in this group will have the greatest impact on the success of failure of a particular implementation.

Do NOT try to find one single camera which will meet all of your imaging needs for all of the different places where you might want to acquire digital images, since different features are probably advantageous for different solutions (Table 8-3). In some cases, the camera will work best if connected directly to a computer. In other cases, a less tethered operation is preferable, but then there needs to be some way to get the images from the camera to a computer. Accept the fact that the camera will probably not last more than a few years, and in some environments like an autopsy suite may not last more than a year. Finally, do NOT buy the camera until you are ready to use it. Avoid the practice of first buying the camera(s), then setting up the storage solution, and then getting everyone on board with the concept of digital imaging, and then buying the computers and software. If the digital camera sits in its box for more than a few weeks, you probably could have bought a much better camera for less money by the time you opened the box. The digital camera marked is turning over very rapidly. Prices are coming down, and quality and features are increasing. However, don't also be sucked into the "megapixel game" of being convinced by someone that you need a 4.5 megapixel camera because it is better than your old 3.2 megapixel camera, or whatever. Remember that a 1024 x 768 pixel image is only 0.8 megapixels.

Table 8-3: Ideal digital camera features are affected by the environment in which the camera will be used.

Feature	Autopsy Suite	Surgical Gross	Photomicroscopy
Image Resolution	1024 x 768	1024 x 768	Perhaps 1280x1024
Ability to operate un-tethered	Important	Not important	Not important
AC Power adapter	Useful, unless have lots of batteries	Important	Important
Removable Media	Important	Not important	Not important
Focusing Range	Broad; macro capabilities	Broad; macro capabilities	Not important
Threaded mount for adapters	N/A	N/A	Very Important
Software to control camera from computer	N/A	Important	Depends on volume
Real time video out to see what image will look like	Useful when mounted on copy stand	Useful; may be part of acqui-sition software	Can be useful; may be part of acquisition software
Remote shutter release (don't have to touch camera)	Important	Useful; may be part of acqui-sition software	Not important

Autopsy Environment

It is often preferable not to have a computer in the immediate autopsy area, since this environment does not support the long term usability of the computer. Therefore, a camera used to acquire digital images in an autopsy suite must function independent of the computer. For *in situ* photography, the camera should be able to operate on batteries, but it also needs to be able to operate with a direct AC power connection when it is on the copy stand, so photography is not frequently interrupted by the need to repeatedly change batteries. The images should be stored on removable media, both to place no limit on the number of images which can be taken and also so that the camera doesn't have to leave the biohazard area in order for the images to be transferred to a computer. The focusing range for the camera needs to be broad (from a few centimeters to a few meters). Also useful are a remote shutter release (to limit user contact with the camera while on the copy stand) and a real-time video-out to assist in framing the images while the camera is on the copy stand.

Surgical Pathology Gross Room

In the surgical pathology gross room, the camera is likely to always remain on the copy stand. Battery operation is not important, but direct AC power is. Because of the larger quantity of images likely to be taken in surgical pathology, and the fact that images will need to be linked to a number of different cases, direct connection to a computer allowing immediate labeling and storage of the images is important to prevent misidentification and misfiling of the images. Again, a broad focusing range is important, but not as broad as for an autopsy environment, and macro capabilities are a must. You may want to even consider a camera which will accommodate a close-up lens. Real-time video-out, either to a separate monitor or directly to camera control software on the computer, are important for proper framing of the images.

Photomicroscopy

The specific camera needs for photomicroscopy will be partially dependent upon the anticipated volume of images at a particular station. At the least, however, the camera needs to have some threaded mount or in some other way support the attachment of adapters, and the appropriate adapters must be available to mount this camera to the microscope. For low magnification photomicrographs, slightly higher image resolution may be desirable. Focusing range is not relevant, since a camera on a microscope should always be focused at infinity. A zoom feature might be nice, both to overcome any vignetting which might occur in the optical system and to allow better control of the framing of the image beyond your choice of objectives. Remember, however, that with a continuous zoom, it may be more difficult to figure out the actual magnification of the resulting image. Avoid "digital" zooms since this simply wastes pixels without providing any more image detail. Finally, if the zoom mechanism extends the lens outward beyond the body of the camera, be sure any attached mounting adapters do not interfere with this mechanism.

Image Storage

Image storage details include not only determining on what hardware the images will be stored (see above), but more importantly how they will be stored. This includes image file format, directory format, and the names of the image files. Obviously, the images are of little value if one cannot find the images for a particular case. There is no *a priori* reason why the image file format for each image has to be the same, but the way in which the images are labeled and electronically filed should be consistent and agreed upon, especially if multiple people are involved in the image acquisition process. Consideration must be given to who will be responsible for managing the storage of the images, including making sure the image files are appropriately backed up.

The ideal image storage solution must, at the very least, reliably file images in a way in which they can be easily located and accessed. It should accommodate multiple image types (gross, microscopic, special stains, radiology, etc.), and accept image formats commonly used by readily available digital cameras. Images acquired from a variety of sources (different manufacturers' cameras, flatbed scanners, slide scanners, etc.) should be accommodated. There needs to be easy access to the images by those who need to access them, and the ability to export images in a format commonly used for other purposes (eg. digital presentations, lectures, conferences, publication, etc.). Finally, the solution should be intuitively easy to use at all steps of the process (storage and retrieval) so that no special training is required.

Complete Clinical Imaging Solutions

Before embarking on clinical digital imaging at a department level, it is important to develop solutions to each of the steps of the imaging process. Numerous options are available, and it is not possible to discuss them all. I will present here two extreme solutions. The best solution for your practice is likely to be somewhere in between.

Integrated Imaging

A number of pathology information system software vendors have begun to address the increasing desire of pathology departments and practices to begin to use digital images. Their software packages provide an integrated, complete imaging solution, from image acquisition to automatic storage and the ability to embed the images in patient reports. The typical approach is case-centric, in that the user brings up the case and then acquires images into that case. There is usually support for a limited number of acquisition options (certain cameras which are supported), but the look-and-feel of the interface is often very similar to that of the laboratory information system itself. Some of the packages support entry of information about the images, such as titles, descriptions, and even annotations. The images are automatically stored, perhaps in a proprietary format, but once acquired they can be viewed from multiple workstations.

These integrated solutions provide both advantages and disadvantages as an overall imaging solution (Table 8-4). If your practice has never done any digital imaging before, and the pathology information system you have has, as an option, the capability of providing a complete solution, you will certainly want to investigate whether or not that meets your need. The relatively higher cost of that approach will likely offset the time required to educate yourself as to the current market, experimenting with several cameras, learning the relevant features, etc. However, in most case, a department/practice is in a different "place" when they contemplate

Table 8-4: Advantages and disadvantages of an integrated imaging solution.

Advantages of Integrated Imaging	Disadvantages of Integrated Imaging
Off the shelf solution; minimal set-up time • It usually works, if recommended configurations are followed • Don't need to research imaging options	Options for image acquisition limited to those thought of/developed by vendor • Need specific software for each capture device • Hardware/software for image capture must be compatible with the workstation needed to access the LIS; limits platform choices • TWAIN standard limits hardware selection • Software availability limits choice of cameras • Software availability lags behind hardware • Many places already have significant hardware investments with which users are familiar; want to be able to leverage that investment • Upgrades to LIS may require upgrade to capture software • Continued support for the integrated software may end before the associated hardware has lost its usefulness
Often consistent user interface; single system	
Images are stored with the current case, decreasing the chances of being misfiled	
Accommodates storage of information (such as when acquired, by whom, etc.) about each image	
Allows access to and use of images within the laboratory information system (LIS)	Acquisition process may conflict with existing workflow • Images acquired one at a time; case centric • Bulk loading is usually not an option • To take one image each for several cases, can spend lots of time navigating software • Case locking – can't get into case at photography station which is locked at the grossing station
	Images may be "trapped" in a proprietary format • Images must be exported for other uses • Exporting has to be done one image at a time • Access to images may be lost if migrate to different LIS • Access to the images is limited to those who have access to the patient data

switching to routine use of clinical digital imaging. Usually, individuals in the group have had some experience with digital imaging, and have a general familiarity with image editing software and use of digital images in digital presentations. More than likely, the practice has already acquired one or several digital cameras, possibly all the same kind but more likely of different kinds. Some method of image storage has been used, although this may be on an individual basis rather than at a departmental level. Each user has enjoyed full control over his/her own images, but is probably starting to wonder how they are going to keep their growing image collection organized in any meaningful way. In this environment, the integrated imaging solutions offered by pathology information software vendors may not be as ideal. The cameras already owned may not be usable, either because they are not compatible with the interface developed for the information system, don't have needed features for the integration, or the vendor's software development team has simply not yet gotten around to developing an integration solution for your particular camera(s). Some of your image acquisition may be occurring on computers which do not even run the pathology information system, and perhaps cannot run that information system because of operating system incompatibilities.

Workflow issues also have to be considered. How does the image acquisition process available through the integrated solution mesh with your department's workflow? Some of the conflicts can be subtle. Are images usually acquired one case at a time, or do you tend to photograph multiple cases at the same time? It is important to consider the number of photography stations available. For example, if your surgical gross room uses one or two shared gross photography stations rather than having a camera at each grossing station, consider the following scenario. At the grossing station, you start on a new specimen. You take some sections from the margins, place them in cassettes, and enter this information into the computer system at the grossing station. You then carry the specimen to the photography station, and want to acquire an image. To do so, you call up the case at the photography station, but cannot get into the case because it is locked, back at your grossing station, so you have to go back to the grossing station to get out of the case so you can go back to the photography station to take the picture, and hopefully remember to get out of the case there so you can get back into it at your grossing station, and then have to repeat the process after you cut into the specimen and want to take a picture of the cut section.

Finally, the format in which the integrated imaging solution stores the images has to be considered, as well as the ease with which those images can be exported for other purposes such as use in digital presentations. Is the level of access provided appropriate for the needs of your practice?

Modular Imaging: "Yale Pathology Solution"

For its clinical imaging needs, the pathology department at Yale Medical School has implemented a modular solution which provides both the advantages of an integrated imaging solution as well as the advantages of flat-file images. This overall solution includes some custom written software, and as such is probably not practical for most departments and/or practices. However, it is presented as an illustrative example of some of the options which can be used to approach this problem.[6]

Yale Pathology is a multiplatform environment, although the vast majority of the desktop machines in the department are Macintosh based. The clinical information system supports integrated imaging, but only runs on Windows machines. The clinical LIS (laboratory information system) is distributed to the Macintosh workstations via a thin-client configuration. Therefore, it is not possible to use the integrated acquisition software from the thin-client workstations.

Solution to the Integrated Imaging Problem

To overcome the hardware and platform issues associated with the integrated imaging solution, while still providing the ability to embed images into patient reports, it was necessary to disconnect the image acquisition from the image filing and storage. A two-step image acquisition process was developed (Figure 8-12). In the first step, images are acquired by any of a number of acquisition devices, and then placed in a holding area. In the second step, the images are removed from the holding area and filed into their ultimate storage locations. To provide greater usability of the images, a dual image storage solution was implemented. One of the storage locations is a repository of standard-format image files, from which JPEG images can be browsed, accessed, and easily downloaded for other purposes. A second location stores the images in the proprietary formatted needed for access by the LIS, just as if the image had been acquired using the integrated acquisition approach.

In the acquisition step, images are acquired by a number of different digital cameras. Depending upon the environment, the camera is either directly connected to a computer, or images are downloaded from a memory card. Images are "addressed" to the correct case before being placed in the "image drop-folder" via their file names, which are set either manually or by

---

[6] For more details on this solution, see Sinard and Mattie (2005) Overcoming the limitations of integrated clinical digital imaging solutions. **Arch. Path. Lab Med.** 2005; 129:1118-1126.

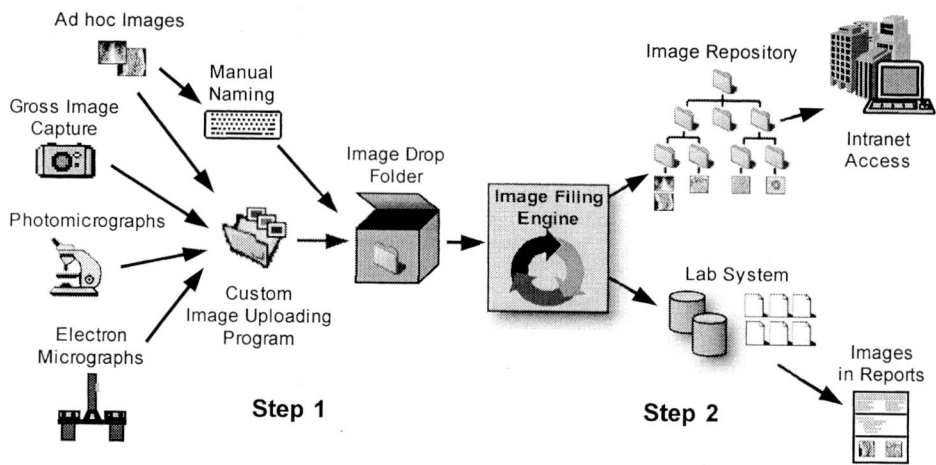

Figure 8-12: Two-step dual storage imaging solution. This solution was developed and deployed at Yale to create significantly greater flexibility with respect to selection of image acquisition devices that the integrated solution offered by our software vendor. The dual storage increased the accessibility of the images for uses other than including in patient reports.

using custom software to automate the naming process and provide some additional functionality.

At Yale, we use a file naming convention for all clinical image files, based predominantly on the accession number assigned the image in the clinical information system (Table 8-5). This allows each image to be

Table 8-5: Naming convention used at Yale to uniquely identify image file.

	PPYYYY-AAAAAAcNN[-dddd].fff
PP	One or two character specimen prefix, in uppercase (e.g., S=surgical, A=autopsy)
YYYY	4 digit year of accession
AAAAAA	6 digit accession number, with leading zeros
c	One character image type code, lowercase (e.g. g=gross photo, m=photomicrograph)
NN	2 digit sequential image number, with leading zero. Numbering restarts at 01 for each image type. Numbers do NOT have to be consecutive, but must be unique within an image type.
-dddd	Optional 4 character description, in lowercase (e.g. for immuno-histochemical stains, can use this to indicate which antibody this image represents)
fff	3 character file extension, indicating the image file format type (e.g. jpg = JPEG)

individually linked to the case to which it belongs, so that if images are misfiled or removed from storage, their origin can still be identified.

After being placed in the image drop-folder, a background process, the image filing engine, moves the standard-format image file into the appropriate directory in the flat-file image repository, which it builds dynamically using a hierarchical directory structure to separate the cases by year and specimen type. The image filing engine also places a second copy of the image in the proprietary format needed for use by the clinical information system. This second step requires a detailed working knowledge of the LIS, and necessitates the involvement/cooperation of the pathology information system software vendor. Care must be taken when images are acquired from multiple acquisition devices to be sure images archived at one point in time do not overwrite images taken previously. One of the responsibilities of this background image filing engine is to renumber the image files, as necessary, to prevent overwriting an already saved image.

Access to the images in the image repository is made possible by additional custom software which provides dynamic web-browser based access into the repository (Figure 8-13). Images can be accessed from any intranet connected desktop workstation, regardless of operating system. Access is password protected since the interface also provides patient names and ages, although individuals who do not have access to the laboratory information system can be granted access to the image repository. Both thumbnail and full resolution image viewing is possible through the web-based interface, and downloading images for other purposes such as printing

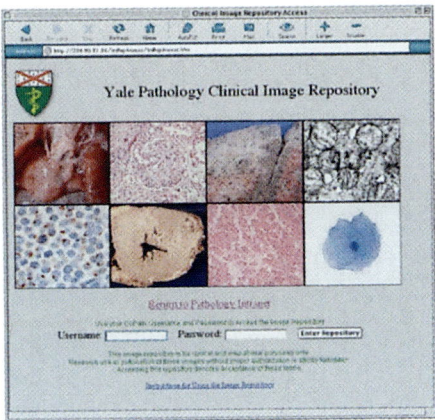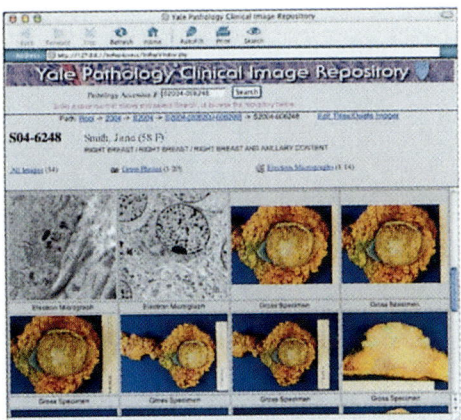

Figure 8-13: Screen shots of the web-based interface to the image repository. Access is password restricted. Images can optionally be viewed a full frame or downloaded to the desktop. (The patient name and specimen number shown are, of course, made up.)

or incorporation into a digital presentation is as trivial as clicking and dragging the image to the workstation desktop.

The dual image storage allows each to serve as a backup for the other, assuring data preservation and availability. As an added safeguard, however, both collections of image files are also backed up independently.

Chapter 9

VIDEO MICROSCOPY AND TELEMICROSCOPY

There are a vast array of technologies and associated applications which share the common end result that a pathologist is able to view a microscopy image not through a microscope but rather via a video display device, either a video monitor or a video projector. All of these, at some point, involve a microscope or microscope-like device, a camera, and a variety of cables and connectors with esoteric names. The terminology for this spectrum of technologies is equally broad: video microscopy, digital microscopy, virtual microscopy, telepathology, remote robotic microscopy, teleconsultation, tele-education, whole-slide imaging, and wide-field digital microscopy. Some of the technologies are "static" (the image is pre-captured), others are "dynamic" (real-time viewing), while still others sit somewhere in between (dynamic viewing of a static image). Some of the technologies are analog, some are digital, and some have elements of both. Strictly speaking, the terminology is not really interchangeable. For example, "video microscopy" generally refers to real-time dynamic viewing of a microscope slide, whether it be a digital or analog signal, whereas "digital microscopy" refers to viewing a digital representation of the image, whether it be static or dynamic. "Virtual microscopy" would seem like a reasonably vague term, but certainly not ideal, since a real microscope is almost involved at some point in the process.

Before embarking on a discussion of video microscopy technology, I should address the question of whether or not this topic even falls within the domain of pathology informatics. Although at the "high end" these forms of microscopy can involve digital image acquisition, compression, and storage, as well as image servers and internet-based image browsers, at the low end we may simply be dealing with a microscope, a camera, and a television monitor. What's digital about that? Well, in the latter case, there is nothing digital about it, but the image is clearly information, and that information has to be managed. Although not all applications involving video cameras may fit well into "informatics", some of them clearly do, and therefore understanding these devices is certainly important to pathology informatics. In addition, if you declare yourself as interested in pathology informatics, I can pretty much guarantee you that someone will ask you to help them put a camera on a microscope.

Video Microscopy Technology

Video Cameras

In a very broad sense, video cameras convert an image into an electronic signal. Portable video cameras have to include some way to store that image (such as on a magnetic tape) or transmit that image (broadcast capable cameras). When used for microscopy, however, since the microscope is generally not portable, there is no need for the video camera to be. When set up, these cameras usually have two cables connected to them: one bringing power to the camera, and the other carrying the video signal away. Some camera manufacturers combine these into a single composite cable.

The core element of any video camera is the device which converts to light signal into an electrical one. This is most commonly done by a Charge Coupled Device, otherwise known as a CCD (*see-see-dee*). A CCD chip is an array of light sensitive elements, referred to as photosites, which produce an electrical signal (voltage) when exposed to light (photons). The greater the intensity of light striking these photovoltaic elements, the more voltage is produced. The photosites on a CCD chip are arranged in an array, and the light entering the camera is focused via the optical components of the camera on the CCD chip, such that each photosite represents a part of the image. Electronics in the camera then scan through the photosites, horizontally, line-by-line, reading the voltages and generating a time-encoded analog video signal (time-encoded means that the signal voltage at any point in time represents light intensity at a particular point in the image).

For monochromatic images, a single CCD chip is all that is needed. CCD chips have different sensitivities to different wavelengths of light, and many are particularly sensitive in the near infra-red range, often requiring a "heat filter" be placed in front of the camera to prevent interference with the visual signal. However, CCD chips cannot actually distinguish colors. For color cameras, color detection is achieved by placing color filters in front of the CCD photosites; only light of one color is allowed to reach that photosite, making it a color specific photosite. As discussed in Chapter 8, all colors of light can be represented by a mixture of red, green, and blue light. Therefore, video cameras need filters for these three colors. Two basic types of cameras exist: three chip and one chip cameras. In a three chip camera, (Figure 9-1) a beam splitting prism splits the incoming light into three "equal" beams. Each is then passed through either a red, green, or blue filter and allowed to strike a CCD chip. Thus, one chip obtains the red "channel", one the green, and one the blue. All three channels are captured at the full chip resolution simultaneously, allowing the highest quality image. Unfortunately, the CCD chip is the most expensive component in a

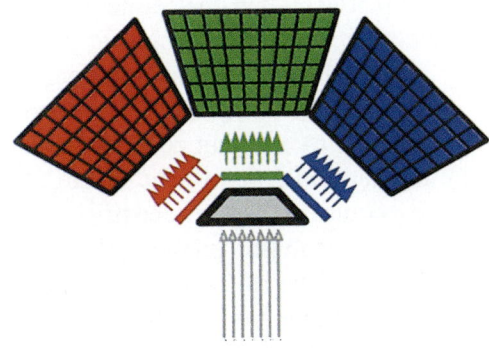

Figure 9-1: Three chip color cameras. A prism splits the incident beam and then passes each through a color filter. Three images are captured simultaneously, one each representing the red, green, and blue signals.

video camera. Having three of them significantly increases the price of the camera. Also, because of the need to split the incoming light into three beams, more physical space may be needed in the camera, so three chip cameras can be larger, further increasing the price. The chips also have to be very precisely aligned.

An alternative to the three-CCD camera is a single chip camera. There are two ways to get three color signals from a single chip camera (Figure 9-2). For still cameras, this can be done with a rotating color wheel. Basically, the same chip is used, in sequence, to obtain the red, then the green, then the blue signal. This approach, however, does not work well for moving or changing images, since the three color channels in the image will not be of the same object. In the second approach, a mosaic of color filters is placed directly on the

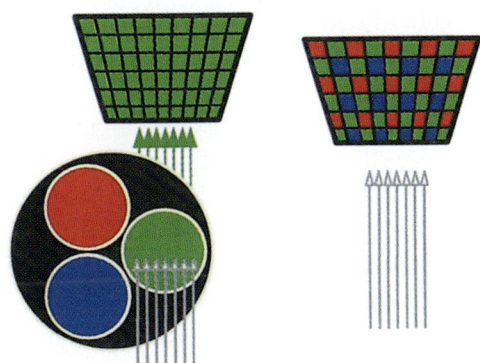

Figure 9-2: One chip cameras. Two options exist for capturing full color with a single chip camera. In one, a color wheel is used to acquire each color channel in succession. This only works well for still images. In the second approach, a mosaic of color filters is placed in front of the CCD chip, and electronics are used to construct the three color channel signals.

CCD chip itself, such that either a red, green, or blue filter sits in front of each photosite. Different mosaic patterns are used, but in general a 2 x 2 array, often with two greens, one red, and one blue, is used. Each photosite detects a single primary color, and then electronics in the camera interpolate the intensities of adjacent color specific cells to determine the actual color of light at a particular part of the image. Single chip CCD color video cameras tend to require a higher density of photosites on the chip to achieve a comparable resolution image, which makes that chip more expensive, but you only need one of them, and you don't need the beam splitting optics, or the precise alignment, so single chip cameras tend to cost about half the price of three-chip cameras.

In an attempt to provide lower cost three-chip cameras, some manufacturers have begun using a different chip technology than the charge-coupled device. An alternative chip, a Complementary Metal Oxide Semiconductor (CMOS, pronounced *see-moss*), is less expensive to manufacture and even uses less power. However, it has more noise at low light levels, and is less sensitive in comparison to traditional CCD chips, and therefore may not work well for all applications.

Video Signals

An analog video image consists of a series of continuous horizontal scan lines, stacked evenly spaced one above the other. The image is drawn on the monitor by starting in the upper left hand corner, drawing a continuous line horizontally with varying intensity along its length until the right edge of the monitor is reached, and then moving on to the next line. In a progressive scan image, each line is drawn, successively, from the top to the bottom of the screen. With an interlaced signal, every other line, say the odd numbered lines, are drawn first, and then the "gun" goes back to the top and fills in the even numbered lines. This all happens very quickly, on the order of 30 times per second, so it is perceived to the eye as a continuous moving image.

A few different standards exist for color analog video signals. Their use varies geographically. The video signal standard most commonly used in North America, Central America, and Japan is the National Television System Committee formatted signal, or NTSC (*en-tee-ess-see*). NTSC signals consist of 525 horizontal lines of information, refreshed at 60 half frames per second in an interlaced fashion as described above. However, only 486 of the lines contain picture information, the others containing closed captioning or a second audio program. Because of incomplete lines and because of the interlaced format, only 480 complete lines of picture information can be reliably obtained from an NTSC video signal. A second video signal format known as Phase Alteration Line or PAL (pronounced like the synonym for "buddy") is used in most European countries, except France. This signal contains 625 lines, refreshed at 50 half frames per second, but again only some of the lines (576 in this case) contain picture information. The two formats are incompatible with each other. A third format, the Systeme Electronique Couleur Avec Memoire or SECAM also exists (although there is not universal agreement as to what SECAM actually stands for). It is similar to PAL in that it also is based on 625 horizontal lines. PAL signals can generally be viewed on SECAM monitors. SECAM is used in France, Eastern Europe, Russia, and Africa.

Video Cables and Connectors

A complete color analog video signal consists of five signal elements, and to display a video signal, the monitor needs to have all five signals. Based upon the above discussion, it is not surprising that three of these contain the red, green, and blue channel signals, respectively. The other two are synchronization signals, one for horizontal and one for vertical. The horizontal synchronization signal marks the end/beginning of each horizontal scan line, and the vertical synchronization signal marks the end/beginning of each frame. To maintain the highest quality image, these five signal elements need to be kept separate from each other. This, however, requires five separate "wires" in the cable (each with its own ground) and thus more expensive cables. Therefore, these signal elements are often electronically combined into a smaller number of signals. They are then separated into the individual signals prior to display. This combining of signals, although a cost savings since it allows for less expensive wiring, does not allow the original signals to be recovered with complete fidelity, resulting in a loss of image quality. Table 9-1 lists the different types of video cabling formats and their corresponding connectors.

RGB

The highest quality video signal maintains the separation of all the elements of the original video signal. Three separate signals contain the

Table 9-1: Video signal standards, cabling and connectors.

Standard	# Signals	Labeling	Connector Type
RGB	4 (or 3 or 5)	R, G, B, S (H, V)	BNC (1 per signal)
Component	3	Y, Pb, Pr	BNC (1 per signal)
S-Video	2	Y, C	S-Video
Composite	1	(yellow)	RCA Phono Jack

luminance (brightness) levels for each of the primary colors, red, green, and blue, each with a connector of the indicated color. Therefore, this type of signal is generally referred to simply as RGB (*are-jee-bee*). In the five "wire" version of this standard, the two other wires are labeled H and V for the horizontal and vertical synchronization signals. (In reality, each of the signals requires two wires, one to carry the signal and one to serve as the ground reference for that signal, so a "five wire" cable actually has ten wires in it.) Occasionally, the two synchronization signals are combined into a single signal, usually with a black or a white connector, creating a four wire connector. This can be done with essentially no loss of quality. Similarly, a three wire connector can be created by combining the two synchronization signals and mixing it in with the green signal, again with essentially no loss of quality since the synchronization signals do not overlap the image content. Traditionally, BNC (*bee-en-see*) connectors (Bayonet Neill Councelman) are used for each of the signal elements in an RGB signal (Figure 9-3), although occasionally manufacturers will use a proprietary connector to carry this information.

RGB cabling can be used with NTSC video signals, as from a standard analog video camera, but are more commonly used between computers and their video monitors, supporting a variety of resolutions. Also, some higher-end video cameras offer RGB output in the form of a standard "VGA" connector, but can support not only the 640 x 480 standard, but also SVGA, XGA, and even SXGA (see Chapter 2 on desktop computer hardware for more details). These outputs can be fed directly into a computer monitor (rather than a television monitor) or into some video projectors for high resolution projection.

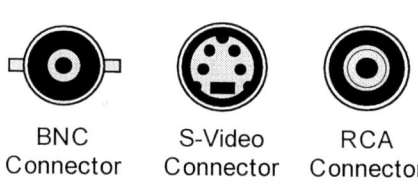

BNC   S-Video   RCA
Connector   Connector   Connector

Figure 9-3: Standard Video Connectors

Component Video

The component video standard uses three signal elements on three wires, each with a ground. The connectors are most commonly labeled Y, Pb, and Pr. The "Y" signal contains the overall luminance or brightness, an essentially black-and-white signal containing the combined brightness of all three color channels. The horizontal and vertical synchronization signals are also combined into the luminance signal. The Pb and Pr signals contain the blue and red color channels. The green color channel can be calculated electronically by subtracting the blue and the red from the brightness signal. Thus, component video is comparable in quality to the RGB standard. Component video signals are used by Digital Video Disc players (NTSC video standard) and High-definition television, and, like the RBG standard, most commonly use BNC connectors.

S-Video

The "Super-video" standard compresses the color video signal information into two signals: luminance and chrominance. The luminance signal, usually labeled "Y", carries the brightness information as well as the horizontal and vertical synchronization signals. The chrominance signal, usually labeled "C", carries all the color information, encoded as hue and saturation. S-Video uses a special 4-pin connector (two signals, two grounds) (Figure 9-3) and was popularized by higher-end video cassette recorders as a higher quality alternative to composite video.

Composite Video

Composite video is the most common type of video signal used, especially for NTSC video signals, because it can be carried on a single wire (plus a ground). In this format, all of the color, brightness, and synchronization information is compressed into a single signal. A yellow colored RCA (Radio Corporation of America) phono-jack is the most common connector used for a composite video signal (Figure 9-3). Occasionally, a BNC connector is used.

RF

The RF (Radio Frequency) standard combines all the video as well as the audio information into a single signal, resulting in significant loss of image quality. It is used for broadcast television, and has no role in video microscopy.

Digital Video

We live in an analog world. Unless you want to get down to the level of quantum physics, the real world involves continuous variations, and that makes it inherently analog. If we want it to be digital, we have to digitize it. Video images are the same. To obtain a digital still or video image from an analog video camera, the signal has to be put through an analog-to-digital (A/D) converter, which samples the various signals at a rapid rate and converts their voltages to digital representations.

The main advantage of digital signals over analog signals is that analog signals are subject to degradation by electrical and magnetic interference, whereas digital signals are not. This is because electrical and magnetic fields can alter the signal voltages on a wire passing through those fields. For analog video signals, the information is contained in the voltages, so any alteration of the voltages degrades the image quality. With digital signals, the information is stored as a series of ones and zeros. Although these ones and zeros are also transmitted along wires as voltages, and therefore subject to the same noise introduced by electrical and magnetic fields (in essence creating the equivalent of a 0.9 or a 0.1 instead of a 1 or a 0), the data is re-converted to ones and zeros on the receiving end, so no data is lost until the interference/noise is so great that a one can no longer be distinguished from a zero. Another advantage of digital still and video images is that they can often be directly loaded into a computer for processing, display, manipulation, and/or storage.

Analog video signals are converted to digital video signals by using an analog to digital converter (actually 3). This electronic device repeatedly samples the incoming analog signals and converts their voltages to a digital representation (Figure 9-4). An 8-bit per channel converter converts each color channel to a series of numbers between 0 and 255. Higher bit-depth converters also exist. When converting the standard NTSC analog output from an analog video camera into a digital signal, remember that the NTSC signal contains 480 continuous horizontal lines of video information.

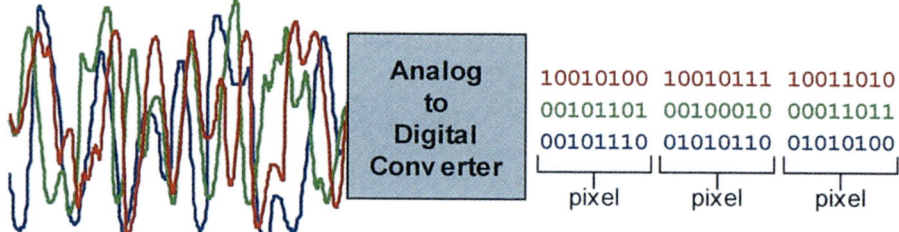

Figure 9-4: Digitizing an analog video signal. A/D converters take an analog video input and convert each channel of color into a sequence of binary numbers. In this example, 8-bit converters are used. Each group of three 8-bit numbers represents the color at one point in the image (one pixel).

Therefore, the greatest vertical resolution which can be achieved is 480 pixels. For the horizontal resolution, one could, in theory, break up the continuous signal into as many packets of data as desired, limited only by the speed of the A/D converter(s). However, when a digital image is displayed, it is almost invariably displayed as square pixels with the same pixel density in both the horizontal and vertical dimensions. Therefore, for the image to look correct, the ratio of the horizontal to vertical pixel resolution has to correspond to the aspect ratio of the original image. For a standard 4:3 video image, that corresponds to 640 pixels in the horizontal dimension. Thus, the output from digitizing a standard NTSC video signal is a 640 x 480 pixel digital image. Similarly, a PAL video signal is digitized to a 768 x 576 pixel digital image.

Since analog video signals are subject to noise and therefore degradation of image quality, if one intends to digitize the analog signal, it is advantageous to do so as close to the camera as possible, to decrease the amount of degradation. Digital still and video cameras use the same CCD chips as found in analog cameras. The difference between a digital and analog camera is that with the digital camera, the analog-to-digital conversion takes place within the camera itself. Although this requires some additional electronics in the camera, the output from a digital camera is digital and therefore immune to electrical and magnetic interference.

Digital Video Signals

Digital cameras have to be able to transfer their images to computers. Digital still cameras usually use a USB connection for this purpose, whereas digital video cameras often use the higher bandwidth IEEE-1394 (Firewire) connection (see Chapter 2 from more details on these digital input/output standards). The two most common signal formats for digital video were both described by the Moving Picture Experts Group and are referred to as MPEG1 (*em-peg-won*) and MPEG2. Both support a combination of video and audio. MPEG1 has a maximum bandwidth of 1.5 Mb/sec and supports images at 352 x 240 pixels, or the equivalent of a wide version of QVGA. MPEG1 is used by Video CDs. MPEG2 supports larger images and better sound, and is used for DVDs. MPEG2 uses up to 15 Mb/sec bandwidth, 9.8 Mb/sec devoted to the picture, allowing wide VGA resolutions of 720 x 480 pixels.

MPEG video signals, although digital, do not yet have much of a role in video microscopy. The resolution is no better than what can be achieved from an RGB analog camera, and almost invariable requires a computer between the camera and any display device in order to view the output. The major advantage it affords is the ability to record the output in a digital form.

Video Microscopy for Pathology Conference Rooms

The most common direct application for video microscopy is in setting up a pathology conference room, to allow a room full of viewers to see what is on the microscope in real time. Multi-headed microscopes are great, but can take up a lot of space and are still limited optically to a little over a dozen viewers. They can also be very expensive. The easy solution to this is to place a video camera on the microscope, and connect that to a video monitor, preferably a large one. Those not at the microscope can now see what is on the microscope, all-be-it not as well as those at the microscope.

As digital images and digital presentation software have become much more commonly used, most modern conference rooms are being equipped with a computer and a ceiling mounted video projector. Depending upon the projector, this provides an opportunity to project the output from the video camera on the microscope. Since these conference rooms will often be used to support visitors from other departments and other institutions, there is also an increasing need to provide multi-platform support (computers with different operating systems) in the conference room, as well as a "hook-up" to allow connection of a laptop computer into the room's projection system.

The two most important components of a pathology conference room set-up are the microscope-mounted camera and the video projector. The key feature to look for in the video camera is the number and type of outputs available (composite video, S-Video, RGB, VGA-like video, USB, Firewire). For the video projector, it is the number and type of inputs available, as well as the maximum projection resolution of the projector. Don't be fooled by projectors which accept multiple input resolutions, including some very high resolutions, but have a maximum output resolution which is limited, indicating that the projector down-samples the input.

If the camera only has a composite video output, you will not, in the long run, be happy with the quality of the image. Although it may be fine at high magnification, and may even be fine at all magnifications for presenting to clinicians in other departments, it will not be acceptable to pathologists at low magnification. This is because the composite video signal is both noisy and limited by the NTSC resolution of 480 visible scan lines. S-Video, at a minimum, is required, and RGB output is by far the best for image quality. A number of cameras are available which provide RGB output. To display these, however, you are going to need an RGB monitor. If you want to project the image, video projectors which take separate RGB inputs are quite rare. Remember also that even if the output is provided as an RGB output in the form of four separate signals, it is likely to still be an NTSC video signal, limited therefore in resolution to 480 visible scan lines. For higher image resolution, one needs to go either with a digital output (eg Firewire), or a high-resolution VGA-like video output. Whereas digital outputs may seem like a better choice, MPEG is also limited to 480 visible scan lines. In addition, with digital outputs, you will probably have to interpose a computer between the camera and the projector. Although there will undoubtedly be a computer in the room, any set up which requires the computer to be running a particular software package, with the appropriate settings to collect the video signal from the Firewire port and send it to some output port which is compatible with the projector is simply going to be too cumbersome to use and will generate a lot of phone calls to ITS, often emergent. I feel that, at the present time, the best solution is video cameras that provide high resolution video outputs using a VGA-like format which can be directly fed into a video monitor or a video projector, without the need for any intervening computer. A number of SVGA (800 x 600), XGA (1024 x 768) and even SXGA (1280 x 1024) cameras are now available. When properly matched with a video projector which will support these higher resolutions, and project them at the higher resolution, the image quality is really quite remarkable. However, there are still a number of signal compatibility issues to address. Not all XGA output cameras, for example, will work with all projectors which support XGA inputs, so don't buy anything until you have had both the camera and the projector set up and working in your conference room.

After several different iterations over the years, we have arrived at a conference room set-up with which we are quite happy (Figure 9-5). In fact, most interdepartmental conferences involving pathology have moved from the remote departments back into our conference room, because of the in-room projection capabilities, and a number of other departments at our institution have begun to use our conference room even for conferences which do not involve pathology. We have a fourteen-headed microscope

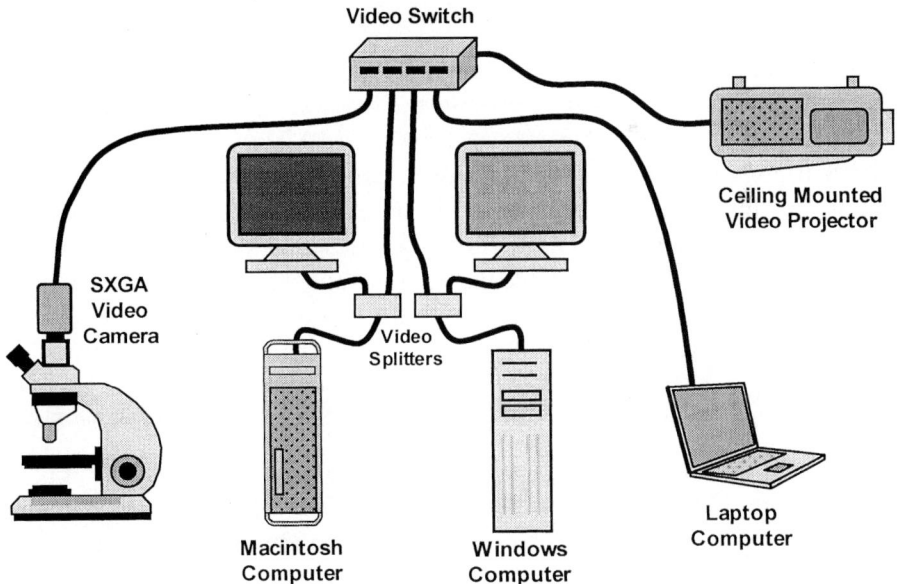

Figure 9-5: Pathology Conference Room Setup. The video switch allows the ceiling mounted video projector to display the current image coming either from the microscope, the Macintosh computer, the Windows computer, or the laptop computer. The video splitters allow the monitors to always display the output from each of the computers, regardless of whether or not that computer's output is currently being projected.

with a SXGA video camera. For computers, we are a predominantly Macintosh department, so we needed to have a Macintosh computer for presentations prepared by departmental faculty and residents. However, some institutional systems, such as radiology, required a Windows operating system for access to on-line digital radiology images, so we decided to add a Windows computer as well. Since we wanted to be able to see what was on each of the computers, regardless of what was being projected, we added a video splitter between each computer video output port and the corresponding monitor. This allows one to "cue-up" what will be projected without having to use the projector. The second output from each of the video splitters, as well as the video output from the microscope mounted camera, are fed into a four position video switch, which sits on the table between the two computer monitors. To the fourth input of the video switch we have connected a long video cable which is used for connecting laptops to the system. The output from the video switch goes to a ceiling mounted video projector.

Telemicroscopy Systems

Once the microscopy image has been transformed into an electronic signal, be it analog or digital, it can be "transmitted" to a remote site, be that a few feet away on a monitor, around the corner, across the building, or across the world.

In sifting through the terminology associated with telemicroscopy systems, an important first step is to separate the terms which identify the technology from those which identify the uses and applications for that technology. Telepathology, teleconsultation, and tele-education are uses, and so I will set those aside for the time being and focus first on the technology: telemicroscopy.

Telemicroscopy Technology

Three different technologies currently comprise the spectrum of telemicroscopy (Table 9-2). All three share the fact that digital microscopic images are transmitted, usually via the internet, to the recipient and viewed on a computer screen.

In the first type of telemicroscopy technology, static telemicroscopy, a pre-selected group of digital images which the person doing the image acquisition feels are representative of the case are transmitted to the recipient. This requires a sufficiently talented person on the sending end to select appropriately diagnostic images.

Table 9-2: Telemicroscopy Technologies.

Technology	Expense of Equipment at the Sending Site	Diagnostic Skill Needed at the Sending Site	Rate Limiting Step in Making a Diagnosis	Special Hardware or Software at the Receiving Site
Static Images	Low	High	Acquisition	None
Dynamic: Non-Robotic	Medium	Moderate	Coordinated Viewing	None
Dynamic: Robotic	High	Low to None	Viewing	? Some ?
Wide Field Microscopy	Very High	Low to None	Acquisition	Some

The second technology, dynamic telemicroscopy, allows the recipient to view live, real-time images from a telemicroscope. Two methods exist: one in which the microscope is controlled from the sending location, and one in which a robotic microscope allows the remote viewer to control field selection, magnification, and focus. Both the these methods require a reasonably high bandwidth transmission. In the non-robotic instance, the only thing being sent to the viewer is the image. A number of "out-of-the-box" solutions exist for this, and some of these are relatively inexpensive. Video servers are devices which take essentially two inputs: a video signal (usually composite video) and an Ethernet connection. Any video signal from any microscope mounted video camera can be used with this configuration. The video server is assigned an IP address, and has built-in software which allow it to be configured with a variety of options. The person viewing the image merely needs to direct his or her web browser to the IP address of the video server and they can see the image on the microscope (Figure 9-6). Usually, no special software is needed on the receiving end. Be sure the video server is connected to the internet (outside the firewall) if you want to enable viewing by anyone. Since only a microscopic image is shown, with no patient identifiers, there are no issues of patient privacy to address. Any clinical information, as well as consultation between the sender and the viewer (such as "move to the left" or "zoom in on that") are conveyed via a telephone call. For this configuration to be effective, the individual sending the image has to be sufficiently talented, diagnostically speaking, to be able to identify the relevant histologic fields, since the viewer has no control over field selection. In addition, both the sender and the viewer have to be available at the same time to use this method of telemicroscopy.

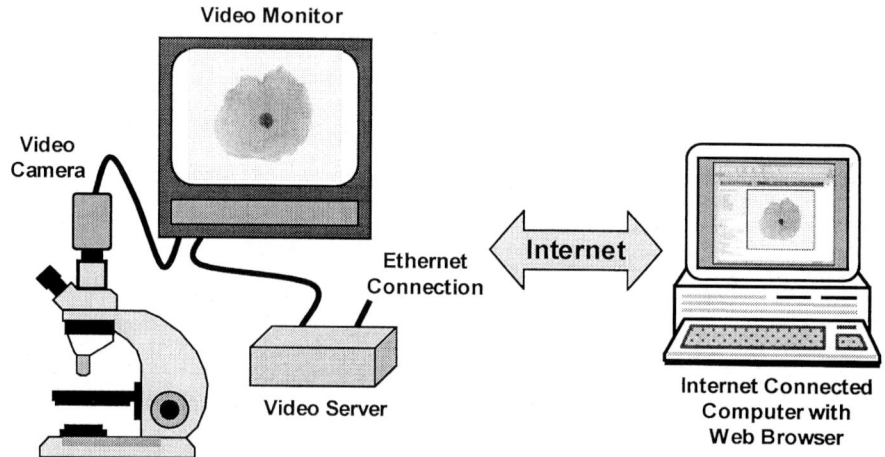

Figure 9-6: Sample dynamic non-robotic telemicroscopy system. The key component of this solution is the video server, a device with built-in web serving capabilities which receives, as inputs, a video signal and an Ethernet connection.

With dynamic robotic telemicroscopy, the image is again sent to the receiving site via the internet, but the viewer has the ability to control the microscope himself/herself from the remote site. This usually requires the viewer to have special software to send the commands for stage movement, objective changing, and focus, and definitely requires an expensive robotic microscope on the sending end. A number of vendors sell such complete hardware and software packages. These usually include not only the video serving hardware, but also the microscope, robotic controls, video camera, and a computer. Some also offer automated slide loading capabilities as well. The advantages of this approach are obvious: the person at the remote site viewing the image has complete control over field selection. No significant diagnostic talent is required on the sending end, so it is possible for a technician to prepare and load slides onto the robotic microscope. The viewing can occur at the leisure of the viewer. The major disadvantage is the cost of the hardware.

The third and newest technology is known as whole slide imaging or virtual microscopy. Neither of these terms are particularly accurate, because one does not have to image the entire slide, and although no microscope is used during the slide viewing process, there is certainly a real microscope or microscope-like device involved in the image capture process. Therefore, the term "wide-field" microscopy has been proposed as a perhaps more accurate alternative. In this approach, a high resolution digital scan of the microscope slide is captured in advance, typically creating an enormous data set (gigabytes of data). This image is made available on a specialized image server which can then deliver portions of the image, as requested, to a remote internet connected computer. At the remote site, the remote pathologist can view this pre-captured image as if he/she were looking at the original microscope slide, including changing the magnification as well as "moving the slide" to select the desired field of view. This is done via a web browser or other internet-linked software interface. As the pathologist "moves" the slide or changes the magnification, this is translated into a request for the new image which the image server addresses by extracting the appropriate information from the image data set and sending it to the viewer. The end result is an interface which more closely approximates the current practice of pathology, and thus is likely to be better received. The viewing interface often provides a low magnification view of the entire slide, and a simple click allows the user to jump to a high magnification, high resolution image of the corresponding part of the data set. This technology requires very expensive equipment to capture the image data set, and additional equipment to serve the images through the internet. The capture process is time consuming, and can take between 10 and 30 minutes to capture an entire slide, although new equipment is being touted to be able to accomplish the entire scan in a few minutes, and undoubtedly future advances will reduce this to seconds.

Uses for Telemicroscopy

Telepathology

Of the various "tele-" terms used in pathology, the one least consistently used is "telepathology". For purposes of this discussion, I define telepathology as the use of any of the telemicroscopy technologies to make the *primary diagnosis* for the specimen (as opposed to consultation or case presentation) from a remote site.

Despite the technical feasibility and numerous "trial studies", telepathology has not caught on except in limited areas. The reasons are multifold. The smaller institutions which are most likely to benefit from electronic consultation are the least likely to have or be able to afford the equipment necessary to request the digital consultation. Most studies into the "success rate" of telepathology have shown about a 98% concordance rate between the telepathology diagnosis and the diagnosis rendered when the actual slides are examined by the same pathologist. Although 98% might constitute good odds for a financial investment, discordance in one out of every 50 cases is not an adequate diagnostic goal. Studies which have suggested that telepathology is more cost effective have almost invariably compared costs to an on-site pathologist. This analysis usually does not take into account that evaluating cases by telemicroscopy takes much longer than routine examination of glass slides – in general 5-20 times as long - because pathologists are simply not used to looking at images on a monitor and making their diagnoses based purely on these images. There are additional costs associated with the remote transcription, remote editing, and remote report distribution which are usually not included in the total cost of the telepathology solution. Plus, the larger specimens which require pathologist examination and therefore have to be sent to the telepathologist's site are often excluded from the study. Finally, and perhaps most importantly, there are very few diagnoses which cannot wait the 12-18 hours needed to send the slides via an overnight delivery service to almost anywhere in the world. As a result, the impact of telepathology, in most practices, has been predominantly as a marketing ploy.

Licensing is also a major issue for telepathology. Many states have already passed laws directly addressing the use of telemedicine, indicating that if the patient is in their state, any physician making a diagnosis on that patient, even if via some telemedicine technology, must be licensed in that state. The ability of the remote telepathologist to bill for these services, and the likelihood of third party payers paying for this service is also an unresolved issue. Finally, medical-legal concerns include such things as the responsibility of the remote pathologist for the content of portions of the slide not shown or available to him or her through the remote technology, as well as documentation of what the remote pathologist actually saw.

Telemicroscopy is evolving, however. The rapidly developing digital acquisition technology, image compression algorithms, inexpensive digital storage media, and higher bandwidth transmissions are making possible the concept of a usable "virtual microscope slide". However, for the time being, the time required to scan the slide, the cost of the equipment, and the fact that one would still be viewing the images on a monitor rather than through the microscope will remain barriers to the general acceptance of this technology for a number of years.

Teleconsultation

In contrast to using the technology of telemicroscopy for primary diagnosis, its use for pathologist-to-pathologist consultation on a small number of difficult cases has much greater utility. When used to replace the informal "hallway" consultation, the pathologist at the sending institution can get essentially an immediate "informal consult" from an expert anywhere in the world. Licensing and liability issues are minimized since the sending pathologist still retains responsibility for the case. Assuming you can find someone willing to render an opinion in this way, this approach can incorporate an outside expert's opinion without delaying the case for the time it would take to send the slide for a more formal reading. This hastens workflow in the practice, allows for rapid and more accurate diagnoses (improves patient care), and can be very educational for the pathologist at the sending institution. Examples of uses for teleconsultation include after hours frozen sections (the resident is on site but the attending pathologist is not), specialty consultations during frozen section (the attending pathologist is on site, but the case requires the input of a colleague with subspecialty expertise), and sharing cases with an off-site clinician.

Tele-education and Teleconferencing

One final use for telemicroscopy which should be mentioned because it will become an increasingly important part of the future practice of pathology is that of tele-education. The same technology which makes telepathology possible can be alternatively leveraged to provide continuing medical education. This is a natural offshoot of the fact that the larger medical centers which are more likely to have access to the hardware necessary to "broadcast" educational conferences are the same centers which have a high concentration of clinical expertise. Using the internet as the communication medium requires that "recipient" stations merely be equipped with a web browser. Tele-education can be accomplished either with pre-packaged training modules which the "student" can view at their leisure, or by real-time conferencing. Video streaming via the world wide web provides the visual information (perhaps two channels – one for a view of the speaker and another for a view of either the projected slides or a through-the-microscope view). The audio information can be provided via a telephone conference call or also through the web interface. The former allows "secure" communication which can preserve patient confidentiality when specific patients need to be discussed. As medical care delivery, especially in pathology, becomes more centralized, tele-education still allows pathologist participation in patient care conferences, morbidity and mortality conferences, tumor boards, as well as didactic conferences for physicians in training.

Wide-field digital microscopy and the future of pathology

Of course, once images of slides have been acquired using wide-field digital microscopy, one does not have to send those images to another institution. They could, in theory, be used in the day-to-day practice of pathology on-site. In fact, there are many pathologists who believe that within another five or ten years, microscopes will be a thing of the past, and pathologists will be sitting in front of their computer screens making diagnoses. Arguments which have been used in support of this belief include analogies to what has occurred in diagnostic radiology, the greater flexibility afforded by being able to view the slides anywhere, and eliminating the need to move glass slides from place to place. Sure, the equipment is expensive, it takes quite a while to scan each slide, and the data sets produced are enormous, posing long-term storage problems as well as network bandwidth bottlenecks. However, technology is advancing at an alarming rate. When I bought my first computer (a Mac Plus) in 1988, it contained a 5 MHz processor, 1 MB of RAM, and a 10 MB hard disk drive. My most recent purchase (a G5 Mac) in 2005 contains dual 2.5 GHz processors, 2 GB of RAM, and 250 GB of disk space. That's a 1000 fold increase in processing capacity, 2000 fold increase in memory, and 25,000 fold increase in disk space, for almost exactly the same cost, in just under 17 years. Network speeds have increased approximately 20,000 fold in the same time period. In addition, these parameters have not been increasing linearly, but rather exponentially. Clearly, the next five to ten years will yield similar advances which will overcome the current hardware limitations of routine wide-field digital microscopy.

Although I am a strong proponent of new technology in general, I am going to take the somewhat controversial position of stating that I do NOT feel that wide-field microscopy will significantly change the day-to-day practice of anatomic pathology in my clinically-active professional lifetime, and by that I mean 10-20 years (hopefully!). Having said this, and even worse having put it in print, it probably will happen long before my prediction, but allow me to defend my current belief.

First, with respect to the analogy to diagnostic radiology, I do not think that this represents a particularly good analogy. Granted, digital imaging has transformed the day-to-day practice of radiology. When computerized tomography began producing the first digital image as the primary data set, radiologists were uncomfortable with the concept of reviewing these on computer screens, and the data was therefore transferred to the more familiar medium of large format film for reading. Eventually, the need to move, file, store, relocate, re-file, copy, and hopefully not lose these films became too much of a burden, especially since computerized tomography and then magnetic resonance imaging starting producing so much film, that a transition was made back to viewing the primary data set – the digital image. Once accepted, the next obvious move was to take the remaining traditional plain films and convert those to digital, and now many radiology practices are entirely digital, with no films to develop, file, or store. By analogy, the argument is that pathologists are currently in that "uncomfortable with reviewing images on computer screens" stage, which time will overcome. Clearly there is some truth to this, and a number of telepathology trials have shown that a pathologist takes significantly longer to review a case by digital imaging than when presented with the glass slides, but with time and practice that difference began to decrease. However, the analogy is far from a perfect one. In most cases, the goal of the radiologist is to develop a differential diagnosis, not to make a definitive diagnosis. This is the reason that the "bottom-line" of most radiology reports is an "impression" rather than a diagnosis. For pathology, in contrast, the goal and in fact the expectation is a definitive diagnosis (although that is not always achieved). In radiology, the image *is* the primary data set (in many cases, the *digital* image is the primary data set), and the "impression" is made based on interpretation of those images. The largest radiology studies may consist of 200-500 images, but the majority are in the range of 2 to 10 images. In contrast, in pathology, the primary data set is the tissue on the glass slide, or more accurately the actual specimen, and the diagnosis is made based on the entire specimen. A typical 40x high power field encompasses approximately 0.25 mm^2 of tissue. Assuming that this could be adequately represented in a single digital image (an issue debatable in itself since the resolution of the eye is much greater than that of a computer screen) the smallest surgical pathology case, a 2x2 mm biopsy viewed at 3 levels, 2 serial sections per level would result in approximately 100 images. A more significant resection producing even as few as 10 slides (one level each) where the tissue area is approximately 2.5 x 1.5 cm would translate into 15,000 images, although I will grant that these are not always viewed, in their entirety, at 40x. Arguing that most diagnoses can really be made from one or two key fields is rather pointless, since that same argument applies at present, yet the need to find those key fields as well as the legal environment in which we operate has not reduced the routine practice of surgical pathology to one section of one representative block for most cases.

Then, there is the issue of image quality. Is a digital image of the slide "as good as" the actual slide? Although the resolution issues have probably been adequately addressed, every pathologist knows that a glass slide is not perfectly flat, and one has to constantly refocus as one scans a slide to compensate for irregularities in the thickness of the glass slide, thickness of the cover-slip, thickness of the tissue, and thickness of the mounting medium. How will the pathologist viewing a digital image of the slide deal with an area which is not quite focused? Does anyone really think it will be considered "acceptable" for the pathologist to miss something in that area because the image was not particularly good? Even when automatic focusing technology at the image capture stage assures adequate compensation of the focus across the imaging field, there is still the issue that the digital image is captured at only a single focal plane, whereas on a glass slide the tissue does have some thickness, and focusing up and down in this "z-axis" can be useful in evaluating nuclear details, nuclear "overlap", and cytoplasmic granularity, and in distinguishing some artifacts from real irregularities in the tissue.

As discussed above, it is likely that the technological limitations on speed will ultimately be overcome, but for the time being, they are a practical reality. Capturing the digital data set corresponding to an entire glass slide takes minutes. This new step is interposed between all of the processing, sectioning, staining, and cover-slipping which currently occurs and the availability of the slides for viewing by a pathologist or resident. For a typical pathology laboratory averaging about 100 cases per day with an average of 10 slides per case (by the time one considers multiple parts and three levels each for biopsies), even a scan time of one minute would require over 16 hours to scan a day's load of slides. This does not include special histochemical stains and immunostains. Clearly, more than one scanner will be needed. Then, there is the image latency time while viewing the digital data set, that is, the time between when the pathologist "requests" a new image, either by "moving" the digital slide or changing the magnification, and when that new image is displayed. During this latency, the request is being sent over the network to the image server, the image server (potentially while also processing other requests from other users viewing other slides) is extracting the appropriate image information from the large data set, transmitting that image back over the network to the viewing station, and then being displayed to the pathologist. Although improving technology is clearly speeding up this process, it is not yet at the speed of light to which pathologists have become quite accustomed. A final practical limitation is the storage of these large image data sets. If one assumes a one gigabyte data set per slide, and we discussed a typical situation of approximately 1000 slides per day, that is a terabyte of disk space per day. Images could be deleted as cases are signed out, but then the record of what the pathologist actually saw is no longer available, and the potential advantage of being able to use these images for other purposes is also lost.

Current practical limitations aside, let us assume that technology advances to the point where whole slide images can be captured in zero time, that the network bandwidth and server processing speed are infinite so that image latency time is also zero, that the long term on-line storage capacity is infinite, and that all of this hardware and technology costs the end user nothing. What are the driving forces for adopting this technology? Even in this very theoretical setting, what real advantages will we achieve?

Telepathology has already been discussed. For those limited instances in which telepathology provides a useful solution, wide-field digital microscopy is one of the best solutions, if the equipment can be afforded. However, the current discussion is focused on the likelihood of wide-field digital microscopy changing the day-to-day routine practice of anatomic pathology.

Wide-field digital microscopy would allow me to view slides without having to actually bring the slides to me. What benefits might this have in the routine practice of anatomic pathology? It would allow me to view slides from my office, which in my particular situation is a couple of buildings away from the main signout area. It would allow me to view slides from home, which could permit home signout, but then I would also have to have easy on-line access to working draft reports for the cases, and potentially be set up for dictation of diagnoses, if this new accessibility is to result in faster signout of cases. For that matter, I could take glass slides home with me, so the only real advantage the digital technology affords is that I could access slides which were not available at the time I left work. Although there might be some minor advantages to multi-site access to the slides, there is nothing here sufficiently compelling to make me consider learning a new way to signout cases.

What about the effect on resident training? Would two or three of us looking at an image on a monitor be very different from reviewing the slides at a multi-headed microscope? Although it might take a little getting used to, I don't see this as a significant advantage or disadvantage. If I am at the computer terminal anyway, I am perhaps more likely to bring up digital images of the gross specimen, so that is a potential plus, but then I already have a computer terminal next to the microscope so there is no new capability there. Also, if I wanted to take advantage of the "anywhere-access" to the digital slides by signing out in my office or at home, the resident is removed from the signout experience, so wide-field digital microscopy is more likely to have a negative effect on resident training than a positive one.

If images from previous cases are kept on-line indefinitely, I potentially could have essentially immediate access to prior material from the same patient whose current material I am evaluating. That definitely would be a nice feature, and save time retrieving old glass slides from the files, but in reality the delay associated with retrieving old material is not a major issue, because other people exist who currently do this for me, and I can work on other cases while I am waiting. Also, as discussed above, the enormous size of the data sets generated by whole slide imaging technology create, at least for the time being, data storage problems which have not yet been resolved, and are unlikely to be resolved in the next 5 years, but perhaps in the next 10.

Once a large number of whole slide images are available on-line, the potential exists to index these by diagnosis, perhaps even annotate them highlighting key diagnostic features, and then allow me to access them when

I am contemplating a particular diagnosis and want to compare my current case to previous cases for which that diagnosis was made. Although this capability, in a different form, exists today (I could search the information system for a particular diagnosis, identify a case, and then pull the slides from that case), it is a cumbersome activity and therefore rarely used. Well indexed whole-slide images could greatly facilitate this process, assuming someone takes the time to do the indexing. Of course, banks of indexed, annotated whole-slide images could be set up for me to access without my having to change the way I do my day-to-day signout, so this is not a particularly compelling reason for me to abandon my microscope in my routine practice of pathology. In addition, there is nothing preventing these indexed image banks from being set up now with static images, but that has not been done at most institutions, suggesting the need is not too great.

There is one potential capability which, if it existed, even I admit would be sufficiently compelling to induce me to consider whole-slide imaging for my daily practice of pathology. If all of my slides were routinely digitally imaged, the potential exists for some computer algorithms to pre-review my slides, comparing cytologic and nuclear features against a bank of previously evaluated and diagnosed digital images, such that by the time the digital slides are presented to me for evaluation and signout, they are accompanied by a ranked list of suggested or likely diagnoses. Perhaps even key areas of the slides would have been annotated electronically to be sure I pay particular attention to those areas. This would clearly be a huge leap forward, and this capability, if it existed, would almost certainly convert the entire practice of anatomic pathology over to wide-field digital microscopy in one or two years. But that capability does not exist, and in fact is not likely to exist within the 10 year time frame under discussion.

In short, I think I'll hold onto my microscope for the time being.

Chapter 10

ELECTRONIC INTERFACES AND DATA EXCHANGE

Electronic data exchange between the pathology clinical information system and other institutional systems can save entry time, improve the accuracy of information, facilitate billing for services, and speed report delivery to clinicians. Electronic interfaces usually run unattended in the background, but do need to be monitored periodically to verify that the connection with the other system(s) is still open, and to process/handle any errors which may have occurred in either inbound or outbound messages. The main disadvantage of input interfaces (in addition to the complexity of setting them up and trouble-shooting problems) is the risk of introduction of duplicate or even erroneous information into the pathology information system.

This section provides an overall introduction to the architecture and components of generic electronic interfaces, as well as an introduction to the more commonly used message formats.

Architecture of an Interface

Interfaces are a combination of hardware and software which allow one information system to send or receive information to/from another information system. The information itself is sent in the form of discrete messages. Interfaces are either "Input" or "Output", depending upon whether the messages are inbound or outbound, respectively. Typical input interfaces for a pathology information system include such things as ADT streams (Admission/Discharge/Transfer), Data Conversion, and Order Entry. Typical output interfaces include results and billing.

Most interfaces consist of two separate software components, a communication handler and a translation processor. Between these two

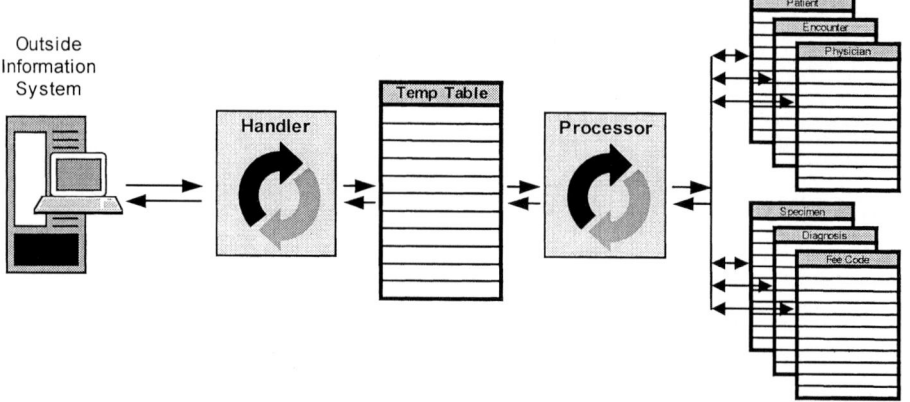

Figure 10-1: Elements of an electronic interface. Most interfaces contain two separate components which run independently. The communication handler deals with data transmission, and the interface processor deals with data interpretation. A "holding table" holds data waiting to be processed or sent.

components sits a temporary storage location, usually a database table (Figure 10-1).

Communication Handler

The communication handler in an interface is the software (and hardware) responsible for receiving the messages from an outside system and placing them in a message-holding input database table, or taking messages from a message-holding output database table and sending them to another system. The communication handler is responsible only for the details of communication, and generally knows nothing about the content of the message (nor does it care).

Different communication handlers are needed for different modes of communication. One of the most common is "real time" communication via a TCP/IP network connection. This is essentially an "always on" connection which provides nearly instantaneous communication between the two systems. This communication mode allows reports on specimens signed out in the pathology information system to appear in the hospital information system literally seconds later. Similarly, orders placed via the hospital information system can appear in the pathology information system before the specimen arrives in pathology. In addition to the actual data messages, the communication handlers of the two computers send and receive control messages which confirm that the communication line is open and which either acknowledge receipt of a message or request that it be sent again.

An alternate communication mode is a batch file. In this mode, multiple messages are placed into a data file. That file is then sent (either physically or electronically) to the recipient, who loads the contents of the file into the receiving system as a batch, and then processes each message individually. Batch files usually contain some error-checking messages which allow the recipient system to verify that the entire batch, and not just a part of the batch, has been received.

Because the duties of the communication handler do not require any knowledge of the content of the messages or of the database associated with the interface, it is the "simpler" of the two components. Once a vendor has written a communication handler for any of its applications, that same handler should work for all of its applications. Very little application-specific issues play a role in designing a communication handler, even for a custom database.

Interface (Translation) Processor

In contrast to the communication handler, whose primary concern is sending/receiving the messages, the translation processor is concerned only with the content of the message, and does not care how it got there or how it is going to get to its destination. For input interfaces, the translation processor is responsible for getting a message from the message-holding input database table, breaking up the message into its component data elements and appropriately filing that information into the database of the recipient system. For output interfaces, the translation processor is responsible for gathering the needed information from the database, packaging it into a properly formatted message, and placing that message into a message-holding output database table.

Clearly, the translation processor requires a detailed knowledge of the database structure and the rules for data storage. As such, translation processors tend to involve a lot more programming than the communication component of an interface. A key element in the design of a translation processor is its underlying matching logic, and this needs to be carefully considered when setting up a new interface, especially an input interface. See the discussion below for the ADT interface for more information.

Interface "Languages"

For two computer systems to be able to "talk" to each other, they need to agree on some common communication method.

Consider the following analogy. All of the employees of company A speak English. All of the employees of company B speak Spanish, and all of the employees of company C speak German. Company A, B, and C decide to work together on a project, and need to be able to exchange information. A few possibilities exist. One of the languages could be chosen as the communication language, and everyone forced to learn that language. That's not particularly fair, and politically impractical if each company feels their language is the best one. Someone at company A could learn Spanish and German and act as a mediator, but if company A backs out of the collaboration, company B and C can't communicate with each other. Finally, some one at each company could learn a new language, say French, and make that the common language for communication. If another company decides to join the group, the rules for being able to communicate are clear. If someone at each company always speaks a common interface language, all of the companies will always be able to communicate.

Pathology information systems need to store information about patients, such as name, address, date of birth, and medical record number. Similarly, the hospital's admission system stores similar information, but probably not quite in the same way (different databases, different table structures, etc.). The hospital billing system also has to store the same information about these same patients, but again, most likely in yet another way. For these machines to transfer information between each other, two of the machines could learn to communicate in the same way as the third, but this requires vendors to work together. The problem gets only more complex as a fourth, fifth, and sixth machine are added. Alternatively, all three machines could learn a single, common language, and if the fourth, fifth, and sixth machines also learn this same common language, each machine only needs to learn a single new language and all of the machines can talk to each other. HL7, described in more detail below, is the "language" most medical information systems use to communicate with each other.

Message Formats

Interface messaging protocols are an attempt to provide a common method for disparate systems to share information. Messages usually consist of a number of different data elements. Two different approaches are used to encapsulate data within a message: syntax and semantics. Syntax identifies data by where it is placed within the structure of the message, and tends to be more precisely defined in messaging protocols than semantics, which addresses how the information is encoded at its pre-defined location.

In early messaging protocols, the data elements in a message were defined not by any labels or identifiers but rather simply by their position. This made for more compact messages and thus more efficient transmission, especially at a time when most communication modalities were slow. As communication speeds have increased, message size is no longer a major concern, and labeling of data elements via markup-tags is becoming more common.

Three main syntactic approaches are used to define storage locations within interface messages. With fixed-length fields, start and stop positions for each data element are predetermined by the rules of the interface, and leading or trailing spaces are added to the data elements so that they completely fill the allotted space. This approach has the advantage that each message will have a previously determined length. Data can be extracted from the message easily by jumping to its storage location at the known offset from the start of the message. The main disadvantage is that any information which might exceed the size of the pre-defined storage location has to be truncated to fit. If there is no data for a particular field, that field's position needs to be filled with spaces to maintain the positions of the other fields.

Another syntactical approach to interface communication is delimited messages. In delimited messages, each data element can be of any length, and its start and stop positions are determined by special characters called delimiters. This eliminates the restriction on field size. However, to extract information from a delimited message, one has to process the message sequentially from the beginning, counting each delimited field until the desired field is reached. With delimited fields, sub-fields can be defined by using a different delimiter within a field. For example, a name field, identified by one delimiter such as the vertical bar ("|"), can be subdivided into last name, first name, and middle name sub-fields using a different delimiter such as the caret ("^"). Although the delimiters add a little to the length of the message, data fields without values take up minimal space. The delimiters still need to be included so that subsequent fields are still preceded by the appropriate number of delimiters. Nonetheless, in settings in which many of the defined data fields lack values, delimited messages tend to be much smaller than equivalent fixed-length field messages.

A third syntactical approach to message formats which is becoming more popular is eXtensible Markup Language, or XML (*ex-em-el*). With XML, data elements are identified by markup-tags, essentially field labels which identify the meaning of each of the data elements. Each tag, which marks the beginning of a data field, must have a corresponding closing tag. For fields with no values for the data, the entire field, including the tags, can be removed from the message. Nonetheless, since a lot of space in the message is used by tags and labels rather than the actual data, XML messages are far less efficient than either delimited or fixed-length field messages. However, XML is far more flexible. Repeating fields are far more easily accommodated with XML, and tags can be embedded within other tags to encode hierarchical relationships.

Health Level 7 (HL7)

HL7 stands for "Health Level 7": "Health" because this is used for exchange of information in the healthcare environment; "Level 7" because this communication occurs in the seventh layer (the application layer) of the Open Systems Interconnect (OSI) model of network communication (see the Network Protocols section in Chapter 4 on Networking). The "7" is not a version number. HL7 was developed by the HL7 working group, a collection of initially 12 volunteers who set out to create a standard for information exchange in the healthcare environment. Version 1 of HL7 was released in 1987, and version 2 the following year. However, it wasn't until 1994 that the HL7 Working Group became an American National Standards Institute (ANSI) accredited standards organization. The most recent ANSI approved version is 2.5, adopted on June 26, 2003. "The HL7 Version 2 Messaging Standard is considered to be the workhorse of data exchange in healthcare and is the most widely implemented standard for healthcare information in the world" (www.HL7.org). Version 2 is a delimited message format.

HL7 messages consist of varying length "segments", each terminated by a carriage return (ASCII 13). Segments can be required or optional, and some may repeat. Each segment begins with a 3-character segment identifier followed by a series of variable length fields separated by field separator characters (delimiters). Fields are separated by a field delimiter, and can be subdivided into components by a component delimiter. Data is identified purely by its position in the segment, and the meaning of those positions is defined in the HL7 standard.

Although the HL7 standard specifies the structure (syntax) of the messages, it provides only minimal specifications for the content and coding (semantics) of the information contained within that structure. The HL7 standards do define encoding for common data types like dates, but do not define how string fields are encoded. Each information system can encode these data elements as it sees fit. Therefore, one computer system might use "I" for inpatient and "O" for outpatient in the "patient type" field, but another system might use "1" for inpatient and "2" for outpatient. These differences are responsible for statements such as "HL7 pseudo-standard" and my favorite "once you've set up one HL7 interface, you've set up *one* HL7 interface." It is unlikely that any HL7 interface set up for communication between two computers will be able to be used, unmodified, for communication between two different computers.

Version 3 of HL7 is XML-based. Although this standard has already been released, few information systems currently support it.

Common Interfaces for Pathology Information Systems

Most pathologists will never have to deal with the details of setting up or maintaining an interface. Pathologists will, however, have to consider the implications of having an interface, and should be familiar with both the advantages and disadvantages of each interface, and be involved in the decision making process for their own practices. Therefore, a brief description of the elements in the most common interfaces is presented here.

Admission/Discharge/Transfer (ADT) Interface

ADT interfaces are used to communicate information about patient "encounters" with the healthcare system. Most ADT interfaces use a real-time network connection (TCP/IP) as their communication method. Each ADT message contains a series of segments, the exact combination of which varies from system to system and with the event which triggered the sending of the message. Typical messages contain segments with information about the event, patient, visit, and the patient's insurance (Table 10-1). A sample ADT HL7 message is shown in Figure 10-2.

Table 10-1: HL7 Segments in a typical ADT message.

Segment	Description	Content
MSH	Message Header	Where is the message coming from, where is it going?
EVN	Event	What event triggered the message (admission, discharge, transfer, update patient info, etc.)?
PID	Patient Identification	Who is this message about?
PVx	Patient Visit	Information about the visit/encounter
GT1	Guarantor	Who has agreed to pay if insurance does not?
INx	Insurance	Insurance information
Zxx	Custom Segments	Anything both parties agree on

ADT interfaces traditionally operate in an "unsolicited" fashion. This means that any information about any patient having an encounter with the healthcare institution will be automatically entered into the pathology information system.

There are many advantages to having an Admission/Discharge/Transfer Interface. The most significant is that, for specimens received from inpatients and often outpatients, patient demographic information, encounter

```
MSH|^~\&|ADT|Link|Hub|SurgPath|20031216141934|YALE1|ADT^A08|20031216^887|P|2.3||
    ||
EVN|A08|20031216141930|||||20031216141930|
PID|1|0005576|700834|||TEST^ONE^^^^|||19650123|F||1|123 MAPLE AVE^^TORRINGTON^CT^0
    6790^|99|||||4|000|4800|023569874||||||||||||||
PV1|1|P|ADMU|3||||SINARD^JOHN^H^^||~~~|135||||2|||SINARD^JOHN^H^^|P|4800|610|60||
    ||||||||||||||||6||||20031212110334||||||  |||
PV2||60^||||||||||||
ZV1|PAIN||||20338|||||135|SURGERY||||||^^^^||||N||||||20338|||||||||||||||||||||||||
    ||||||||||||
GT1|1|R2843911|TEST^ONE^^^^||123 MAPLE AVE^^TORRINGTON^CT^06790^||||19650123|F||1
    |023569874||||||||||
IN1|1|STANDARD|5|MEDICAID CONNECTICUT|1000 STANLEY DRIVE^^NEW BRITAIN^CT^0605200
    00^|||(800)842-
    8440||||||19610819|20061225||3|TEST^ONE|1|19610819|123 MAPLE AVE^^TORRING
    TON^CT^06790^|||||||||||||||||123654789||||||1|F||2840611
IN2||023569874||||||147852369||||||||||
IN1|2|STANDARD|1|SELF-PAY|^^^^^|||||||||||5|TEST^ONE|1|19610819|123 MAPLE AVE^^TOR
    RINGTON^CT^06790^|||||||||||||||||||||||||||F||2840611
IN2||023569874||||||||
```

Figure 10-2: Sample HL7 formatted ADT message. In this example, each segment is started on a new line. In standard HL7 messages, the segments would be contiguous.

(visit) information, and insurance information are already in the computer system before the specimen arrives in pathology. This both saves time in data entry and increases the accuracy of the data. This information is also updated automatically, as the institution acquires updated data. Encounter information can include the names of clinicians, clinical teams, and admitting diagnoses, aiding in interpretation of the often illegible scribbling present on requisition forms accompanying specimens. Finally, as patients move from unit to unit during their stay in the hospital, this information is updated in the hospital information systems, and via the ADT interface can be updated in the pathology information system. Thus, when the pathology report is ultimately signed out, if the pathology system has the ability to sort reports by unit for distribution, the reports will go to the unit the patient is on at the time the report is printed, rather than where the patient was at the time the specimen was originally received.

Unfortunately, no good thing is without its downsides, and the often overlooked downsides of an ADT interface can be very significant, to the point that pathologists should seriously consider, based on the particulars of their practice and the source of any potential ADT data streams, whether or not the advantages outweigh the disadvantages. Having an ADT interface exposes the accuracy of the information in the pathology information system to the potential inaccuracy of the information coming from the hospital information system. Because there are generally more individuals entering information into the hospital information system than the pathology information system, many of whom may not be particularly vested in the accuracy of that information, the information in the ADT data stream can be filled with inaccuracies. We were particularly surprised by the frequency with which the gender information in the incoming data is inaccurate (we are pretty confident that we have the correct information in many of these instances, based on prior receipt of a PAP-smear or a prostate biopsy). Without proper filtration of the incoming data, a carefully curated patient data set in the pathology information system can rapidly become fraught with erroneous data.

Because ADT interfaces tend to be unsolicited, the vast majority of patients who are entered into the system represent patients from whom the pathology department will never receive a specimen. The situation would be different for a clinical pathology system, where essentially every patient gets some sort of blood work, but only a small fraction of the patients who have an encounter with the healthcare system produce an anatomic pathology specimen. This means that either these patients fill up the system, increasing the possibility of accidentally accessioning a subsequent specimen to the wrong patient, or these patients need to be deleted from the system.

Great care has to be given to understanding the matching logic used by the interface processor for the ADT interface. As new messages containing patient demographic information are received from the outside system, the interface processor needs to decide whether this is a new patient, in which case it should add a new patient to the database, or whether the incoming information relates to a patient which is already in the database. In the latter case, the information in the database should be updated with the "new" information about this patient. One can readily imagine the consequences of a mistake in this matching process. If the interface processor mistakenly thinks that the "Mrs. A. Jones" in the incoming message is the same as the "Mrs. B. Jones" already in the database, and changes the information on Mrs. B. Jones to that of Mrs. A. Jones, then not only is the information on Mrs. B. Jones lost, but Mrs. A. Jones has just inherited all of Mrs. B. Jones' medical history. On the other hand, if the matching logic is too restrictive, the pathology information system will rapidly end up with twenty or thirty instances of Mrs. A Jones, perhaps with elements of her history spread out amongst her various instances. Understanding and controlling the balance of this matching logic is the crucial element which will determine whether this interface is a time saving benefit or a horrendous management nightmare.

Using the patient name as the only basis for matching logic in an ADT interface is clearly not a good idea. Something more unique is needed. Many ADT interfaces use a presumably unique field such as the medical record number to perform its matching logic (although we are all, undoubtedly, familiar with patients who have more than one medical record number from the same institution). This can help prevent duplicate entries of the same patient, but only if EVERY specimen in the pathology information system comes from the institution which provides the ADT interface. Medical record number based matching logic can be a significant problem for practices which have an outreach program. If the pathology department has previously received a specimen on this patient, perhaps review of an outside biopsy, then that patient will be in the information system, but may not have a medical record number associated with it. When the new message is received, with a medical record number, the interface processor will not be able to find an existing patient with that medical record number and will create a new instance of the patient. The visit account number information will be associated with the new instance. Now, imagine a specimen arrives in pathology from that patient. The accession team has two choices. If they put the specimen with the new instance of the patient, the previous material remains with the old instance, so a working draft report for the new specimen will indicate that there is no old material on that patient. On the other hand, if the new specimen is added to the original instance of the patient, the old material will be identified, but the new specimen will not be able to be linked to the visit information (including the account number) because that information is associated with a "different" patient, so the billing will not go smoothly. The only solution is to merge the two instances of the patient, and to do so in a timely fashion. One must be careful, however, about how many users are given the ability to merge patients, since inappropriate merges can have tremendous medical consequences and can be very difficult to undo.

Billing Batch Interface

Because the vendors of pathology information systems do not want to take on the responsibility of keeping their system up to date with all the most recent rules and regulations associated with billing insurance carries for medical procedures, most pathology LIS's do not produce files that are sent to payers. Rather, the billing interface routines collect the billing data from a period of time, often one day, and assemble it with patient demographic and insurance information and transfer it to some other billing system which handles the details of the billing logic associated with payers. This transfer of information occurs through a billing interface.

Billing interfaces usually operate in batch mode. Rather than sending a billing message as each specimen is signed-out, batches are generally compiled once a day for all charges posted since the previous batch was complied, and then an HL7 formatted batch is created and saved as a text file. This file is then transferred, either electronically or by some other method, to the billing system which reads the file and processes the information.

Billing batch files typically contain, in addition to the segments described above for ADT messages, the segments listed in Table 10-2.

Table 10-2: Additional HL7 segments contained in billing batch files.

Segment	Description	Content
BHS	Batch Header	General info about batch (batch #, date, etc.) [occurs once per batch; usually at beginning]
MSH	Message Header	Same as ADT. Marks start of new patient in batch.
FTx	Financial Transaction	Fee codes and quantities [once per fee code]
BTS	Batch Trailer	Summary data to check completeness of batch [once per batch; usually at end]

Billing messages tends to vary more than ADT information because of the greater diversity of billing systems in general. However, it is difficult to imagine managing the billing needs of a busy anatomic pathology practice without relying on the information system to produce some sort of billing files. The information system should have the ability to specify a billing type for each specimen accessioned, and based on that billing type, the billing interfaces should assemble the information into appropriate batches for proper subsequent handling. This routing allows, for example, separation of professional from technical charges.

Results Interface

Results interfaces allow the information from a signed out case to be exported to another hospital information system, ideally one to which the clinicians have access. Results interfaces are generally real-time, so that the results are sent as soon as the case is signed out.

Results messages, as with the ADT messages, begin with MSH segments and contain EVN, PID, and PVx segments. They also contain additional segments with the result information (Table 10-3).

The advantages of some sort of results interface are obvious. Clinicians would like to get their results as soon as possible. They often have access to some centralized hospital information system, but generally not direct access to the pathology information system. By transferring the results of signed out anatomic pathology reports to an institutional electronic medical record (EMR) system, clinicians with appropriate access can look up this

Table 10-3: Segments present in many HL7 results interfaces.

Segment	Description	Content
ORC	Common Order	If the result is in response to the order, this provides the link back to the order
OBR	Observation Request	Identifies the test whose result is being sent
OBX	Observation/Result	The result; in AP, the text of the report

information as soon as it is available. This can save numerous phone calls to the pathology department. In addition, if the EMR system has appropriate auditing capabilities, many of the responsibilities for compliance with HIPAA regulations requiring monitoring of access to protected healthcare information can be transferred to the institution, out of the pathology department. These EMR systems may also have document archiving capabilities (the ability to store original as well as amended versions of reports), making up for a deficiency which may be lacking in the pathology information system.

For the most part, results interfaces are a win-win situation. However, care needs to be taken on the part of the pathology department to assure that the information is appropriately stored and displayed in these systems and therefore is not misinterpreted by reason of being ambiguously presented. A one or two line "window" is generally not sufficient for the multi-line, often quite long anatomic pathology results (see discussion in Chapter 6). Also, since HL7 is an ASCII text communication method, it is generally not possible to send formatting information or images via this interface. (Although modifications to the HL7 standard can accommodate an ASCII encoded binary image as part of the HL7 message, few systems currently support this.) This means that formatted data which might look quite nice in the pathology information system may look very different and almost unreadable once received into the EMR system. It is important for pathologists to take an active role in determining how results of pathology evaluations are displayed in EMR systems. As these systems become more and more common, the data in the EMR system, rather than the printed patient report, is becoming the primary means by which pathology results are communicated to clinicians.

Recipient electronic medical record systems usually have a limited number of generic "containers" into which it will insert the results for access and display by hospital clinical staff. One of the key fields, generally a required field, is the type of test for which the result is being reported. This "list of tests" goes by a variety of different names, often containing the word "master" like "master test directory" or "charge master list". In laboratory medicine, there is a long but defined list of available tests. In anatomic pathology, however, anything can be received for evaluation, and in almost any combination. This concept can be difficult for the interface programmers in the EMR system to grasp, since they need to build a dictionary of tests and want to know what to put in that dictionary. Most EMR systems will not accept simply a free text description of what was received. Therefore, it is often necessary to define the anatomic pathology "tests" by a handful of very generic terms like "Surgical", "Cytology-GYN", "Cytology-FNA", "Consult", and "Autopsy", or even just one very generic "Anatomic Pathology". The consequence of this is that it can be harder to locate a particular anatomic pathology result in the EMR system. When a clinician calls up the patient in the EMR system, they are generally presented with a list of tests. If they want to look up the glucose, or the bilirubin, they can click on these test names to get the result they are looking for. If they want to look up an anatomic pathology result, however, it is likely to simply say "Surgical Specimen" or "Anatomic Pathology". This in general is not a problem, since most patients have a relatively limited number of anatomic pathology specimens, and these can often be further identified by the date of the procedure. However, if a particular patient has a liver biopsy and a bone marrow biopsy and a lymph node biopsy and a thyroid FNA, the clinician looking for a particular result may be presented with four "Anatomic Pathology" listings, and have to access each one to find the one they are looking for.

One final issue to be considered concerning results interfaces relates to amending reports. If a pathologist notices an error in a report just after signing it out, some pathology information systems may allow the pathologist to "un-signout" the case without formally amending it, since the report has not yet been mailed to anyone. However, with a real-time results interface, it is very possible that, seconds after issuing the signout command in the pathology information system, someone is viewing that result in a recipient system. Therefore, any changes to the report after signout, even if only a minute after signout, must be done via a formal amendment.

Results Interfaces and Outreach Material

The presence of a significant amount of outreach material in an anatomic pathology practice can also have implications for the setup and operation of a results interface. Most commonly a practice receives the majority of its material from a single "client", the institution housing the practice, and has an ADT interface from that client. However, the practice also receives, as an outreach laboratory, material from a number of other physician practices and/or surgical centers in the geographical region. The pathology information system has a results interface to the housing client. If the specimen being reported out of the pathology information system came from the housing institution (either an inpatient or an outpatient visit/encounter), the result is sent to the institution's electronic medical record system. If the specimen being reported was received as an outreach specimen from a physician treating a patient who is not and never was a patient of the housing institution, that result is not sent to the institution's electronic medical record system, since that patient will not be in the EMR. These two situations are pretty straightforward.

However, how should the pathology information system's results interface handle a result on a patient when the specimen was received in the pathology laboratory as an outreach specimen from a clinician not affiliated with the housing health care institution, but because of a prior encounter between that patient and the institution, the pathology information system knows that patient's institutional medical record number? This will not be a rare occurrence, since much of the outreach material will come from the same local vicinity and many of the patients will have been seen at the housing institution. The choice is binary: send the result to the institutional EMR, or don't.

Strong medical arguments can be made for sending the result. One of the rare definitive statements which can be almost considered a universal truth in medicine is that it is always better for physicians to have the most complete medical history possible for the patients they are treating. Sending the outreach results enhances the electronic record for that patient, and this can be directly relevant to subsequent therapy. From a medical perspective, all physicians would advocate this practice. In fact, if the outreach physician also happens to practice at the institution and the institution's EMR allows web-portal-based access to results, the clinician may have more rapid access to the result by this route rather than waiting for the report to arrive in the mail. Most patients would also advocate this practice as well, and probably many would consider this an added benefit of having chosen a clinician who happens to use the institution's pathology practice for processing and evaluation of their material.

So why not always send the results whenever possible? Consider another scenario. A patient receives most of his care at the hospital which houses your pathology practice. This patient, perhaps an employee of the hospital, is concerned he has a problem, but for whatever reason decides he is not ready to share that concern with his routine physician. Therefore, he drives thirty miles away to a private clinician's office for a biopsy, not realizing that that clinician sends his biopsy specimens to your pathology practice for evaluation. You evaluate and signout the case, and since you have that patient's hospital medical record number from a previous specimen, your pathology information system sends this to the hospital's EMR, where the patient's routine physician sees the result when reviewing the patient's medical history prior to his next routine visit. The pathology information system has done something that the patient was specifically attempting to avoid. This is likely to be an uncommon event, and as physicians we can argue that patients should not try to withhold potentially relevant medical information about themselves, but then that is really not our decision to make. A possible solution is some sort of query on the pathology requisition form, asking the submitting clinician to indicate whether or not the patient wants the information included in the hospital medical record for the patient, but then the pathology information system has to have the ability to record this choice and appropriately send or not send the result to the hospital's EMR.

One final issue to consider is that even if the pathology information system has the institutional medical record number on a patient for whom they are reporting an outreach result, and you have decided to send this result to the institutional electronic medical record system, this may not be sufficient for the institutional EMR system to file the result. Some institutional EMR systems store patient information not by medical record number but by encounter/visit number. In this case, there will not be an institutional encounter/visit number corresponding to the external patient-clinician encounter, so to file this result, either the pathology information system or the institutional EMR system will have to "make up" an encounter, and that may not be technically possible.

Chapter 11

CASE IDENTIFICATION BY DIAGNOSIS

Michael Krauthammer and John Sinard

Health care is an information-rich environment. Notes, reports and documents are used to communicate medical findings, procedures and recommendations. Discharge summaries document a patient's medical history and establish the context for a patient's current condition. Test results and imaging give a detailed picture of a patient's health status. Integrating such diverse information is an essential prerequisite for successful patient management. Given an ever-increasing volume of patient data, information integration is facilitated by computer systems that rapidly retrieve, present and process relevant patient data. However, without data standardization, computers would not be able to properly access medical data. This is because computers are notoriously bad at interpreting unstructured data, and unlike health care professionals, they do not have the intrinsic capacity to translate unstructured data into information, as in recognizing a test print out as a whole blood count, or in determining from the text of an anatomic pathology report whether or not the patient has a malignant neoplasm.

In order to translate medical data into structured and machine-readable information, it is necessary to code medical data according to an agreed-upon reference standard. In essence, each data point is paired with an identifier that unambiguously links a data value to a defined medical concept, as in labeling a potassium value as a 'potassium test result', or in defining "malignant neoplasm of the lung" as 162.9. These labels or codes are computer-readable, and enable the proper interpretation, routing and processing of the data value. Given the multiple roles and tasks of computer systems in health care, different reference standards exist. In Chapter 10, we discussed standards for communicating medical data between computer systems, such as HL7. This chapter introduces coding standards for the proper recognition and interpretation of medical concepts across computer systems, which is crucial for many basic and advanced functions of electronic health care systems. The focus here will be on the use of coding standards for retrieving data from anatomic pathology information systems, and includes a discussion of "free text" searching and auto-coding of medical documents.

Evolution of Coding and Information Retrieval

Coding of medical information was established long before the advent of computers. Classifying and categorizing diseases have been essential tools in the arsenal of public health officials for improving the health status of the general population. Three major needs drove the development of coding systems. The most obvious was that of dealing with synonyms: the terms "myocardial infarction" and "heart attack" refer to the exact same disease process, yet the actual phrases themselves bear no resemblance to each other. Assigning the same code to each of these terms allows them to be treated as equivalent in the categorization process. A second and related driving force was that of concept permanence. As our understanding of disease has evolved, terminologies have changed, yet the actual disease process, the "concept", remains the same. For example, purely scanning the text of the medical literature for the past couple of centuries would suggest that the disease "dropsy" has been completely cured – no new cases have been reported for decades. However, over the same period of time when dropsy was disappearing, congestive heart failure rapidly spread throughout the population. These are the same disease. Assigning each of these the same code allows persistence of the concept over time, despite changes in the terminology. Finally, the third major driving force for the development of coding was the need for statistical analysis of large amounts of medical data. If different institutions used the same coding system, thus creating a coding standard, data from one institution or study could be combined with data from another institution.

Computers both expanded and challenged the traditional use of medical coding standards. The inherent capacity of such standards to enable mapping between different expressions of the same medical concept is increasingly being used in integrated health care systems, where coding systems serve as common communication standard between departmental information systems. Thus, information can be transferred from one system to another without loss of its inherent meaning. Advanced medical coding systems include features for establishing relationships between medical concepts, which can be exploited by automated decision support applications.

However, for document retrieval, the speed of computers seemed to challenge the need to code every single document. Traditionally, the sheer impossibility of reading every document in vast medical archives fostered the use of master indices that contained summary codes of each available medical document. The index listed the medical record numbers of medical cases with the same or related medical codes. However, as more and more of these documents became available in electronic form, computers were able to quickly search the contents of vast numbers of medical documents for specific medical keywords, even when no codes were available. As we will discuss below, such keyword queries (also called free text queries) have both advantages and disadvantages over code-based document retrieval. Additionally, advanced free text processing, also called Natural Language Processing (NLP), enables computers to auto-code medical documents, thus potentially abolishing the need for manually coding every single document while retaining the clear advantages of coded medical information.

The Terminology for Terminologies

Not surprisingly, experts in the field of coding systems are somewhat particular in their use of terms to describe what they do. Unfortunately, the rest of us are not, and as such these terms have been widely used, and misused, in a variety of ways such that, when you see them, they could mean almost anything. However, we will try to shed some light here on the more common trends.

The first observation is that often the words "terminologies" and "coding systems" are used interchangeably. This is because terminologies, especially controlled terminologies, offer a formal way of defining medical concepts that can be uniquely identified by a concept code. Controlled terminologies (also referred to as controlled vocabularies) emphasize the important distinction between "terms" and "concepts". A concept is a thing or a process. A term is a name given to that concept. Several terms can be used to describe the same concept. We have already discussed this, using the example of "myocardial infarction" and "heart attack" as two terms which describe the same concept. Controlled vocabularies recognize this problem and employ pre-designed terms that are used consistently to describe the same set of concepts. This implies that users can't simply add new terms to the controlled vocabulary on-the-fly. Addition of new concepts and terms requires a process, review, approval, and formal release of a new "version" of the vocabulary. Similarly, the same process can be used to retire concepts or terms from the controlled vocabulary. Elements of a good controlled vocabulary are discussed below.

The term "nomenclature" is also used to describe a collection of terms, but with some subtle differences. Nomenclatures allow terms (or their corresponding concepts) to be combined according to pre-established rules, assembling more complex concepts from atomic ones. This results in a large number of possible concepts, and can accommodate inclusion of concepts not originally included in the terminology

Essentially all medical terminologies use some sort of a classification system for ordering their concepts. In its broadest sense, "classification" is the process which divides objects and/or concepts into different classes or groups based on attributes which they share and which distinguish them from members of other groups. This process results in a specific concept hierarchy, where concepts are in a parent-child relationship: the parent concept represents the more general (e.g. "neoplasm"), and the child concept the more specific entity (e.g. "lung cancer"). A generic classification system can be as simple as two groups (gender) or incredibly complex (dividing all living organisms up into species). Concept hierarchies can be quite extensive. This means that the objects or concepts are divided not only into groups, but those groups are divided into subgroups, and sub-subgroups.

Terminologies that employ a sophisticated classification system have many advantages. The grouping of related concepts within a specific branch of the hierarchy facilitates the lookup of a particular entity of interest, which can be located by drilling down from the more general concept. This is especially true if the codes used for these terminologies have a similar hierarchical structure themselves. In such a code, each successive digit or character of the code corresponds to a specific branch or sub-branch of the hierarchy. For example, "neoplasms" might be identified by codes in the 1000 to 1999 range, with "lung cancers" being coded from 1000 to 1099 and "colon cancers" being coded from 1100 to 1199. As a consequence, a simple search pattern such as "11**" (where the asterisk represents a wildcard character for any digit) would retrieve all colon cancers, while the more general search pattern "1***" would retrieve all neoplasms.

Terminologies are often distinguished by the classification system they use. A classification, in its strictest sense, often denotes a terminology with a uni-hierarchical classification: every concept has one, and only one, parent. A good example is the International Classification of Diseases (ICD). A "taxonomy" is a classification which is fully instantiated. Fully instantiated means that it is exhaustive, incorporating all members/concepts of the domain being classified. The most classic example of a taxonomy is that published in the *Systema Naturae* by the Swedish naturalist Carolus Linnaeus in the middle of the 18th century, in which he classified all of the then known organisms in the world, including 7700 plants and 4400 animals, into a hierarchical sequence of kingdom, phylum, class, order, family, genus and species. His taxonomy used a controlled vocabulary, which consisted of Latin terms rather than codes.

In contrast, an "ontology" is a knowledge classification system for concepts in a particular domain with some additional features. Ontologies may contain multiple hierarchies (a member can have multiple parents) and they support inclusion of concept properties and a variety of relationships between the concepts. This allows logical inferences to be drawn across members of the ontology. An example of a medical ontology is GALEN (Generalized Architecture for Languages, Encyclopedias, and Nomenclatures in medicine), which includes biomedical concepts such as diseases and symptoms.

A final term worthy of mention in this context is "nosology", the science of classifying diseases or the signs and symptoms related to those diseases. Any classification system used in medicine falls within the scope of nosology.

There are a number of factors which make development of stable medical terminologies very difficult. Classifications work best when there is a single principle by which members of the classification are ordered. This single ordering principle allows for a single hierarchy. However, human diseases can be and have been ordered by a large number of different principles. They can be grouped by the organ systems which they involve, or the etiologic agent, or the primary symptoms they produce, or by the method of treatment. For example, does a bacterial pneumonia get classified under infectious diseases, or under pulmonary disorders, or community-acquired diseases, etc. No one system is superior to another, as each is inherently useful in different situations. Another difficulty in building classification systems for medical concepts is that our understanding of diseases is constantly evolving. For example, many of the cases of what was formerly known as non-A, non-B hepatitis have since been discovered to be due to hepatitis-C, but not all of them. The concept "non-A, non-B hepatitis" needed to be divided. As a second example, Kaposi's sarcoma was originally known to be a malignant neoplasm which occurs in the setting of acquired immunodeficiency syndrome. Should it be classified as a neoplasm, or as a sign of a serious immune disorder? When it was subsequently learned to be secondary to Human Herpes Virus 8 infection, should it be reclassified as an infectious disease? All of the prior associations are still valid. How is the new information added? These issues significantly complicate classification systems in medicine, and that is before we even introduce the problem of concepts for which there is disagreement among the medical specialties as to the "correct" associations.

Elements of an "Ideal" Controlled Vocabulary

Terminology researchers have compared the usefulness of different classification systems and medical vocabularies (or terminologies) and started to think how such systems can represent medical knowledge for decision support and other knowledge-driven applications. To adapt medical classification systems to this end, they began to include ideas originally developed in ontology research that deal with conceptualizing and formalizing domains of interest, employing tools from several disciplines including philosophy, computer science, and linguistics. The core insights of this research have been spelled out in an already "classic" work by James Cimino[1] who described twelve necessary components for an ideal controlled vocabulary (Table 11-1), which he referred to as "desiderata". Designed to ensure proper

Table 11-1: **Required elements of a controlled vocabulary for medicine.**

Desiderata	
I	Content
II	Concept Orientation
III	Concept Permanence
IV	Nonsemantic Concept Identifiers
V	Polyhierarchy
VI	Formal Definitions
VII	Reject "Not elsewhere classified"
VIII	Multiple Granularities
IX	Multiple Consistent Views
X	Representing Context
XI	Graceful Evolution
XII	Recognize Redundancy

encoding of medical documents, these required elements included measures to formally represent medical knowledge and to ensure a smooth integration of terminologies into clinical information systems. We will discuss these required elements in the context of searching coded documents to retrieve specific medical information of interest.

The first required element, content, deals with the expressiveness of a terminology. There has to be sufficient breadth and depth of content to allow sophisticated coding of the medical documents, and thus a higher precision of document retrieval. Increased content can be achieved either by adding concepts as they are needed, or by encoding atomic concepts and combining them to obtain greater complexity.

Concept orientation highlights the difference between concepts and terms discussed above. The vocabulary should be built on concepts, each unambiguously defined and allowing for synonymous terms to refer to the same concept. This helps prevent the same concept from being encoded with two different codes, which would hamper document retrieval by creating uncertainty as to which codes were used in the first place. A non-

---

[1] James J. Cimino, Desiderata for Controlled Medical vocabularies in the Twenty-First Century. Originally presented at the IMIA WG6 Conference, Jacksonville, FL Jan 19-22, 1997; subsequently published in Methods Inf Med 1998 Nov; 37(4-5): 394-403.

vagueness requirement discourages the use of solely generic codes such as "diabetes", which may refer to several different diseases and thereby retrieve unrelated documents.

Concept permanence refers to the persistence of the meaning of a term which was present in a legacy version of a terminology. This requirement prevents the reassignment of codes from one concept to another when issuing a new version of a terminology, which would result in incorrect retrieval of documents that were coded previously. In practice, terminology designers are urged to "retire" codes that are not carried into a new version of a terminology. Retaining and renaming such concepts, such as renaming non-A, non-B hepatitis to hepatitis-C could incorrectly group legacy documents of unknown hepatitis type as hepatitis-C cases.

Nonsemantic concept identifiers is a departure from the traditional hierarchical codes in which the codes themselves have meaning. Such semantically meaningful codes exhibit some clear advantages in that they are somewhat human readable and easily allow for searching at different levels of detail. However, this benefit is offset by problems with concepts which do not fit into a single hierarchy and problems with expanding existing terminologies with novel concepts (one may not have enough unused numbers for a particular region of the terminology). What is recommended is a meaningless code, usually an integer, which can be assigned sequentially as new concepts are added to the terminology. Although this can complicate searching for related concepts, in the long run it allows for the greatest flexibility and longevity of the vocabulary.

Multiple hierarchies have already been discussed. Many concepts are appropriately classified in two or more categories, created by different ordering principles. This results in some concepts having multiple parents. As another example, "retinitis pigmentosa" may be classified as a genetic as well as an ocular disorder. Given an intelligent interface, a query for genetic disorders should be automatically expanded to include any child concepts and codes of that concept, including retinitis pigmentosa.

The desiderata also spell out requirements that are not directly related to coding medical concepts. The requirement for formal definitions deals with encoding different types of relationships between concepts, and are useful for formally representing medical knowledge (think of a "caused by" relationship of the concept "Pneumococcal pneumonia" to another concept "*Streptococcus pneumoniae*"). These relationships are useful for decision support and other knowledge-driven applications for triggering appropriate actions (such as sending an alert for the possibility of a bacterial pneumonia in the case of a sputum culture positive for *Streptococcus pneumoniae*). Context representation adds another layer of relationships and concepts that encode the contextual facts about a domain of interest, which can be tremendously helpful in assuring that concepts are used and handled properly.

Some of the remaining required elements directly related to the coding of medical concepts include desideratum VII, rejecting "not elsewhere classified" (NEC). NEC is a "back-up" concept for not yet classified medical concepts. The problem created by the use of this concept is that of semantic drift: as newer version of the terminology introduce novel concepts which previously may have been included under NEC, the scope and thus meaning of the NEC code changes over time. This negatively affects the retrieval of NEC-encoded documents. The requirements for multiple granularities and multiple consistent views recognize the fact that vocabularies are used by different user groups, each of which may require access to different depths (details) of a terminology. A general practitioner may not need access to concept codes that are regularly used by a neuro-radiologist to describe vascular brain abnormalities. Designers should ensure that these levels are actually present in the terminology, that is, that general concepts as well as detailed concepts are equally represented.

The two final requirements of an ideal vocabulary, graceful evolution and recognition of redundancy, are concerned with the evolution and growth of terminologies over time. While terminologies usually become more expressive as they evolve, due to newly added concepts, this expressiveness may actually cause problematic redundancies with regard to how something can be coded. Examples include the introduction of pre-coordinated concepts, replacing the need to code with two or more atomic concepts. As seen before, document retrieval may suffer as a result from uncertainty with regard to how the concept was coded in the first place.

Coding Systems used in Anatomic Pathology

Having discussed a number of the design elements of terminologies, let us now turn to terminologies used in anatomic pathology. Medical terminologies come in various shapes. Some terminologies encode medical concepts at a very broad level (such as discharge codes), others at a very granular level (such as codes for medical tests). There even exists a "mother" terminology that enables the translation and mapping of other medical terminologies.

Current Procedural Terminology (CPT)

The current procedural terminology was originally released in 1966 and is currently in its fourth formal edition (CPT-4), although new versions are released each year and have begun to be identified simply by the year of release (e.g., CPT 2005). The CPT codes are a set of codes with associated descriptions which identify procedures and services which can be performed by physicians and other health care providers. More than any other code, these are often referred to, in slang, as the "billing codes". CPT is maintained and copyrighted by the American Medical Association. It has been a standard code set used by the Health Care Financing Administration (renamed the Centers for Medicare and Medicaid Services in July 2001) for many years. In 2000, the Department of Health and Human Services designated the CPT Code Set as a national standard for coding physician services, as designated by the Health Insurance Portability and Accountability Act (HIPAA) (see Chapter 12 for more details).

CPT is a numeric, partially hierarchical coding system. Base codes consist of 5 digits. The largest group of codes are for surgery, and encompass all codes beginning with a 1, 2, 3, 4, 5, or 6. These are further divided by organ system. All pathology and laboratory codes begin with an "8". Anatomic pathology codes all begin "88", with autopsy codes beginning "880", cytopathology codes beginning "881" and surgical pathology codes beginning "883". Multiple two character alphanumeric modifier codes can be added to the base codes, separated by a hyphen.

Only six base codes exist for surgical pathology, namely 88300, 88302, 88304, 88305, 88307, and 88309. Therefore, for report retrieval by diagnosis, CPT codes are not very helpful. However, they could be used, as a first approximation, to try to distinguish a biopsy from a resection specimen, since these are usually coded differently (although not for all specimens, e.g., skin resections).

International Classification of Diseases (ICD)

One of the most widely used medical terminologies is the International Classification of Diseases (ICD). Descended from the London Bills of Mortality from the seventeenth century, it was originally published with the initials "ICD" in 1900 as the International List of Causes of Death (by the International Statistical Institute), and its sole purpose was the categorization of causes of death so that data could be compared and combined for statistical purposes. In 1948, the World Health Organization (WHO) added codes for morbidity to the mortality codes, and renamed the classification system as the International Classification of Diseases. The ICD has been through several revisions, the most recent of which is the 10th edition, published in 1993.

In the middle of the last century, the US Public Health Service and the Veterans Administration investigated expanding the use of ICD for indexing hospital records by disease and operations. This expanded use was formally codified with the release of an adapted version of ICD-8 in 1968. Additional modifications were made, but use within the United States was sporadic. In the late 1970s, a multi-organizational working group convened by the United States National Center for Health Statistics began developing a "clinical modification" of ICD-9, and in January 1979, ICD-9-CM was released to be used throughout the United States. It was adopted by the Health Care Financing Administration (now the Centers for Medicare and Medicaid Services) in April, 1989, and became a HIPAA designated code set in 2000. ICD-9-CM, although fully compatible with ICD-9, contains greater detail than its parent code, added to allow greater ability to index medical records, morbidity data, and the reasons for medical encounters. Most diseases processes (as well as causes of death) can be coded using ICD-9-CM. One of the most common uses for ICD codes is to "justify" the CPT codes used to bill a case. Therefore, although ICD codes are not billing codes per se, it is unlikely that a bill will be paid by a payer unless accompanied by appropriate ICD codes. Most payers have complex tables and algorithms by which they compare the CPT and ICD codes for a submitted claim to attempt to determine whether or not a particular procedure (CPT code) was appropriate given the patient's diagnosis (ICD code).

Although ICD-10 was released over a decade ago, it has not been widely used in the United States, although a clinical modification for ICD-10 is being prepared, and a switch is predicted in or after 2008. The switch will not be easy, as ICD-10 uses a completely different coding format than ICD-9 and has twice as many categories. Therefore, for the time being, ICD-9-CM remains the most commonly used version.

ICD-9 uses predominantly a 3-digit numeric base code to hierarchically group disorders according to major disease categories (Table 11-2). Where greater subdivision was desired, a fourth digit was added, usually separated from the base code by a period. The clinical modification to ICD-9 added additional fourth-digit subdivisions, as well as some fifth-digit subdivisions to increase the clinical detail. For each of these subdivisions, numbers 0 to 7 are used for specific items. "8" indicates "other" (not elsewhere classified) and is used for coding rare, no specifically listed disorders. "9" indicates "unknown" (not otherwise specified) and is used where the information available is incomplete.

ICD-9-CM is a true diagnosis coding system, and can be very useful for document retrieval. Although the rather general nature of the coding system does not permit retrieval of specific pathologic diagnoses (e.g., "Adenocarcinoma of the Lung"), broader categories of diseases can be relatively easily and accurately retrieved (e.g., 162 = "Malignant neoplasm of trachea, bronchus, and lung"). The broad nature of the categories

Table 11-2: ICD-9 Categories by Base Code

Code	Disease Category
001-139	Infectious/Parasitic Diseases
140-239	Neoplasms
240-279	Endocrine, Nutritional, Metabolic, Immune Disorder
280-289	Diseases of Blood/Blood-Forming Organs
290-319	Mental Disorders
320-389	Nervous System and Sense Organ Disorders
390-459	Diseases of the Circulatory System
460-519	Diseases of the Respiratory System
520-579	Diseases of the Digestive System
580-629	Diseases of the Genitourinary System
630-677	Complications of Pregnancy
680-709	Diseases of the Skin
710-739	Diseases of the Musculoskeletal System
740-759	Congenital Anomalies
760-779	Conditions Originating in Perinatal Period
780-799	Symptoms, Signs, Ill-Defined Conditions
800-999	Injury and Poisoning
V01-V84	Factors Influencing Health Status and contact with Health Services
E800-E999	External Causes of Injury and Poisoning

promotes more accurate coding, and personally we have found that when one wants a high sensitivity search, at the expense of specificity, searching by ICD code is often the best choice. The hierarchical nature of the code also allows searching over a range of codes to retrieve related diseases.

There are, nonetheless, several deficiencies with ICD-9. Most strikingly for pathologists, there is no inherent mechanism to specify the histologic subtype of a tumor, beyond indicating whether it is benign or malignant, and primary or secondary. ICD-9 also offers a limited ability to accurately code mental disorders, and most clinicians rely on the American Psychiatric Association's Statistical Manual of Mental Disorders (DSM-IV) for assigning appropriate codes.

For those involved with tumor registries, another ICD system, the International Classification of Diseases for Oncology (ICD-O) exists. First released in 1976, the third edition went into effect in 2001. Unlike the standard ICD system, the ICD-O classification allows specification of the type of neoplasm, not just its location. ICD-O is a bi-axial classification system, including both a topography and a morphology code. The four character topography code includes a "C" followed by two digits, a decimal point, and then a third digit. The third digit further localizes the topography within the anatomic region specified by the first two digits, using ".9" for "not otherwise specified". ".8" is used for lesions which cross a boundary between two different sites. In some listings, the decimal point is omitted. The morphology code has two components: an "M" with a 4 digit numeric histology code, and a one digit behavior code. The histology and behavior codes are separated by a "/". The histology codes range from M8000-M9999, are hierarchical, and define the histogenesis and/or differentiation of the tumor. The one digit behavior code is either a 0 (benign), 1 (uncertain or borderline malignancy), 2 (non-invasive), 3 (malignant), 6 (metastatic or secondary site), or 9 (malignant, but uncertain as to whether primary or secondary).

The greater degree of specificity of the ICD-O system for malignancies make it a far more effective code for retrieving reports on malignant neoplasms. As such, this is the classification used by tumor registries. Coded information is reported to the state, and in many cases to the National Cancer Database (NCDB) maintained by the American College of Surgeons, and has allowed aggregation of cancer data nationally.

Systematized Nomenclature of Medicine (SNOMED)

The Systematized Nomenclature of Medicine (SNOMED) is one of the most advanced controlled biomedical terminologies to date. Its rich history reflects the investments of the College of American Pathologists (CAP) in the development of a terminology that meets the challenges of the modern health care enterprise. The code set is copyrighted and maintained by the CAP. Starting as the Systematized Nomenclature of Pathology (SNOP) in 1965, its name was changed to SNOMED in 1974 with the addition of expanded content which cut across medical specialties. A second revision, SNOMED-II, was published in 1979, and is the one currently integrated into most pathology information systems. Nonetheless, SNOMED continued to evolve. SNOMED-III, also known as SNOMED International, was released in 1993. A collaboration with the Kaiser Permanente organization resulted in the development of SNOMED Reference Terminology (RT), which was released in 2000 and featured many innovations such as the use of description logic and a relational database structure. 2002 saw the release of SNOMED Clinical Terms (CT), which represented a merger of the contents of the UK Read codes (named after James Read), which focused on primary care, with SNOMED RT. In 2003, the United States National Library of

Medicine signed a five year license agreement with the CAP allowing use of SNOMED CT throughout the United States. With the signing of this agreement, it is generally believed that SNOMED CT will become a universal standard for computer interoperability and exchange of medical information.

All of the versions of SNOMED are multi-axial (multiple hierarchies). The first edition had 6 axes, the second 7, and the third 11. SNOMED CT now supports 15 (Table 11-3). SNOMED CT follows most of the "desiderata" for controlled medical terminologies discussed above. Its content is impressive, featuring over 350,000 unique concepts with close to one million English-language synonyms. The codes themselves are non-semantic, allowing for future expansion. Over one million semantic relationships link SNOMED concepts among themselves. It is cross-mapped to several other vocabularies, including ICD-9-CM, Nursing Interventions Classification (NIC), Nursing Outcomes Classification (NOC), North American Nursing Diagnosis Association (NANDA) and Peri-operative Nursing Data Set (PNDS).

For document retrieval, documents are coded by using as many of the axes as appropriate for the medical data contained within the document. By combining codes for multiple concepts,

Table 11-3: Axes (hierarchies) supported in SNOMED CT.

Findings
Disease
Procedure and Intervention
Observable Entity
Body Structure
Organism
Substance
Pharmaceutical/biological Product
Physical Object
Physical Force
Events
Environments and Geographic Locations
Social context
Context-dependent categories
Staging and Scales

essentially any medical situation can be coded. In general, all of the axes will not necessarily be used for all documents. The usefulness of SNOMED is limited only by the accuracy and compulsiveness of the coder. This is, however, a real limitation. The existence of the code creates the capacity for very detailed coding, but at the current time no usable automatic coders exist for SNOMED CT, and developing one will not be a trivial process due to the complexity of the coding systems and, more importantly, to the complexity of medical records.

Unified Medical Language System (UMLS)

The Unified Medical Language System (UMLS) is maintained and distributed by the United States National Library of Medicine, and is one of the most comprehensive coding systems available. It represents a coding system in itself with over 1 million concepts and 5 million concept names (synonyms) that are derived from more than 100 source vocabularies. The UMLS Meta-thesaurus, the prime repository for these concepts, cross-maps similar concepts from different source vocabularies via unique non-semantic UMLS concept identifiers.

Often, there is a need to translate one coding schema into another. For example, one is interested in conducting a statistical analysis on some documents coded in ICD-9 and ICD-10. Automatically translating ICD-9 codes into ICD-10 codes would resolve the problem of merging the two datasets for the common statistical analysis. The Unified Medical Language System (UMLS) can be used to perform this code translation.

The idea behind UMLS is to foster the construction of information systems that incorporate the ability to process diverse types of coding schemas currently employed in the biomedical field. It is a resource for developers who are working at incorporating codes and coding schemas into health information systems, representing a one-stop solution for accessing any of the important biomedical terminologies (such as ICD, SNOMED and LOINC). It is also a research tool for the academic researcher interested in building intelligent systems in biomedicine. The UMLS provides several tools for these purposes, such as the Semantic Web, a small ontology of very generic biomedical terms that serves as a semantic bridge between the Meta-thesaurus concepts. Further, there are specific tools (SPECIALIST tools) for research and development in Natural Language Processing (NLP). NLP is concerned with mapping the free text of biomedical documents to structured information within the UMLS. One of these NLP tools is the Meta-Map Transfer (MMTx) program. MMTx is essentially an auto-coding tool, which maps lexical variants of document terms to their corresponding UMLS concept IDs.

Despite the tremendous utility of the UMLS for informatics research, it currently has a limited role in the day-to-day practice of pathology.

Information Retrieval and Natural Language Processing

The goal of searching through documents is to retrieve the subset of those documents which refer to a particular concept. This constitutes information retrieval. If the documents have been previously coded, prereducing each document to a list of coded concepts, then the search for a particular concept can be performed simply by looking through the lists of extracted concept codes for the code(s) corresponding to the concept(s) sought. If these codes happen to be pre-indexed, the searches can be performed much more quickly. As discussed above, information retrieval was one of the main driving forces behind coding in the first place.

Keyword-based information retrieval

The move from paper charts and documents to electronic archives challenged the pre-eminence of coding as the primary means of information retrieval in the health care field. The enormous processing power of current computers can be used to quickly search a large number of electronic documents for particular keywords, even when the documents are not coded in the first place. This process has been variably termed "free-text" searching, natural language searching, and keyword searching. Of these, keyword searching is probably the most accurate term. Searches are usually referred to by what you are looking for (keywords) rather than what you are looking at (free text), and "language" implies a greater degree of sophistication than is generally employed.

At its simplest level of implementation, computers can perform a word-by-word search through all of the documents in an archive, looking for a particular word or phrase. However, the time it takes to perform these searches increases proportionally with the number and size of the documents being searched, and this becomes an inadequate solution for any reasonably sized document archive.

The process of keyword searching can be greatly facilitated by building indices. In much the same way as indexing concept codes allows for concept based indexed searching, the building of word indices in which each word in all of the documents is pre-indexed permits rapid keyword based indexed searching. (In practice, the computerized word indexing usually ignores a pre-defined collection of noise words such as "is", "a", and "the", which would otherwise fill up the index.)

Indexed-based document retrieval usually uses Boolean operators (such as AND or OR) to identify appropriate word or code combinations in documents. However, formulating an adequate Boolean query can be quite difficult, and many users prefer to use simple lists of keywords and codes instead. This can be clearly seen in many online search services, which by default offer keyword-centric user interfaces. For users with more specific search needs, these services often offer advanced search pages, where users can access Boolean search options via clearly structured search forms.

There is a trade-off between code and keyword based document retrieval. The advantages of code-based document retrieval have already been discussed, and included the fact that a word is not necessarily a concept, and that lexical variations (including spelling variants and synonyms) will map to the same concept code. However, many studies have shown that the most commonly used codes in the health care field (mostly ICD-9 CM codes that are manually extracted for billing purposes), are inadequate for document retrieval (such as for research purposes). One of the key problems is the limited expressiveness (content) of ICD-9 CM, resulting in a high sensitivity but low specificity retrieval. Employing more comprehensive terminologies may alleviate this situation, including the use of nomenclatures such as SNOMED CT that offer atomic terms for creating any number of post-coordinated expressions. However, the latter strategy may introduce code redundancies that are difficult to track (see above).

The advantages of keyword-based queries lie in their ability to search for user-defined terminological expressions, and they are therefore very efficient at retrieving very targeted document instances. However, keywords fail to ensure complete retrieval of available document instances, as simple keyword searches do not address the lexical variations of free text. Usually issues such as capitalization are easily addressed, single vs pleural versions of words is sometimes addressed, and spelling variations as well as synonymy are rarely addressed. In addition, keywords searches ignore the semantic peculiarities of words (such as words with several meanings) and usually do not account for contextual cues that modify word meaning (such as negation of words).

Given the advantages and limitations of code and keyword-based queries individually, the two approaches can be used, in combination, to complement the respective strengths. The combination of keyword and code-based queries can actually retrieve documents with a higher precision than queries based on keywords or codes alone. Inclusion of codes ensures that lexical variations are addressed, and the inclusion of keywords ensures the retrieval of documents based on very specific terminological expressions.

As a side note, neither code nor keyword-based queries provide a means to rank retrieved documents. Documents are selected based on the presence or absence of some keywords or codes, leaving it up to the user to determine the relevance of each retrieved document. This is especially problematic in the case of literature searches (such as searches via PubMed), where adequate selection from a pool of millions of publications is crucial. This limitation of keyword and code-based document searches can be addressed by more advanced Information Retrieval approaches, such as word-statistical retrieval. Instead of treating each word in each document as equivalent, these techniques apply statistical approaches to weigh each word (or code) in the document according to the so-called "Inverse Document Frequency times Term Frequency" (IDF*TF) measure. This measure assigns more weight to "specific" rather than general words. What determines the final document rank is the sum of weights of each query word within the document. Word statistical approaches thus provide a better way to map query terms and codes to documents of interest.

Natural Language Processing

Often, we do not have the luxury of searching previously coded documents. Under these circumstances, we usually resort to the use of keyword-based searches. However, we identified several limitations that hamper keyword-based queries: the inability to recognize lexical variants as well as the inability to uniquely identify the semantics (meaning) of words. Natural Language Processing (NLP) offers several approaches to overcome some of these limitations. NLP should not be confused with natural language searching. NLP is not an information retrieval method per se, but rather a formalized process for extracting information from what, in the perspective of the computer, is simply a sequence of words.

The main aim of NLP is to add a syntactic and semantic layer to a free text document. Syntax describes various aspects of words in a sentence, including their part of speech (whether a word is a noun, an adjective, etc.), their constituency (whether a word belongs to a noun phrase, a verb phrase etc.) and their grammatical relations (the role of the word in the sentence, such as subject or object). In contrast, semantics refers to the *meaning* of words, sentences or paragraphs, and is usually expressed in annotating sentence constituents with defined word-categories from some domain ontology, or, more fitting for our discussion, from some controlled terminology. NLP is most often employed in "Information Extraction", the transformation of unstructured (so-called free) text (discharge summaries, pathology or radiology reports) into structured information that is machine-readable. Examples include the extraction of medication names, treating physicians, vital signs or diagnoses from discharge summaries. NLP also plays an important role in mapping natural language expressions to controlled vocabularies, as well as in advanced applications such as machine translation. NLP approaches range from very simple to very complex. It is therefore crucial to clearly understand the goal of a specific NLP application. For example, extracting the patient weight from a discharge summary may be accomplished via a simple regular expression such as "[\d\.]+ pounds" (any number and periods followed by the word 'pounds'), ignoring further syntactic or semantic aspects of the problem. However, if the goal is a higher-level understanding of a document, more sophisticated NLP approaches are needed.

NLP in the Clinical Domain

Natural language processing research and tools usually target everyday English, such as the English found in newspaper articles. Such English is quite different from medical English, and applying NLP tools to medical documents introduces some unique problems. Medical or clinical English is a so-called *sublanguage*, i.e., a language with fixed patterns of word compositions. It uses words from a few basic word classes (such as disease, patient, treatment), fixed word co-occurrence patterns (ways in which words or word classes can be combined) and omission of words, all of which have a profound impact on the use of NLP in the medical domain. Often, medical reports leave out whole sentence parts, without compromising the understandability of the report. This is possible because the context of medical reports and documents is well established. A radiology report saying nothing more than *"small calcified mass in left upper lobe"* is perfectly clear to any health care professional that deals with such types of reports. Expanding the phrase to a grammatically correct, complete sentence such as *"I observed a small calcified mass in the upper lobe of the left lung of the patient"* is not necessary. These omissions of sentence elements, although not always present, influence the use of NLP in the clinical domain. Indeed, for many medical NLP applications, it is sufficient to concentrate on the so-called noun phrases (basically a sequence of words surrounding at least one noun, such as the *"small calcified mass in left upper lobe"* above) and ignore the rest of the medical document. This is especially true for document retrieval, where the main goal lies in mapping a user query to document concepts. Such concepts are usually expressed within noun phrases. There exist more sophisticated NLP approaches that use fully developed grammars for complete parsing of sentences. These systems are able to extract biomedical concepts that are expressed beyond simple noun phrases (such as extracting the concept *"gallbladder operation"* from the phrase *"we immediately operated on the patient's gallbladder"*, which contains both verb and noun phrases).

Concept negation is another factor that calls for the application of natural language processing tools when searching clinical documents. Medical texts, for a variety of reasons, contain numerous negative findings. An individual word search for "lymphoma" will match not only "Large B-Cell Lymphoma" but also documents containing the phrases "negative for lymphoma" and "the differential diagnosis would include a number of different things, but it is definitely not a lymphoma". Negation itself can be expressed in a variety of different ways, including "no evidence of", "rule out", "without", "not", and "negative for". In any case, there exist grammar and heuristic rules to spot negated phrases. The simplest approach for negation detection is to define a word window in which to look for any of the above expressions. NLP is also useful for recognizing semantic issues that run across several sentences. This includes anaphoric expressions, such as pronouns that refer to document elements from previous sentences. This is exemplified by a sentence such as "*a CT scan was performed to search for signs of pulmonary embolism. It was negative.*" Here, "signs of pulmonary embolism" could mistakenly be interpreted as an instance of a positive finding. However, the correct and complete parsing of the medical report reveals that "pulmonary embolism" was actually ruled out. NLP approaches to resolve such issues are not trivial and are beyond the scope of this book.

Term Identification in Biomedicine

The identification of document concepts is a very fundamental NLP task. A string of one or more words is usually referred to as a *term*, and the mapping of such terms to some controlled terminology is called *term identification*. A controlled terminology by definition attaches a unique meaning to a term, and thus establishes term identity. The process basically consists of three steps, term recognition, classification and mapping. Many term identification approaches do not necessarily follow these steps, but for the sake of this discussion the subdivision into three subtasks is very helpful.

Detection of term boundaries (such as the words *small* and *lobe* in "*small calcified mass in the left upper lobe*") results in **term recognition**. Term recognition basically is a way of saying that a string of words corresponds to a biomedical concept without knowing anything about the true identity of that concept. What are the different approaches to term recognition? One approach is to start with recognizing base noun phrases in sentences. Base noun phrases are the basic sentence chunks that divide a sentence into objects and subjects, and, unlike more "non-terminal' noun phrases, can not be nested (i.e., such noun phrases do not split into other noun-phrases). NLP tools that identify base noun phrases are accordingly called "chunkers". In a sentence such as "*the physician ordered a CAT examination for staging the metastatic tumor*", a sentence chunker would recognize *the physician*, *a CAT examination*, and *the metastatic tumor* as noun phrases. The simplest way of recognizing such sentence chunks is to specify part of speech patterns. For example, a pattern such as <DT ADJ* NN> (determiner [DT] followed by any number of adjectives [ADJ*], followed by a noun [NN]) would conveniently recognize "*the metastatic tumor*" as a noun phrase.

Next, one needs to identify the terms within these noun phrases. An obvious approach is to use a list of controlled terms, and match it against the identified noun phrases. If there is a direct match between the terminology and the words within the noun phrase, one has effectively mapped a term to a controlled terminology. More commonly, however, there will be no exact match, or, equally problematic, no one-to-one match. These situations arise with lexical variants (such as term spelling variants) and ambiguous terms (term with several meanings). For example, UMLS (release 2005) has several entries for the term *cat,* including cat the animal, CAT the protein (chloramphenicol acetyl-transferase) and CAT the medical examination (computerized axial tomography); there is no UMLS entry for the compound term *CAT examination*, which would unambiguously identify the term in our example sentence. In such situations, the use of a controlled terminology is helpful to *recognize* the term *cat*, but is not sufficient for final term identification. **Term classification** approaches identify broad term categories, and help to select from within multiple matches for a given term. Machine-learning algorithms can be trained to recognize specific contextual clues (such as neighboring words) to permit term classification. In our example, the word *physician* might constitute a sufficient clue to classify the term *CAT* as a *diagnostic procedure*, the UMLS semantic category that is linked to the UMLS concept *computerized axial tomography* (alternative UMLS semantic categories are *mammals*, which is linked to the concept cat the animal, and *amino acid, peptide, or protein*, which is linked to the concept CAT the protein). The classification of CAT as a diagnostic procedure in the example above enables the definitive mapping to the appropriate UMLS concept.

Finally, **term mapping**, which is obviously linked to term classification, is mostly concerned with transforming a text string to some form that corresponds to an entry in a controlled terminology. Consider our example in which *CAT examination* was not included in the current UMLS release. However, the term *CAT scan* is included, and it is the latter term that unambiguously identifies this term as a diagnostic procedure. In such situations, we can use extensive synonym lists to capture the different lexical variations of terms. Alternatively, we can use *variant generators* to automatically generate all possible lexical term instantiations. Such a tool might decompose *CAT examination* into its word constituents, and generate variants for each of the constituents separately. Resulting term variants would include *CAT exam*, *CAT inspection* and *CAT scan* (*exam, inspection and scan* being synonyms or near synonyms of the term *examination*). Thus, a variant generator might be able to uniquely map CAT examination to the correct UMLS concept. Variant generators are also useful for producing "spelling variants" of terms (such as interleukin-6, interleukin 6), which hampers term mapping especially in the molecular biology domain. Variant generators employ diverse NLP methods to generate the variant terms. Extensive lists of synonyms and abbreviations are combined with basic rules to generate derivational, inflectional and spelling variants from word stems. Derivation is the process of creating terms with similar meaning from a common word stem, such as *ocular* and *oculus,* or *ophthalmitis* and *ophthalmia.* Inflectional variants are syntactically different expressions of a term, such as *oculus* and *oculi.* Equivalence rules between terms are also useful to generate spelling variants. For example, it has been shown that, in most instances, omission of dashes is acceptable when generating protein names. So both, interleukin-6 and interleukin 6 are viable alternatives.

NLP-assisted information retrieval

Although natural language processing is not a searching or information retrieval process itself, the techniques of NLP can be used to enhance our ability to retrieve information from archives of un-coded documents. These techniques can be employed "on-the-fly" at the time of the query, or in advance to pre-extract concept identifiers from documents.

Expansion of keyword queries

Query expansion is one way to use NLP to improve keyword queries. Term variants are added to the query term to ensure more complete document retrieval. A query term, such as *ocular tumor*, could be expanded to include *ocular tumors, eye tumor, eye tumors, ocular neoplasm* etc. The search is then performed in a logical "OR" fashion against all of these terms. Using a set of terms rather than a single term guarantees a better retrieval of documents. Query expansion can also take the form of adding search terms that are derived from the initial set of retrieved documents. In this case, a user retrieves a set of documents based on some initial keyword query. At this point, the user selects the most appropriate documents among the pool of retrieved entities. A query expansion algorithm then examines the set of selected documents, and extracts keywords that are likely to be the most useful for finding similar documents. These keywords are then added to the initial query terms, and the search is re-run.

Auto-coding of Medical Documents

The advent of electronic documents, high performance computing, and computerized document searching has not replaced the need for coded documents. Retrieving coded documents is still more expressive and precise than the use of simple keyword searches.

Term identification as discussed in the previous sections can be used to extract conceptual information from electronic documents. In many ways, this process mirrors the manual coding task, where human coders read and interpret the content of medical documents. When these NLP-extracted concepts are mapped to a particular terminology, the end result is automated coding of electronic documents, with a list of codes that represent the content of some electronic document. Given the high labor costs of manual coding, there is likely to be a role for automatic document coding in medicine, especially in non-critical sections of the health care enterprise. Examples include the use of auto-coders in clinic-wide data repositories. Data mining and knowledge discovery across documents in such repositories can be successfully performed even in the absence of perfect auto-coding performance. Of course, other sections of the health care industry are less fault-tolerant. Examples include the coding of discharge summaries for billing purposes, where suboptimal coding could have a profound impact on the reimbursement total for a hospital. Therefore this process is still routinely performed manually, or at least semi-automatically with human supervision.

Because many medical documents are still coded manually, and because both the documents themselves and the manually assigned codes are often available electronically, these can provide a potentially rich source for development and testing of new auto-coding algorithms using complex natural language processing techniques. Tumor registries represent an example of the type of environment in which this can be performed. Such new algorithms and NLP systems may eventually obviate the need for manual coding.

Chapter 12

EXTERNAL REGULATIONS PERTINENT TO LIS MANAGEMENT

More and more, what we can do, what we have to do, and what we can't do is being determined not by our experience or judgment but rather by externally imposed regulations. Some of these regulations are "voluntary", to the extent that we can choose whether or not to be accredited or to be eligible to receive Medicare payments, while others represent Federal law. Information systems have not escaped notice, and a number of external regulations specifically apply to procedures for the management of these systems. Most of the regulations are not particularly objectionable, because they represent good and ethical practice. In many instances, meeting the regulation is not nearly so hard as documenting that one is meeting the regulation. Of course, in order to meet a regulation, one has to understand it. This chapter will discuss some of the key external regulations impacting upon pathology information system use and management.

I should mention at the outside that this is a somewhat tricky chapter to write, because while I would like to provide "up-to-date" information, the topic is a bit of a moving target. External regulations change frequently, and sometimes dramatically. Therefore, as a disclaimer, consider that by the time you read this, some of the details of these regulations may have changed. I will focus on the underlying principles rather than the details, in the hopes that those are less mutable.

Health Insurance Portability and Accountability Act

Few rules or regulations have sent so great a ripple through the health care industry as those following the enactment of the Health Insurance

Portability and Accountability Act (HIPAA). Following closely on the heels of the "Y2K preparedness" (perhaps one of the most anti-climactic moments in electronic history), HIPAA preparedness has rapidly surpassed even the most pessimistic initial concerns about complexity and cost of implementation. Nonetheless, with the growing use of computers to store and transmit personal health information about individuals, a need existed for formal legislation protecting the rights of patients. Although onerous and at times simply annoying, the need to protect health information goes well beyond the importance one might associate with keeping a credit card number or a bank account number secure. If someone learns my credit card number, I can always cancel that credit card and get a new one. Sure, this may be very inconvenient in the short term, but this is a problem which can be solved. However, if someone inappropriately learns personal health information about me, I cannot get a new medical history.

In order to receive proper medical care, patients have to share personal information about themselves with their health care providers. Additional personal information about the patient is also obtained during the process of providing that care, for example in the form of test results. This information, as well as the rights of the patient, must be kept protected. There are three closely related but nonetheless distinct abstract principles which need to be considered: privacy, confidentiality, and security. Privacy is the right of an individual to freedom from unauthorized intrusion; simply stated, your right to be left alone. Privacy is violated when, for example, a physician or employee contacts a patient to obtain information for a purpose other than the health care of that patient, such as for a research study. Confidentiality is the right of an individual to have personal information about them, either provided or otherwise obtained during the process of health care delivery, kept private and not disclosed or used for any purpose other than to provide health care. Confidentiality is breached when a person who is authorized to have access to information either uses that information for a purpose other than that for which it was provided or discloses it to a person NOT authorized to have access to it. Security refers to the physical, technical, and procedural safeguards used to prevent unauthorized access to information stored either electronically or in any other format. Security is breached when someone who is NOT authorized to have access to information seeks to obtain it. Two other less frequently considered elements of security include preserving the integrity of the data (assuring that the information is both accurate and complete) and preserving the availability of the data (assuring that the information is available to authorized individuals when needed). Privacy, confidentiality, and security are clearly inter-related. To protect a patient's privacy, one must keep information about them confidential. To maintain confidentiality, one must make sure information about the patient is kept secure.

Contrary to popular belief, the privacy and security regulations resulting from HIPAA are not simply an information technology problem. It was soon realized that protecting only the information stored electronically did not make much sense, so the regulations were expanded to include any individually identifiable health information about a person, regardless of how it was stored. Thus, compliance with HIPAA is really more of a workflow policy-and-procedure issue than an "ITS problem".

Background: Privacy, Confidentiality, and Security

The privacy and security regulations associated with HIPAA did not arise *de novo*. They were based on a number of principles and legislation which have been around for quite some time.

In July 1973, the Secretary of Health, Education, and Welfare's advisory committee on automated personal data systems issued a report entitled "Records, Computers and the Rights of Citizens". In this report, recommendations were put forth to protect individuals against arbitrary or abusive record-keeping practices by the government in the computer age. These recommendations were referred to as "The Code of Fair Information Practice", and became the basis for the Privacy Act of 1974 (Public Law 93-579, incorporated into the United States Code as 5 U.S.C. 552a). The Code consisted of five basic principles:

- There must be no personal data record keeping systems whose very existence is secret.
- There must be a way for an individual to find out what information about him is in a record and how it is used.
- There must be a way for an individual to prevent information about him that was obtained for one purpose from being used or made available for other purposes without his consent.
- There must be a way for an individual to correct or amend a record of identifiable information about him.
- Any organization creating, maintaining, using, or disseminating records of identifiable personal data must assure the reliability of the data for their intended use and must take precautions to prevent misuse of the data.

These recommendations, as well as many other elements of this report, formed the basis for the privacy and security regulations eventually promulgated in response to the HIPAA legislation.

History, Elements, and Implementation of HIPAA

The Health Insurance Portability and Accountability Act of 1996, also known as the Kassebaum-Kennedy Bill, or the far less glamorous Public Law 104-191, was enacted on August 21, 1996. As stated in the preamble to the bill, this act was designed "to improve portability and continuity of health insurance coverage in the group and individual markets, to combat waste, fraud, and abuse in health insurance and health care delivery, to promote the use of medical savings accounts, to improve access to long-term care services and coverage, to simply the administration of health insurance, and for other purposes."

Title II, Subtitle F of HIPAA, ironically entitled "Administrative Simplification", was what set into motion the regulations we all know today. As stated in Section 261 of this subtitle, "It is the purpose of this subtitle to improve the Medicare program under title XVIII of the Social Security Act, the Medicaid program under title XIX of such Act, and the efficiency and effectiveness of the health care system, by encouraging the development of a health information system through the establishment of standards and requirements for the electronic transmission of certain health information." Section 262 of HIPAA modified Title XI of U.S. Code 42.1301, and required the adoption of standards for:

a) transactions, and data elements for such transactions, to allow health information to be exchanged electronically

b) unique health identifiers for each individual, employer, health plan, and health care provider

c) code sets for appropriate data elements for the transactions referred to in subsection a)

d) security policies and procedures and safeguards to ensure the integrity and confidentiality of health information

e) electronic transmission and authentication of signatures

f) transfer of information among health plans

Section 262 also indicated that such standards should be adopted "not later than 18 months after the date of the enactment of the Health Insurance Portability and Accountability act of 1996" (which would be Feb 21, 1998), and that compliance by health plans should be achieved within 24 months of the date on which the standard is initially adopted (36 months for small health plans). Penalties for non-compliance were also defined: a general penalty of $100 for each violation, limited to $25,000 per person per regulation per year. However, a person who knowingly improperly uses, obtains, or discloses individually identifiable health information is subject to a $50,000 fine, and/or one year imprisonment, increasing to $100,000 and 5 years if done under false pretenses, and to $250,000 and 10 years if done with the intent to sell or use for commercial advantage, personal gain, or malicious harm.

Another important part of the Administrative Simplification subpart (Section 264) was the statement that "if legislation governing standards with respect to the privacy of individually identifiable health information ... is not enacted by the date that is 36 months after the date of the enactment of this Act, (which was Aug 21, 1999) the Secretary of Health and Human Services shall promulgate final regulations containing such standards not later than the date that is 42 months after the date of the enactment of this act" (which was Feb 21, 2000). Congress failed to pass such legislation in the time period indicated, so the department of Health and Human Services, after publishing proposed regulations and soliciting comments, ultimately put forth final regulations relating to patient privacy protection. Other regulations have also been finalized, and their compliance dates and locations in the Code of Federal Regulations are shown in Table 12-1. (A brief note about United States Law: when congress passes a law, otherwise known as an Act or Statute, it becomes part of the United States Code (U.S.C.). HIPAA was such a law. Often, these laws authorize specific government agencies to promulgate regulations to "fill in the details" about a general principle set forth in the law. These regulations are compiled in the Code of Federal Regulations, or CFR. Both the USC and CFR are divided into "Titles", which are divided into numbered Parts, which are divided into

Table 12-1: Publication and compliance dates for HIPAA standards.

Standard	Final Rule Date	Regulation	Compliance Date
Transactions and Code Sets	Aug 17, 2000	45 CFR 162 I-R	Oct 16, 2002
Privacy Regulations	Dec 28, 2000	45 CFR 164 E	Apr 14, 2003
National Employer ID	May 31, 2002	45 CFR 162 F	July 30, 2004
Security Regulations	Feb 20, 2003	45 CFR 164 C	Apr 21, 2005
National Provider ID	Jan 23, 2004	45 CFR 162 D	May 23, 2007
National Health Plan ID	[pending]		
National Individual ID	[on hold]		

Note that these regulations have moved around a bit in the Code of Federal Regulations (CFR) since they were originally published, and may move again. The compliance dates for "small health plans" are generally one year after the dates indicated here.

lettered Subparts. 45CFR164E refers to title 45 of the Code of Federal Regulations, part 164, subpart E.)

It is well beyond the scope of this book to provide a complete documentation of the details of the regulations resulting from the Health Insurance Portability and Accountability Act (sorry). However, some of the major issues pertaining to information systems, including some controversial ones, will be discussed.

General Provisions

45 CFR 160 provides some general provisions applicable to all of the regulations promulgated in response to HIPAA. Among these are definitions of terms, relationship to state law, and rules for compliance and enforcement. Definitions of key terms such as business associate, covered entity, disclosure, electronic media, health care, health plan, individually identifiable health information, protected health information, transaction, and use are included. The most important of these are:

Covered entity: "(1) a health plan, (2) a health care clearinghouse, (3) a health care provider who transmits any health information in electronic form". Basically, if you practice pathology and both store AND transmit heath information electronically, HIPAA applies to you. An entity can be as small as a single independently practicing pathologist, or as large as a major academic medical center. Definition of the entity is important since it determines whether an exchange of health information is a use or a disclosure.

Use: "the sharing, employment, application, utilization, examination, or analysis of information within an entity that maintains such information"

Disclosure: "the release, transfer, provision of, access to, or divulging in any other manner of information outside the entity holding the information"

Protected health information: "individually identifiable health information... that is (i) transmitted by electronic media; (ii) maintained in electronic media; or (iii) transmitted or maintained in any other form or medium."

Individually identifiable health information: "information that is a subset of health information, including demographic information collected from an individual, and: (1) is created or received by a health care provider, health plan, employer, or health care clearinghouse; and (2) relates to the past, present, or future physical or mental health or condition of an individual; the provision of health care to an individual; or the past, present, or future payment for the provision of health care to an individual; and (i) that identifies the individual; or (ii) with respect to which there is a reasonable basis to believe the information can be used to identify the individual."

Business Associate: "a person or organization not part of the workforce of a covered entity who assists that covered entity in the performance of any function or activity involving individually identifiable health information. A covered entity may be the business associate of another covered entity." This definition is important because if you are part of an independent pathology practice who gets information from a hospital, you need to have a business associate agreement with that hospital. If you outsource your computer system management, or even if your computer system vendor has access to your computer system which contains protected health information, you need a business associate agreement with that vendor.

With respect to state law, in brief, the regulation states that any standard contained within these regulations which is contrary to a provision of State law preempts that State law unless the State law is more stringent.

Electronic Transactions and Code Sets

The first standards to go into effect were those relating to the electronic exchange of health information, usually for purposes of filing claims, establishing coverage, or enrolling in health plans. Most of these regulations pertain to details which are routinely handled by billing services (health care clearinghouses) and therefore are not directly pertinent to a practicing pathologist. Of note is that use of the standards is not optional: "if a covered entity conducts with another covered entity (or within the same covered entity), using electronic media, a transaction for which the Secretary has adopted a standard under this part, the covered entity must conduct the transaction as a standard transaction."

The code sets adopted as standards which pertain to pathology are, fortunately, two of the coding sets with which we are most familiar, namely:

International Classification of Diseases, 9th Edition, Clinical Modification (ICD-9-CM) Volumes 1 and 2 for diseases, injuries, impairments, other health problems, and causes of the above

Current Procedural Terminology, Fourth Edition (CPT-4) for physician services, physical and occupational therapy services, radiologic procedures, clinical laboratory tests, and other medical diagnostic procedures

More detail on these coding systems is provided in Chapter 11.

Privacy Regulations

The privacy regulations have already undergone several modifications and amendments since initially published in their "final" form on December 28, 2000. Many of these changes were in response to the fact that compliance with the initially published regulations was impractical or simply impossible to achieve. The modified regulations are far more reasonable, but it would probably be naive to assume that further modifications will not be made. As of the October 2004 versions, the privacy regulations filled 43 pages of text much smaller than the print you are reading now. I will not attempt to cover them in full, but rather emphasize those issues of particular pertinence to pathologists and information systems. The privacy regulations formally went into effect on April 14, 2003.

Both the privacy and security regulations allow for the definition of a "hybrid entity", stating that "legally separated covered entities that are affiliated may designate themselves as a single covered entity". This is directly applicable to the distinction between "uses" and "disclosures" of health information, as defined above in the section on general provisions. This allows large medical centers or affiliated hospitals to designate themselves as a single entity, converting sharing of information amongst themselves from disclosures to uses. The distinction is important because, as will be discussed, disclosures need to be tracked for accounting purposes, but uses do not. To be affiliated, the legally separate covered entities must be under "common ownership" (defined as equity interest of 5% or more) or "common control" (defined as one entity having "the power, directly or indirectly, significantly to influence or direct the actions or policies of another entity".

Covered entities may use or disclose health information "for treatment, payment, or health care operations". The latter term is rather broad, and includes quality assessment and improvement activities, education and training, business planning and development, and management activities. An original restriction was placed on the use and disclosure of information to the "minimum necessary" for the purpose for which the information was being used or disclosed, but that minimum necessary requirement was dropped when used or disclosed for treatment purposes. The limitation was not, however, dropped for other permitted uses or disclosures. Additionally, specific authorization may be required for psychotherapy notes and for marketing purposes.

When first published, the privacy regulations made special reference to physicians who had what was termed an "indirect treatment relationship" with the patient. Pathologists were specifically mentioned as meeting this criteria. Such physicians had certain exemptions from elements of the privacy regulation, such as the need to obtain patient consent prior to using information about the patient to provide health care. The requirement for a formal written consent to use information about the patient for health care purposes related to that patient was subsequently dropped from the amended regulations, so a special exception for providers with an indirect treatment relationship (e.g. the pathologist) was not longer needed. However, providers with an indirect treatment relationship retain the exemption from the requirement to provide patients with a written notice of their privacy practices.

Section 164.512 lists a number of uses and disclosures for which no authorization is required. This includes such things as disclosures required by law, for public heath activities (for example, mandatory reporting of some diagnoses to the State Public Health department or the Centers for Disease Control), for health oversight and judicial activities, and for law enforcement purposes. There are also special exemptions from authorization for disclosing information for organ or tissue donation purposes, and information about deceased individuals may be disclosed to coroners, medical examiners, and funeral directors, as needed for them to perform their duties. Finally, no authorization is required to disclose information for research purposes when previously approved by an institutional review board. More on this in a bit.

Section 164.522 allows the patient to request a restriction on the use or disclosure of information about themselves, even for treatment, payment, or health care operations. Although the covered entity is not required to agree to this restriction, if it does, it is obligated to abide by the agreement. For example, our autopsy service once was granted permission to perform an autopsy on the condition that the report was NOT sent to the patient's community physician. The difficulty is in communicating any agreed upon restrictions to other members of the entity who might otherwise be able to disclose the restricted information. Most pathology information systems do not have any mechanism of recording that the entity has agreed to any particular restrictions.

Individuals are allowed access to health information about themselves. However, there is a specific exclusion of access which would violate the Clinical Laboratory Improvement Act of 1988 (CLIA). CLIA regulations (42 CFR 493) specifically state that for covered laboratories, which includes all pathology laboratories, "test results must be released only to authorized persons", and "authorized persons" is defined as "persons authorized under State law to order tests or receive test results, or both". Thus, patients are not allowed access to pathology results directly from the pathology laboratories, unless State law specifically permits that. They are, however, allowed access to those results contained within the medical records, but pathology laboratories do not need to establish mechanisms or procedures to allow patients direct access to their results in the laboratory.

Section 164.526 allows individuals to request that protected health information about themselves be amended. The only instance of this which I have encountered so far in pathology is when a family member requested that an autopsy report be amended because they did not like the fact that the autopsy report suggested that findings of a cirrhotic liver and bleeding esophageal varices, and thus the patient's death, was related to his chronic alcohol consumption. Covered entities have the right to deny a request for amendment if, among other things, they feel the information as held is accurate and complete. However, the patient (in this case the family member) can still provide a formal "statement of disagreement" and require that the entity designate the record as disputed and provide the statement of disagreement along with any subsequent disclosures of that record. Here, again, the potential difficulty from an informatics perspective is in the capabilities of the information system to record that a dispute exists.

One of the most onerous tasks associated with the HIPAA privacy regulations is addressing the patient's rights to request an accounting of any disclosures of health information about themselves. Remember that a disclosure means release of information outside of the entity holding that information. The accounting of disclosures includes disclosures which are permitted to occur without any prior authorization. Although some disclosures do not need to be accounted for (for example, disclosures for treatment purposes do not require accounting), disclosures of information to coroners/medical examiners and to funeral directors DO need to be included in disclosure accounting. This represents a new administrative requirement for pathology departments/practices which run morgue operations for their institutions. If some sort of information system is in use to manage morgue patients, it may be possible to electronically extract this information, but most commercially available pathology information systems do not include morgue management capabilities, and therefore a separate stand-alone informatics solution or a manual paper solution to this regulation will be required.

Research Use of Anatomic Pathology Information Systems

Research use of an anatomic pathology information system is perhaps the most vulnerable aspect of the information system with respect to compliance with the privacy regulations. Anatomic pathology information systems contain a tremendous wealth of information of potential use for health care research. Many of the tools available within these systems for management and quality control purposes, such as case finding by diagnoses, can be used to identify cases for research studies. However, doing so without appropriate prior authorization or institutional review board approval constitutes an ILLEGAL use of the information system under the privacy regulations. Although it is tempting to significantly limit user access to these capabilities in order to curtail the illegal use of these features, the same tools are also useful for educational and quality improvement activities, which are allowable uses by HIPAA. This is a dilemma for which I have not yet found a good solution.

Research use of health care information about patients has traditionally been covered under 45 CFR 46, otherwise known as the "common rule". The HIPAA privacy regulations to not replace those requirements and restrictions, but rather add to them. In the 1980's, each Federal agency had its own set of regulations pertaining to the protection of human subjects. On the recommendation of the ad hoc Committee for the Protection of Human Research Subjects, a unified federal policy was developed based on the then current standards in use by the Department of Health and Human Services. This "common rule" was published for public comment in June of 1986, modified and republished as a proposed rule in November 1988, and ultimately published in final form on June 18, 1991, with an effective date of August 19, 1991. A "human subject" was defined as "a living individual about whom an investigator obtains either (1) data through intervention or interaction with the individual, or (2) identifiable private information." Research is defined as "a systematic investigation designed to develop or contribute to generalizable knowledge." There is some inconsistencies between institutions as to whether or not a single case report constitutes research. Many take the position that a report consisting of three or fewer cases in which no systematic investigation or qualitative analysis is performed also does not constitute research. However, any systematic, hypothesis based collection of a series of cases certainly does. Using the anatomic pathology information system to identify these cases therefore constitutes a research activity, and cannot be legally performed without prior institutional review board (IRB) approval.

From an informatics perspective, there are a few issues to consider. First, do the managers of the information system assume any responsibility for inappropriate use of the system by its users, and if so, what safeguards or auditing activities should be in place to regulate that use? This is clearly an institutional decision. (However, the security regulations, discussed below, require that a risk analysis be done of each information system, and that the managers of the system should protect against any reasonably anticipated uses which are not permitted under the privacy regulations.) Secondly, assuming the system is used with appropriate IRB approval, if any of the investigators are considered external to the HIPAA entity holding the information, providing access to that information constitutes a disclosure which must be included in the accounting of disclosures held by that entity. There are two ways to exempt the release of information from the need to account for disclosures. One is to completely de-identify the information, so that it no longer is considered protected health information and therefore no longer subject to HIPAA regulations. A code can be maintained which would allow potential re-identification of the data, but the key for the code cannot be held by any of the researchers and the code cannot be based on any of the patient information. This solution is generally not viable, since in most cases the researchers will need to know the specimen accession number for the cases (for ordering recuts or special stains), and that is considered a unique identifier. The second solution is to create what is termed a "limited data set", and enter into a data use agreement with investigators. A limited data set could contain a specimen accession number, but could not contain any names, addresses, medical record numbers, or other account numbers. Again, this is generally not practical, because most anatomic pathology information systems are not designed to provide de-identified information. Therefore, if the pathology information system is used for research purposes and information is disclosed to individuals outside of the HIPAA defined entity, a mechanism needs to be established to account for all of these disclosures.

A word about research on deceased individuals. The common rule, by defining a human subject as "a living individual", specifically exempts research solely on deceased patients from the requirement for IRB approval. HIPAA, however, does not. For the most part, all of the HIPAA requirements, restrictions, and regulations about patients apply to deceased individuals as well. Any person authorized to act on behalf of a deceased individual or his/her estate is afforded the status of "personal representative" and entitled to the same protection as would otherwise be appropriate for the deceased individual. To achieve greater consistency with the common rule, however, HIPAA does include a special exemption allowing information on deceased patients to be used for research purposes without prior authorization and without IRB approval, provided the researcher provides appropriate representation that the information will only be used for research on deceased individuals and that the information is necessary for the research. Release of this information outside of the holding entity, however, still constitutes a disclosure and still must be included in disclosure accounting.

Note that even if the research is properly deemed exempt from IRB review, either because the data is not individually identifiable or involves only deceased patients, most institutional assurance agreements require the

IRB to specifically review the proposed research to determine that it is, indeed, exempt from review.

Security Regulations

Whereas the privacy regulations pertain to both the electronic and non-electronic information, and compliance with those regulations requires more policy and procedural changes than any specific changes to the information systems themselves, the security regulations apply specifically to information systems. As with the privacy regulations, these standards were also "softened" after initial release, because some of the recommended features were simply not within the technical capabilities of many of the information systems currently in use in health care today.

The HIPAA security standards define three elements to security. The one we all think of is prevention of unauthorized access. Two other dimensions of security, however, are the integrity of the data (assuring the information has not been altered, lost, or destroyed, in whole or in part) and the availability of the data (assuring that the information is accessible, on demand, by an authorized person), since data which is potentially incomplete or unavailable cannot reasonably be considered to be "secure". All three elements of security are addressed by the HIPAA security regulations.

The security regulations are divided into three types of safeguards: administrative, physical, and technical. Within each category are standards, and each standard has one or more implementation specifications. Each specification is defined as being either "required" (self explanatory) or "addressable" (which means that each institution must assess whether the "specification is a reasonable and appropriate safeguard in its environment", and implement it if so, and if not, document why not and implement an equivalent alternative, if appropriate. Each of the standards and the required and addressable implementation specifications are indicated in Tables 12-2, 12-3, and 12-4.

The administrative safeguards (Table 12-2) refer to policies and procedures to promote proper security practices. Each information system must undergo a risk analysis, and steps must be taken to reduce the security risks identified. The regulation is silent as to who is to do this analysis, but the regulations do allow the covered entities to take into account factors such as "the size, complexity, and capabilities of the covered entity", "the covered entity's technical infrastructure, hardware, and software capabilities", and "the costs of the security measures". Specific written policies need to exist for how violations by members of the workforce will be handled, and there must be written documentation of regular review of information system activity, "such as audit logs, access reports, and security incident tracking

Table 12-2: Administrative safeguards.

Standard	Required Implementation	Addressable Implementation
Security Management Process	Risk Analysis Risk Management Sanction Policy System Activity Review	
Assigned Security Responsibility	Identify Responsible Official	
Workforce Security		Authorization/Supervision Clearance Procedure Termination Procedures
Information Access Management	Isolate Clearinghouse Functions	Access Authorization Access Establishment and Modification
Security Awareness /Training		Security Reminders Anti-Virus Protection Log-in Monitoring Password Management
Security Incident Procedures	Response & Reporting	
Contingency Plan	Data Backup Plan Disaster Recovery Plan Emergency Mode Plan	Testing/Revision Procedure Applications and Data Criticality Analysis
Evaluation	Periodic Technical & Non-technical evaluations	
Business Associate Contracts	Written Contracts	

reports". The workforce security standard deals with restricting those members of the workforce whose job responsibilities do not require information system access from obtaining that access, including providing supervision and terminating access when employment is terminated. Formal policies for how information system access is granted or modified should be documented. Security awareness training is needed for all members of the workforce. Security incident monitoring is required, as is mitigation, as practical, of any harmful effects of a security breach. Required elements in the contingency plan category include data backups, disaster recovery plans, and a plan to enable continuation of critical business processes in the event

Table 12-3: Physical safeguards.

Standard	Required Implementation	Addressable Implementation
Facility Access Controls		Contingency Operations Facility Security Plan Access Control/Validation Maintenance Records
Workstation Use	Policies for Appropriate Use of Workstations	
Workstation Security	Restrict Access to Authorized Users	
Device and Media Controls	Disposal Media Reuse	Accountability Data Backup and Storage

of a system failure. Addressable elements include testing of the contingency plans, and analysis of how critical each system and its data is to ongoing operations.

The physical safeguards (Table 12-3) all pertain to measures to protect the equipment used to store and manage protected health care information from environmental hazards and unauthorized intrusion. This includes access policies to secure areas. Of relevance to every pathology practice is policies addressing appropriate (and therefore inappropriate) use of workstations, the physical attributes of the workstation surroundings, and restricting access to authorized users. Any devices or media which is to be discarded or re-used must be appropriately stripped of any protected health information before release. Note that it is usually not sufficient to simple delete the files.

The technical safeguards (Table 12-4) refer to technological capabilities of the information systems themselves to protect the information contained within them. Each user with access to the system must have their own user-name. It is inappropriate and in fact illegal for two or more users to share a user-name, or for an administrative assistant to use the log-in identity of one of the physicians which they assist. Each person accessing the information system must first authenticate themselves, either by a unique user-name and password or some biometric process (e.g. thumbprint scanner). The system must be monitored for inappropriate use (for example, monitoring for after-hours access by individuals who do not work after-hours). The security regulations also call for a procedure for emergency access to the system. This is for settings in which a treating physician needs to access health care information on a patient for potential life saving treatment, but does not

Table 12-4: Technical safeguards.

Standard	Required Implementation	Addressable Implementation
Access Control	Unique User Identification Emergency Access Procedure	Automatic Logoff Encryption & Decryption
Audit Controls	Examine System Use	
Integrity		Authenticate Electronic Health Information
Person/Entity Authentication	Authentication prior to granting Access	
Transmission Security		Integrity Controls Encryption

currently have the needed security clearances to access that information. This is sometimes referred to as "break-glass" access, akin to pulling a fire alarm. For anatomic pathology information systems, this need generally does not exist. However, one still needs an official policy stating that fact.

In addition to the actual safeguards, the security regulations require that appropriate policies and procedures be documented for each of the implementation standards. The phrasing used is "Implement reasonable and appropriate policies and procedures to comply with the standards, implementation specifications, or other requirements of this subpart, taking into account those factors specified (the size, complexity, and capabilities of the covered entity, the covered entity's technical infrastructure, hardware, and software capabilities, the costs of the security measures, and the probability and criticality of potential risks)". This would appear to give entities some flexibility in assessing and managing the risks of their systems. Documentation must be available, updated as needed, and old/replaced policies must be maintained for at least six years from the date when it was last in effect.

Rules pertaining to electronic signatures, originally part of the security regulations, were dropped from the final published regulations.

National Identifiers

The standard unique employer identifier regulation went into effect on July 30, 2004. This was the most anticlimactic of all the standards promulgated, since a decision was made to adopt the unique employer identifier used by the internal revenue service.

The National Provider Identifier (NPI) will be a 10-digit numeric identifier (the 10th digit is a check digit) which will be assigned to each provider and will replace all previous provider identifiers, including the UPIN and Medicaid numbers. The regulations provide for establishing a National Provider System which is to being processing applications for NPIs in 2005. All providers are to begin using the new identifier by May 23, 2007.

As of the writing of this chapter, final regulations for a National Health-Plan (payer) identifier are still pending. Health plans are defined as any individual or group plan that provides or pays the cost of medical care, and therefore this includes a large number of entities, including health insurance companies, health maintenance organizations, Medicare, Medicaid, employee welfare benefit plans, military health care plans, the veterans health care program, etc.

The concept of a Unique Health Identifier for Individuals is far more controversial and has, for the time being, been put on hold. Much of the administrative cost savings benefits hoped to be achieved by HIPAA require such an identifier, but ongoing concerns for individual privacy have hampered and in fact at least temporarily halted plans to develop such a system. The National Committee on Vital and Health Statistics recommended to the Department of Health and Human Services that "it would be unwise and premature to proceed to select and implement such an identifier in the absence of legislation to assure the confidentiality of individually identifiable health information and to preserve an individual's right to privacy."[1] This recommendation supported the concept of the identifier in principle, but recommended waiting. In a dissenting opinion authored by two members of the Committee, a far more conservative stance was taken: "Public and congressional concern about identification numbers and about privacy is at an all time high. Any decisions about a new number should be made directly by the Congress. This is not a issue to be decided administratively on technical or economic grounds alone. It is a political choice that should be made only by elected representatives in a public fashion."[2] Further information about a universal patient identifier is provided under the discussion of electronic medical record systems in

---

[1] Letter to Donna Shalala, Secretary of the Department of Health and Human Services, from Don Detmer, MD, Chair of the National Committee on Vital and Health Statistics, dated September 9, 1997.

[2] Letter to Dr. Don Detmer, Chairman of the National Committee on Vital and Health Statistics, from Robert Gellman and Richard Harding, two members of the Committee, dated September 19, 1997.

Chapter 6 on the relationship of Pathology laboratory information systems to institutional information systems. Whether regulations for such an identifier are promulgated by the Secretary of Health and Human Services, or result from legislation passed by Congress, or never appear at all, is yet to be seen.

College of American Pathologists' Checklists

The other major set of regulations directly addressing requirements of information systems used in pathology are those put forth by the College of American Pathologists (CAP) as part of their inspection checklists. Since these regulations pre-dated the HIPAA security regulations, there is some overlap between the two, the CAP providing guidelines at a time when there were no specific external regulations addressing electronic information system management. Since the practice of the CAP has been, in general, to avoid specific rules which overlap Federal regulations, so as not to run the risk of inconsistent requirements or to be deemed interpreting/enforcing Federal law, it is likely that the CAP checklist composition as it relates to information system management will change over the next few years.

The CAP checklists consist of a series of questions which describe minimum requirements which pathology departments are expected to meet to be accredited. Each checklist question is categorized as Phase I or Phase II. Phase II deficiencies must be corrected for a laboratory to become accredited. Phase I deficiencies are strongly recommended, but some allowances are accepted for unique institutional situations. The questions are edited by the CAP resource committees on an on-going basis, and revised checklists are posted approximately quarterly to the CAP web site (www.cap.org). The questions pertinent to laboratory information systems are included in the "Laboratory General" checklist.

Table 12-5 lists the pertinent checklist questions as of the March 2005 release. The questions have been recently updated to reflect the understanding that some laboratories outsource their information management to external organizations. For those with in-house facilities, a number of the questions address the physical environment of the facility. Result reporting questions address accuracy of calculated and electronically transmitted information, format and content of reports, and procedures for amending and reporting amended test results. All three elements of security (protection from unauthorized access, data integrity, and data availability) are addressed. Documentation in the form of policies, procedure manuals, and numerous logs are stressed throughout the checklists.

Table 12-5: College of American Pathologists' Checklist Questions.

GEN	Phase	Question
42165	II	If components of the LIS are located at a facility other than the one under this CAP accreditation number, is there evidence that the remote facility complies with CAP requirements for host LIS functions?
42457	II	In the judgment of the laboratory director, is the functionality and reliability of the computer system (hardware and software) adequate to meet the needs of patient care?
Computer Facility		
42750	I	Is the computer facility and equipment clean, well-maintained and adequately ventilated with appropriate environmental control?
42800	II	Is fire-fighting equipment (extinguishers) available?
42850	I	Are all wires and computer cables properly located and/or protected from traffic?
42900	II	Is the computer system adequately protected against electrical power interruptions and surges?
LIS/Computer Procedure Manual		
42950	II	Are LIS/computer procedures clearly documented, complete and readily available to all authorized users?
42975	II	Is there a procedure for the support of the computer system?
43000	II	Is there documentation that laboratory computer procedures are reviewed at least annually by the laboratory director or designee?
Hardware and Software		
43011	II	Is there documentation of all hardware modifications?
43022	II	Is there documentation that programs are adequately tested for proper functioning when first installed and after any modifications, and that the laboratory director or designee has approved the use of al new programs and modifications?
43033	II	Are customized programs appropriately documented?
43044	II	Is there an adequate tracking system to identify all persons who have added or modified software?
43055	II	Is there documentation that all users of the computer system receive adequate training initially, after system modification, and after installation of a new system?
43066	II	Is there a responsible person (e.g., Computer System Manager) in the laboratory who is notified of significant computer malfunction?
43077	II	Has the laboratory information system been validated for blood banking/transfusion medicine activities?
43088	II	Is there a documented system to verify the integrity of the system (operating system, applications and database) after restoration of data files?

(continued)

GEN	Phase	Question *(continued)*

System Maintenance

GEN	Phase	Question
43099	II	Is downtime for maintenance scheduled to minimize interruption of service?
43110	II	Is there a documented schedule and procedure for regular maintenance of hardware and software either by maintenance contracts or documented in-house procedures?
43121	II	Are service and repair records available for all hardware and software?
43132	II	Is there evidence of ongoing evaluation of system maintenance records?

System Security

GEN	Phase	Question
43150	II	Are there explicit documented policies that specify who may use the computer system to enter or access patient data, change results, change billing or alter programs?
43200	I	Are computer access codes (security codes, user codes) used to limit individuals' access to those functions they are authorized to use, and is the security of access codes maintained (e.g., deleted when employees leave, not posted on terminals)?
43262	I	Are policies and procedures in place to prevent unauthorized installation of software on any computer used by the laboratory?
43325	II	If the facility uses a public network, such as the Internet as a data exchange medium, are there adequate network security measures in place to ensure confidentiality of patient data?
43387	II	Does the laboratory have procedures to ensure compliance with HIPAA?

Patient Data

GEN	Phase	Question
43450	II	Is there documentation that calculations performed on patient data by the computer are reviewed annually, or when a system change is made that may affect the calculations??
43600	I	Are data tables set up to detect absurd values before reporting?
43750	II	Does the system provide for comments on specimen quality that might compromise the accuracy of analytic results (*e.g.,* hemolyzed, lipemic)?
43800	II	Is there an adequate system to identify all individuals who have entered and/or modified patient data or control files?
43812	I	Does the laboratory have a process to ensure appropriate routing of patient test results to physicians?
43825	II	Are manual and automated result entries verified before final acceptance and reporting by the computer?
43837	II	Are there documented procedures to ensure reporting of patient results in a prompt and useful fashion during partial or complete downtime and recovery of the system?

(continued)

GEN	Phase	Question	*(continued)*

Autoverification

43850	II	Is there a signed policy by the Laboratory Director approving the use of autoverification procedures?
43875	II	Is there documentation that the autoverification process was validated initially, and is tested at least annually and whenever there is a change to the system?

Data Retrieval and Preservation

43900	II	Can a complete copy of archived patient test results be reprinted, including original reference ranges and interpretive comments, and any flags or footnotes that were present in the original report?
43920	I	When multiple identical analyzers are used, are they uniquely identified such that a test result may be appropriately traced back to the instrument performing the test?
43933	I	Does the laboratory have a process to monitor computer system performance, to ensure that the data storage capacity and performance of the system are sufficient to meet the patient needs of the organization?
43946	II	Are there documented procedures for the preservation of data and equipment in case of an unexpected destructive event (*e.g.*, fire, flood), software failure and/or hardware failure?
43972	II	Is emergency service for both computer hardware and software available at all necessary times?
44000	II	Are storage data media (*e.g.*, tape reels, disk cartridges) properly labeled, stored and protected from damage and unauthorized use?
44100	II	Are computer error messages that alert computer users of imminent problems monitored and is the error message response system tested periodically?
44150	II	Is there documentation of responses to any error messages during the system backup?
44200	II	Is there a documented record of unscheduled downtime, system degradation (response time), or other computer problems that includes reasons for failure and corrective action taken?

Interfaces

45500	I	If the system uses an interface to populate data into another computer system, is a documented encoding and transmission scheme such as HL7 utilized?
46000	I	As applicable, are reference ranges and units of measure for every test transmitted with the patient result across the interface?
46500	I	Are acceptable transmission limits established for data throughput by the interface engine, and is this parameter periodically monitored and recorded?

(continued)

GEN	Phase	Question *(continued)*
Interfaces *(continued)*		
47000	II	If data in other computer systems can be accessed through the LIS (*e.g.,* pharmacy or medical records), are there documented policies to prevent unauthorized access to that data through the LIS?
48500	II	Is there a documented system in operation to periodically verify that patient results are accurately transmitted from the point of data entry (interfaced instruments and manual input) to all types of patient reports (both paper and video displays)?
48750	II	Are there procedures for changes in laboratory functions necessary during partial or complete shutdown and recovery of systems that interface with the laboratory information system?
Networks		
49000	I	Is there periodic monitoring of network performance and availability to all sites?
49500	I	Is the network equipment accessible, well-maintained, and adequately labeled, showing which devices are using a specific port?

NOTE: From the Laboratory Accreditation Program Checklists, S. Sarewitz, MD, (ed.); Published by the College of American Pathologists, 325 Waukegan Road, Northfield, Illinois 60093-2750; March 30, 2005 version. Reprinted by permission.

From having been on both sides of the inspection process, I can personally attest to a certain amount of "arbitrariness" associated with the inspection of clinical information systems. Although the checklist questions themselves address important issues and standards, there is sometimes little guidance for the inspectors as to what is required to meet the standard. This can leave the "inspectee" subject to the inspector's interpretation of the standard. The expertise of the inspectors in evaluating clinical information systems can also vary significantly from one inspection to the next. To address these issues, an increasing number of "notes" are being added to the questions by the CAP Informatics Committee to provide guidance as to how to assess whether or not a laboratory is meeting the standard. In addition, consideration is being given to specially trained teams of inspectors for specific technical areas like laboratory information systems.

American College of Surgeons

For those pathology practices which serve institutions which have elected to seek approval of their cancer program from the American College of

Surgeons' Commission on Cancer, there is an additional regulation which anatomic pathology departments must meet. Although this is not a computer issues per se, it is an informatics issue, because it concerns the information which must be included in patient reports.

The Commission on Cancer (CoC) sets standards which it feels institutions striving to provide high quality multidisciplinary care for cancer patients should meet. These standards include requirements for administrative leadership, data management (in the form of tumor registries), research, community outreach, professional education, and quality improvement, in addition to requirements for clinical management. The 2004 edition of their Cancer Program Standards (effective date January 1, 2004) lists 36 standards which institutions must meet for full approval status. Standard 4.6 is "The guidelines for patient management and treatment currently required by the CoC are followed". As originally published, this standard states that "90 percent of pathology reports that include a cancer diagnosis will contain the scientifically validated data elements outlined on the surgical case summary checklist of the College of American Pathologists publication, *Reporting on Cancer Specimens.*"[3] Interestingly, this is the only "guideline for patient management and treatment" listed. However, this standard generated some controversy, in particular because it was unclear as to precisely which pathology reports were included in the standard and how the information was to be included in pathology reports. Therefore, the Commission on Cancer released a document entitled "Clarifications and Modifications Made Since the January 2004 Implementation", available from their web site[4], which clarified that this standard applied only to pathology reports for therapeutic resections, specifically excluding cytologic specimens, diagnostic biopsies, and palliative resections. They further specify that although all of the data elements enumerated in the checklists needed to be included in the pathology report, there was no requirement as to where in the report the data was to be included: they could be included in the final diagnosis, the gross description, the microscopic description, or in the special studies sections of the reports. No specific order is required, and in fact, at least for the time being, no specific format is required (e.g. synoptic vs. narrative), although synoptic reporting is specifically mentioned as preferred, and there is reason to believe that a future iteration of these standards may ultimately require the synoptic format.

---

[3] American College of Surgeons (2003) *Commission on Cancer: Cancer Program Standards 2004*, p 38.

[4] www.facs.org/cancer/coc/standardsclarifications.html

Some pathologists feel that they should merely be required to provide the data elements in the report, and assign someone else the responsibility of extracting this information to build the appropriate American Joint Commission on Cancer (AJCC) stage assignment. Not only does the CoC require that the pathologist assign the pathologic stage, to the extent to which the needed information is available to the pathologist, I also think it is important that pathologists not "step-back" from this responsibility and be content with simply providing data elements. We must remain in our role as consultants, and not slip into a role of simply a data provider. A more detailed discussion of this philosophy is included in Chapter 13.

In response to this requirement, the major anatomic pathology information system vendors have begun to include synoptic reporting capabilities in their information systems, and a number of independent software companies have devised stand-alone solutions to meet this need and are aggressively marketing their products to pathology departments. Chapter 7 includes a discussion on the issues associated with the use of checklist-based/itemized/synoptic reporting, as well as some of the features of different implementations. The checklists themselves can be downloaded from the College of American Pathologists web site (www.cap.org). Similar checklists are also available from Association of Directors of Anatomic and Surgical Pathology (ADASP) web site (www.adasp.org).

Clinical Laboratory Improvement Amendments of 1988

The Clinical Laboratory Improvement Amendments of 1988, otherwise known as CLIA-88, are itemized in Title 42 of the Code of Federal Regulations, Section 493 (42 CFR 493). These regulations apply to any laboratory falling into their rather broad definition of a laboratory, namely "a facility for the biological, microbiological, serological, chemical, immuno-hematological, hematological, biophysical, cytological, pathological, or other examination of materials derived from the human body for the purpose of providing information for the diagnosis, prevention, or treatment of any disease or impairment of, or the assessment of the health of, human beings." Most anatomic pathologists, especially cytopathologists, are very familiar with CLIA. Among other things, CLIA defines test complexity, requirements for laboratory certification, and a number of quality control and proficiency regulations.

Although the regulations contained in CLIA do apply to anatomic pathology laboratories (as well as clinical pathology laboratories), there are no standards which directly relate to pathology information systems. In fact, the word "computer" only occurs a few times (predominantly in reference to electronic signatures), "information system" occurs only once (stating that if data is entered into an information system, the laboratory must ensure that it is entered correctly), and the term "database" does not occur at all.

Nonetheless, pathology information systems can assist in meeting several of the quality control requirements set forth in CLIA. Included among these are keeping track of the number of slides reviewed by cytotechnologists on a daily basis, selection of cases for random review and documenting that review, and meeting the requirements for annual statistical evaluations of cases.

There are a few elements of CLIA which do indirectly impact the capabilities and management of the pathology information system. However, these are currently in flux. Section 1109 of 42 CFR 493 used to define standards for the test reports produced by pathology labs. That section has subsequently been deleted and replaced by Section 1291, with some important changes. For those pathology practices using information systems to generate their reports, these standards need to be considered. Some of these are very straight forward: the test report must include the name and address of the laboratory where the test was performed. However, the original standard also stated that the laboratory must retain and be able to produce, for a period of at least ten years after the date of reporting, the original report or exact duplicates of test reports. Many pathology information systems do not store the actual final report exactly as formatted when originally printed. Rather, the report is generated each time it is printed or viewed by inserting case specific data elements into a report template. This means that if the report template is modified, any report printed subsequently, even from old cases, will be formatted using the new template, and therefore will not represent an "exact duplicate" of the original report. Perhaps for this reason, the most recent (as of Oct, 2004) version of the regulation now states, in section 1291(j), that "all test reports or records of the information on the test reports must be maintained by the laboratory in a manner that permits ready identification and timely accessibility." Clearly, storage within the information system meets this standard. However, section 1105 still states that the laboratory must "retain or be able to retrieve a copy of the original report at least 2 years after the date of reporting". Many pathology departments address this by treating the copy of the report in the medical record as the "official" report, thereby transferring the responsibility for retention of the report to the medical records division, but this does not pertain to reports on outreach patients, for whom no medical record may be present in the institution. It is likely that this internal inconsistency will be corrected; it would be wise to keep track of which direction that correction takes. One report retention issue which is clear pertains to amended reports. Section 1291(k) states that "when errors in the reported patient test results are detected, the laboratory must … (3) maintain duplicates of the original report, as well as the corrected reports".   Although many pathology information systems store, internally, the un-amended version of the final diagnosis field, most cannot produce a copy of the report as it appeared before it was amended. Procedures need to be in place to meet this standard manually with either a printed or electronic archive of reports which have been amended.

Another regulation pertinent to result reporting which has to be considered by those managing the information system is contained in section 1291(f), which states "test results must be released only to authorized persons and, if applicable, the individual responsible for utilizing the test results and the laboratory that initially requested the test." Where this comes into play is for those pathology information systems which manage specimens from both hospital patients and outreach patients. Many of the outreach specimens will be received from patients who have been or will be hospital patients. Should the results on these outreach specimens be made available, formally or electronically via a results interface, to hospital physicians or hospital information systems? This issue is discussed in greater detail near the end of Chapter 10 on Electronic Interfaces. What is "right" or "wrong" in this case is certainly not black or white, and each practice should adopt a policy with which it is comfortable.

Clinical and Laboratory Standards Institute

There is another standards creating organization with which pathologists should be familiar. Originally founded in 1967 under the name of "National Committee for Clinical Laboratory Standards", their acronym, "NCCLS", was often confused with "NACCLS", the "National Accrediting Committee for Clinical Laboratory Sciences", which develops accreditation standards for cytotechnologists and more recently pathologist assistants. Perhaps in part because of this confusion, in 2004 "NCCLS" changed their name to the "Clinical and Laboratory Standards Institute" or "CLSI". At their web site (www.clsi.org), this organization described themselves as "a globally recognized voluntary consensus standards-developing organization that enhances the value of medical testing within the healthcare community through the development and dissemination of standards, guidelines, and best practices." The keyword here is "voluntary". Although they became an American National Standards Institute (ANSI) accredited standards creating organization in 1977, they do not have the legislative authority to impose any of the standards they create. However, other accrediting organizations (for example, the CAP) not infrequently adopt their standards, and many of the suggested rules they put forth are quite simply good ideas.

CLSI produces three types of documents[5]. "Standards" are documents which have been through their consensus process and include "specific, essential requirements for materials, methods, or practices for use in an unmodified form." These represent their "strongest" recommendations. The consensus process includes making a proposed standard available for comment by relevant specialty groups in the field, and then taking into account their comments and suggestions. "Guidelines" have also been through the consensus process, and "describe criteria for a general operating practice, procedure, or material for voluntary use. A guideline may be used as written or modified by the user to fit specific needs." Finally, CLSI also produces "reports", which include information and perhaps suggestions but which have not been through the consensus process. These documents are available for download, for a fee currently ranging from $100 to $120 per document for non-members, through their web site. Proceeds from the sales of the documents are used to fund the organizational structure, including covering expenses for volunteer committee members participating in project development.

CLSI documents are produced by one of their ten "area committees", groups of individuals who focus on specific areas of laboratory practice. One of these groups is the Area Committee on Automation and Informatics". Some of the documents produced by this committee are listed below.

AUTO 01: Laboratory Automation: Specimen Container/Specimen Carrier

> Standards for the design and manufacture of specimen containers and carriers used for collecting and processing liquid samples, such as blood and urine, for clinical testing in laboratory automation systems.

AUTO 02: Laboratory Automation: Bar Codes for Specimen Container Identification

> Specifications for use of linear bar codes on specimen container tubes in the clinical laboratory and for use on laboratory automation systems.

AUTO 03: Laboratory Automation: Communications with Automated Clinical Laboratory Systems, Instruments, Devices, and Information Systems

> Standards to facilitate accurate and timely electronic exchange of data and information between the automated laboratory elements.

AUTO 04: Laboratory Automation: Systems Operational Requirements, Characteristics, and Information Elements

> Operational requirements, characteristics, and required information elements of clinical laboratory automation systems. This information is used to determine the status of a clinical specimen within the clinical laboratory automation system, as well as the status of the actual components of the clinical laboratory automation system.

---

[5] Information obtained from the CLSI web site at www.clsi.org

AUTO 05: Laboratory Automation: Electromechanical Interfaces

Standards for the development of an electromechanical interface between instruments and specimen processing and handling devices used in automated laboratory testing procedures.

AUTO 07: Laboratory Automation: Data Content for Specimen Identification

Specifications for the content of linear bar codes on specimen container tubes in the clinical laboratory and for use on laboratory automation systems.

AUTO 08: Protocols to Validate Laboratory Information Systems (Proposed Guideline)

Guidance for developing a protocol for validation of the Laboratory Information System (LIS) as well as protocols for assessing the dependability of the LIS when storing, retrieving, and transmitting data.

AUTO 09: Remote Access to Clinical Laboratory Diagnostic Devices via the Internet (Proposed Standard)

Standard communication protocol for instrument system vendors, device manufacturers, and hospital administrators to allow remote connections to laboratory diagnostic devices. The remote connections can be used to monitor instruments' subsystems; collect diagnostics data for remote system troubleshooting; and collect data for electronic inventory management.

In addition, the CLSI web site also distributes other documents pertinent to pathology informatics, some produced by other area committees, and other "Laboratory Information System" documents formerly produced by the American Society for Testing and Materials. These include:

GP19-2: Laboratory Instruments and Data Management Systems: Design of Software User Interfaces and End-User Software Systems Validation, Operation, and Monitoring (Guideline)

Important factors that designers and laboratory managers should consider when developing new software-driven systems and selecting software user interfaces. Also included are simple rules to help prepare validation protocols for assessing the functionality and dependability of software.

LIS01: Standard Specification for Low-Level Protocol to Transfer Messages Between Clinical Laboratory Instruments and Computer Systems

Specification for the electronic transmission of digital information between the clinical laboratory instruments (those that measure one or more parameters from one or multiple samples) and computer systems (those that are configured to accept instrument results for further processing, storage, reporting, or manipulation).

LIS02: Specification for Transferring Information Between Clinical Instruments and Computer Systems

Covers the two-way digital transmission of remote requests and results between clinical instruments and computer systems. It enables any two such systems to establish a logical link for communicating text to send result, request, or demographic information in a standard and interpretable form.

LIS03: Standard Guide for Selection of a Clinical Laboratory Information Management System

Covers the selection, purchase, use, enhancement, and updating of computer technology supplied by a vendor as a complete system in the clinical laboratory. The purpose of the guide is to assist hospitals, clinics, and independent laboratories through the entire automation project in order to minimize the risks and maximize the benefits. It also includes checklists of items and design aids to be considered at each stage of planning to assist in carrying out the project.

LIS04: Standard Guide for Documentation of Clinical Laboratory Computer Systems

Covers documentation (defined as the information needed to install, use, maintain, or modify the system) for a computer system operating in a clinical laboratory.

LIS05: Standard Specification for Transferring Clinical Observations Between Independent Computer Systems

Details how clinical observations can be transferred between independent computer systems.

LIS06: Standard Practice for Reporting Reliability of Clinical Laboratory Information Systems

Describes a system for collecting data, maintaining records, and reporting on the reliability of operating clinical laboratory computer systems. The reliability measure will be achieved by documenting the number, severity, cause, impact, and duration of the failures that a system experiences. This practice can be implemented with paper forms or computer records.

LIS07: Standard Specification for Use of Bar Codes on Specimen Tubes in the Clinical Laboratory

Identifies the way bar coded sample identification labels are applied to clinical specimen containers. It documents the form, placement, and content of bar code labels on specimen tubes that are used on clinical laboratory analyzers. It enables Laboratory Information System vendors to produce reliable bar coded symbols that are readable by any complying clinical laboratory analyzer vendor.

LIS08: Standard Guide for Functional Requirements of Clinical Laboratory Information Management Systems

Covers the capabilities needed for a Clinical Laboratory Information Management System (CLIMS). It was written so that both vendors/developers of CLIMS and laboratory managers would have a common understanding of the requirements and logical structure of a laboratory data system. This guide will also provide more uniformity in the way that requirements are expressed from one laboratory to another.

LIS09: Standard Guide for Coordination of Clinical Laboratory Services Within the Electronic Health Record Environment and Networked Architectures

Covers the process of defining and documenting the capabilities, sources, and pathways of data exchange within a given network architecture of a Health Information Network (HIN) serving a set of constituents.

Chapter 13

PATHOLOGY INFORMATICS AND THE FUTURE OF MEDICINE

It is often useful, every decade or so, to step back and re-examine why we do what we do. The pathologist's role in patient care is often described as making tissue diagnoses. However, in a more general sense, we provide information necessary to direct the clinical care of patients. Every pathologist is at least subconsciously aware of this. We choose the wording of our reports in order to trigger the appropriate clinical response. Examination of tissue specimens has traditionally been the primary mechanism by which we make our clinical decisions. The histologic image is one of the richest data streams in medicine today, and the ability of the pathologist to synthesize and interpret this information is unlikely to be duplicated electronically for some time. The process we use is one of classification – putting this patient's lesion into some subcategory (or sub-subcategory) which will best allow prediction of outcome and determine the appropriate treatment. Yet, pathologists also incorporate into our classification process other information derived from the tissue via other techniques such as immunohistochemistry, flow cytometry, and electron microscopy (Figure 13-1). We also incorporate non-tissue derived information, such as presenting signs and symptoms, duration of illness, clinical impression, and past medical history.

A Look Ahead Into the Future

The practice paradigm depicted in Figure 13-1 has worked for decades. Sure, some advances such as immunohistochemistry and newer molecular tests have come along which have added improved discriminating tools to our repertoire of data sources. However, our underlying practice philosophy

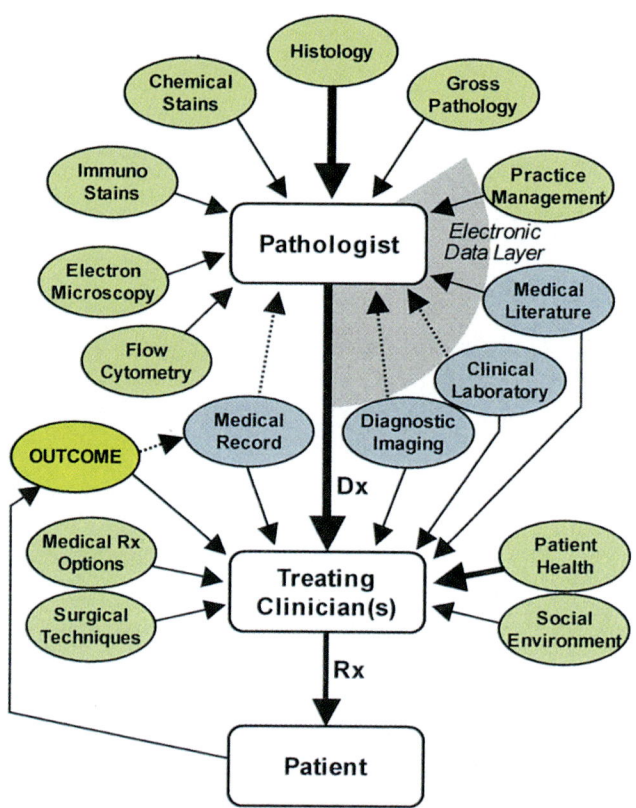

Figure 13-1: Model of the current practice of pathology. Information systems are used predominantly for practice management and access to medical literature. Conspicuously absent is any direct connection between patient outcome and the pathologist.

has not changed. But the practice of medicine, as a whole, is changing in response to a number of external forces. It would be more than just a little naïve to assume that the practice of anatomic pathology will survive this revolution unchanged.

Forces Reshaping Medicine

Sometimes changes to a profession are driven by internal forces. New technology is a good example of this, because it is adopted by the profession and is used to enable better performance or new opportunities. We are a little more comfortable with internal changes, because we have some control over the pace and direction of the resulting changes. When change is driven by external forces, there is significantly less control, less of a clear understanding of where we are going, and less overall comfort with the process. Nonetheless, the major forces currently driving changes in the practice of medicine, including pathology, are external. These can be categorized into a few major inter-related fronts.

Information Availability

The internet, with its myriad of search engines, has made a tremendous amount of information available to anyone and everyone. Whether it be medical or popular literature, opinions and commentary, or life-style choices, it is continuously and instantly available on-line. Before long, each individual's medical record will be as well, although this will hopefully be secure. Among the millions of data pages and databases filling the world wide web are vast amounts of medical information. All physicians, including pathologists, will be expected to be current in the latest developments in their fields. Increasingly sophisticated informatics tools will be needed not only to deliver such information on demand to the pathologist but, more importantly, to integrate and present such information in ways that improve the accuracy and consistency of patient care decisions. Such systems should provide computer assisted and statistically accurate decision support, data mining capabilities, and presentation technologies that enable the pathologists to rapidly identify from a vast ocean of data all information relevant to a specific clinical situation.

Consumerism

The ultimate consumer in the health care industry is the patient, and our consumers are getting more involved in their own care. Fueled by the increased access to medical information, they want greater control of their diagnostic and treatment decisions, and they have expectations for consistency, quality, and value. Now, search engines can deliver highly detailed information to individuals without requiring them to acquire the perspective of context which comes from immersing oneself in a discipline. (I once had a patient phone me to ask if I had done a keratin stain to confirm my diagnosis of their squamous cell carcinoma of the larynx because they had read on the web that squamous cell carcinomas are supposed to be keratin positive.) Public concern about quality to care, media attention over "medical errors", and pure economics has forced the medical industry to place a greater emphasis on process design and the development of error-resistant protocols, so as to make the whole system less susceptible to "human" errors. Information systems will be instrumental to most such processes, and in many cases will drive these processes. Experts in information management will be called upon to participate in these process designs. Pathology information systems house the majority of the objective patient specific information, and will be integral to the development of new pathways and solutions.

New, Complex, Data Streams

The completion of the sequence of the human genome, our better understanding of genetics and the role somatic genetics plays in disease, new diagnostic and prognostic molecular markers, and new technologies producing vast data sets are already changing how we think about, diagnose, and respond to disease. Pathologists will be expected to digest, interpret, and draw conclusions from enormous data sets. New informatics solutions will be needed to turn the vast amount of "data" now becoming available into usable "information". Previously, the only really "information rich" data stream came from viewing histologic tissue sections, but its preeminence is being challenged by the massively parallel data acquisition strategies of genomics and proteomics. New data presentation tools will be key in enabling the success of this process. Other efforts in the emerging field of pharmacogenomics seek to understand individual differences in drug susceptibility and responsiveness in terms of each individual's unique genetic composition. Personalized medicine has made its appearance in the form of individual screening for susceptibility to particular drugs prior to treatment, and this trend is going to become even more popular. Pathologists are likely to be integral in making decisions about the appropriateness or likely effectiveness of different treatment regimens.

Two Views of the Future

The need for informatics tools to assist in future medical decision making processes is clear. It is equally clear that these tools and solutions will be demanded and will be developed. What is unclear is who will be the first to most effectively mobilize, capitalize, and leverage the informatics resources necessary to secure professional "ownership" of the decision making role in medicine, and whether the pathologist will be central or peripheral to this role.

Pathologist as a Data Provider

In one possible scenario (Figure 13-2), the pathologist restricts his/her evaluation to the tissue submitted, and provides an interpretation that becomes data in someone else's decision support system, perhaps that of the treating clinician, who integrates it with other information about the patient and draws upon outcomes databases to make treatment decisions. In this model, the pathologist is protected from mastering new diagnostic modalities, and continues to utilize information systems geared largely to

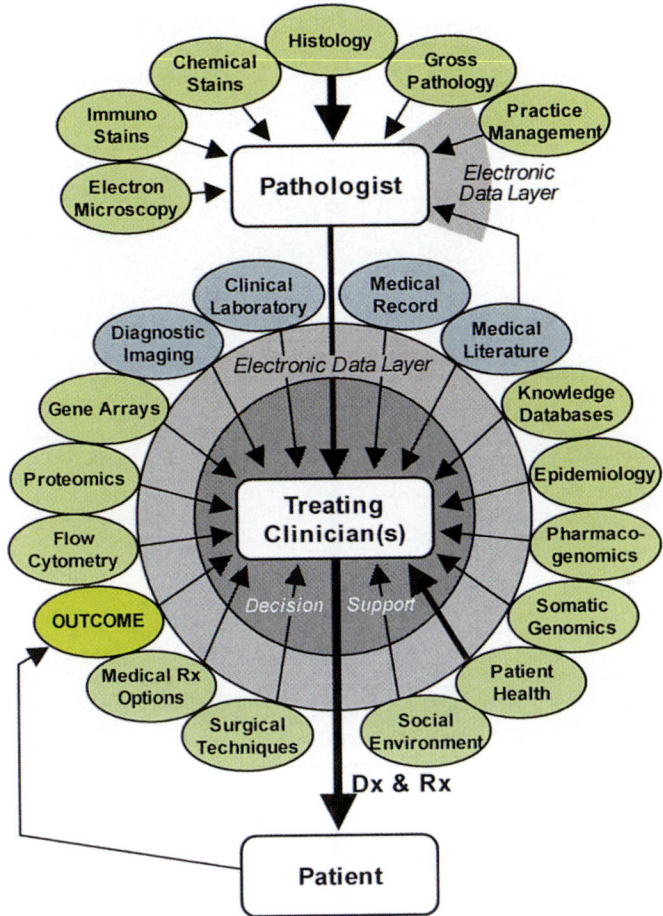

Figure 13-2: Pathologist as a data provider. If pathologists restrict their role in patient care to the histological evaluation of tissue, treating clinicians will increasingly draw upon other diagnostic modalities to make patient care decisions, and the relative contribution of the pathologist will diminish.

practice management. However, as new information sources proliferate, our relative contribution to patient care diminishes. In this future, the anatomic pathologist will function increasingly as a data provider, and less as a provider of professional consultation, a fate similar to what has already largely happened in the clinical laboratory.

Pathologist as the Diagnostic Specialist

In an alternate scenario (Figure 13-3), the pathologist is at the center of the information circle. Here, with the aid of an advanced pathology information decision support system, the histologic interpretation of the case

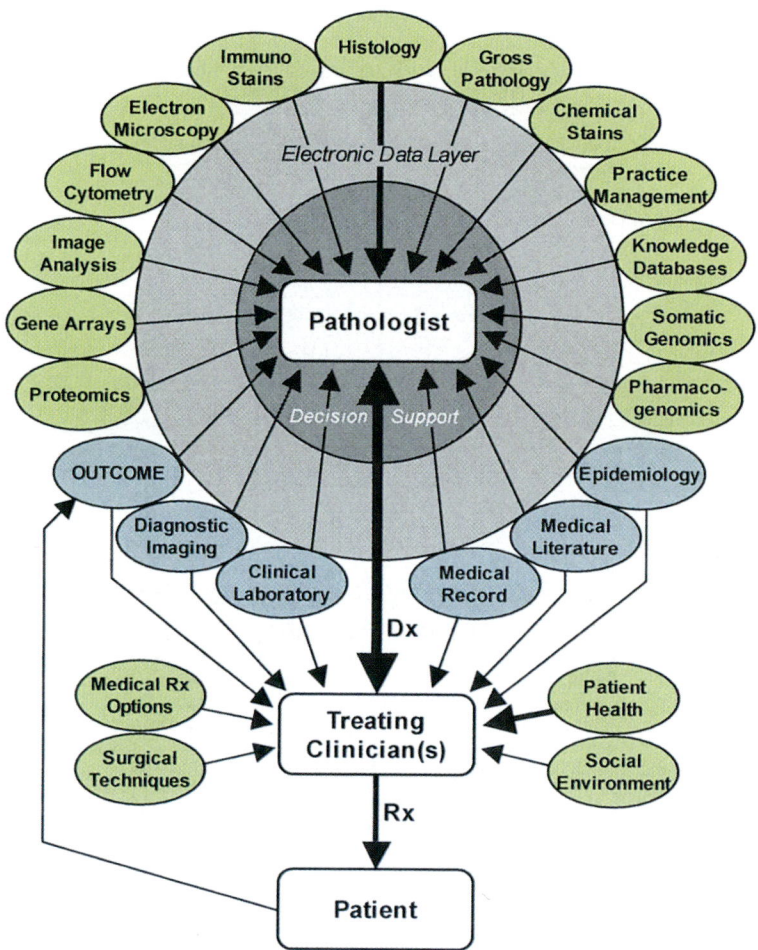

Figure 13-3: Pathologist as the diagnostic specialist. In this possible future, pathologists use informatics tools to leverage access to data from emerging technologies and secures their role in patient care.

is integrated with electronically accessible information from the clinical findings, past medical/surgical history, laboratory data, immunohisto-chemistry, flow-cytometry, genetic studies, data on pharmacogenetics, proteomic studies, and multiple knowledge databases including outcomes data, all to derive an optimal therapeutic decision. The output of this process is an outcomes based treatment recommendation, one reproducible, rationalized on the basis of sound statistical methodologies, and tempered by the wisdom and insight of the pathologist. Treatment decisions are made in collaboration with the other members of the clinical team. To this collaboration, the treating clinician(s) bring knowledge of the patient's current medical status and social environment. Combined with an understanding of recent medical therapy options and surgical techniques, the appropriateness of various treatment options can be assessed. In this future, the pathologist must be an early adapter of new diagnostic and information system methodologies. As a discipline, we must take the lead in validating and integrating the contributions of every appropriate information stream into the diagnostic process. The use of information systems to advance our diagnostic capabilities will have to become as common in the day-to-day practice of pathology as is immunohistochemistry.

For a number of reasons, the "Pathologist as the Diagnostic Specialist" seems the more attractive of the two views of the future. Pathologists, largely freed from the task of routine day-to-day patient-care delivery, have traditionally been well positioned to fulfill the role of data integrator. In fact, there are already many examples of the pathologist filling this role. Few pathologists will sign out a bone neoplasm without knowing what the radiology showed, or sign out a liver biopsy without knowing the patient's liver function test values, or sign out a bone marrow core biopsy without knowing about the results of the smear or the flow cytometry. These ancillary "test results" are already being integrated into our decision making process, and sometimes even into our reports. As a hospital-based specialty, pathologists also have typically enjoyed greater access to capital resources and information system infrastructure when compared to many other specialties. Arguably, this vision of the future is more in keeping with the current roles of the respective players, and perhaps even the personalities and interests for which the two disciplines have traditionally selected. By broadening our role to rigorously encompass many information modalities in the rendering of a consultative opinion, pathologists will secure their continued role as the profession providing the most definitive diagnostic consultation.

Building a Path – Making a Future

Of course, it is one thing to paint lofty visions of the future, arguing on and on about why things should be one way or another. It is quite a different thing to offer realistic suggestions as to how we might actually get there, or at least start down a path which might lead there. Let me propose a few areas where I think greater attention needs to be focused. Building a path to our future will require advances on multiple fronts, all focused on the common goal of defining and securing the pathologist's role as diagnostic specialists.

I should say at the start that I do not feel that a new quantum-leap in technology which revolutionizes the practice of pathology is going to be needed to start us down the right path. Rather, it will be the management of existing technology. Technology has already outpaced the translation into usable systems so far that the actual practice of pathology will be years catching up. This "catching up" will occur within pathology departments themselves, pushed forward by individuals and groups who appreciate the capabilities and limitations of those technologies, who thoroughly understand the practice of pathology and the barriers to adopting new practices, and who have a vision of what the role of the pathologist will be 10-20 years in the future.

Whole-slide Imaging

A number of individuals have suggested that whole slide imaging will fundamentally change the day-to-day practice of pathology, and that within a few more years pathologists will no longer have microscopes at their workstations but rather just computer monitors. Interestingly, most of the people I have heard make this claim are individuals who do not practice anatomic pathology on a regular basis. For a number of reasons, delineated in Chapter 9, I do not personally feel this is likely to happen any time soon. I will not repeat all those arguments here. However, for some limited applications, whole-slide imaging may play a role in the practice of anatomic pathology. This will become especially true once image analysis tools are available which can provide computer assisted diagnosis on the scanned images. When this happens (also quite a few years off), pathologists will want to have maintained control of the management of these images at their institutions. Therefore, to the extent to which pathology practices begin using this technology, it is important that they not turn over stewardship of these images (for example, to institutional PACS systems), without securing unrestricted access to them so that they will be able to explore the use of these diagnosis-assisting tools as they become available.

Create Pathology Informatics Programs

I well remember the advice given to me by a very prominent figure in American anatomic pathology when I asked how they became the "world expert" in their subspecialty field. His advice was simply "the first step in becoming an expert in a field is to declare yourself the expert." He then went on to explain that by declaring yourself the expert, everyone will send you cases, seeking your opinion, and before long you will have seen more cases of that type than any other person in the world, and will become the expert. I must admit that this approach runs somewhat counter to my personality, but the basis for the advice is sound. In a vacuum, the appearance of validity is often as good as the validity itself. Granted, that appearance has to rapidly be backed up by some substance, and the persistent lack of substance will do irreparable harm to any claims one may make in the future, but when one is prepared to provide that substance, a strong show can be a good first step.

Nearly every pathology practice and department has members with special interests in information management. Pathologists are just far too compulsive a group for that not to be the case. But in many instances, these interested parties are scattered about, working independently, and although certainly respected for their technical abilities are often not taken seriously as a decision making body. Coalescing these interests and abilities into a more formal structure can add significant validity to the group, and by coordinating their efforts, they can accomplish a lot more.

Choosing appropriate leadership for the pathology informatics program is important. There might be a tendency to assign a technical manager to this position. However, this will change the perception and focus of the group to that of a technical unit which exists to solve technical problems. Rather, the senior leadership of the informatics group should be a pathologist who can keep the direction and philosophy of the unit aligned with the clinical needs of the department and who is attuned to the future role of the pathologist in the practice of medicine, and how informatics will be key in achieving that goal. This professional vision is more important than technical knowledge and skills. Of course, if one can get a pathologist with the correct vision who also is well versed in informatics technology, that is truly ideal, and hopefully the department/institution will recognize the value of these unique individuals (I say this in case my chairman happens to read this section!).

The scope of a pathology informatics program can vary significantly from institution to institution (see Chapter 1 for a more lengthy discussion). However, three important responsibilities for almost any program should include 1) supporting existing departmental informatics tools; 2) providing specifications for and/or directly developing informatics solutions to meet departmental needs; and 3) training current and future pathologists in the use and integration of informatics tools.

An extension of pathology informatics programs is the position, championed by some, that pathology informatics should be made a formal subspecialty of pathology. However, as discussed in Chapter 1, I would not favor this evolution, and recommend, instead, that pathology informatics continue to be considered a tool to be adopted by all pathologists in their day-to-day diagnostic practice.

Pathology and Computerized Patient Records

Anatomic pathology information systems often function as an island, perhaps with one bridge which allows only inbound admission-discharge-transfer data traffic and outbound final results data. Unfortunately, we often know or care little about what happens to this data once it has left our systems. This is a bad choice, because more and more clinicians are getting our diagnoses through these systems. As this evolution continues, the primary product of our pathology practice shifts from the printed pathology report to the information contained in and displayed by these external systems. Not only must we maintain ownership of that data and assure that it is being communicated, presented, and interpreted correctly (a number of issues pertinent to this are discussed in Chapter 6), but these systems will evolve into true electronic medical records systems, and pathology must have a stake in that process.

Institutional Electronic Medical Record Systems

Electronic medical records are coming. They are a natural extension of the spread of information management tools throughout health care, and represent an ideal opportunity for medically trained individuals interested in information management. Pathology needs to be involved in the evolution of these systems. The biggest volume data generator for centralized clinical data repositories is the clinical pathology laboratories, and related issues pertinent to the clinical pathologist include not only data display but also the mechanisms by which physicians can access that data. Computerized provider order entry (CPOE) is also becoming a major component of the early computerized patient records (CPR), centered largely around drug orders and driven by concerns over patient safety. However, CPOE systems are also being used for ordering laboratory tests, and offer the opportunity to introduce decision logic to assist in selecting the correct tests to order and to prevent the unnecessary duplication of tests. While these systems need to be designed to facilitate test ordering, they also need to have the appropriate checks and balances to prevent an inexperienced clinician from ordering an expensive, difficult test which is not likely to provide usable information but which can be ordered as easily as clicking in a checkbox on the computer screen.

Anatomic pathologists have largely been protected from computerized order entry, since we can't do an evaluation until we have a tissue specimen, and the type of examination required generally comes either explicitly or implicitly with the specimen rather than being ordered in advance. However, pre-approved "reflex tests" are becoming more popular, and as decision logic is created to support these, pathologists need to be key players in the design process. An appropriate balance needs to be achieved between the increasing battery of molecular tests available and the potential abuse of our "self referral" testing privilege.

If pathologists hope to position themselves to be the data integrator in the practice of medicine, the electronic medical record is going to be the source of the data to be integrated, and we need to be major decision makers in the design and availability of these emerging electronic medical records systems. Although many of the issues discussed in this section are somewhat peripheral to the goal, they are certainly more than enough justification for the involvement of pathologists as these medical records systems are introduced. Pathologists need to secure positions on decision making committees at their institutions, and need to make it clear that we need early access to the information in these systems to integrate that information into our diagnoses. Perceptions that the pathologists are simply providers of data for these systems but don't actually need to access them must be corrected.

Longitudinal Electronic Patient Records

Of course, the ultimate goal of the electronic medical record is that each patient will have a portable, secure, complete electronic medical record which will grow over their lifetimes and be fully and immediately available to any current and future treating physician, either being accessed from some central, secure storage location or carried by the patient in some portable, universally readable format. Not only are there security issues to be addressed, but the number of technical standards which must be developed and adhered to in order to assure this portability are significant. Currently, at many institutions, there are significant technical barriers to integration of multiple internal systems (e.g. radiology and laboratory and anatomic pathology), with disagreements over shared formats and methods of access. Imagine the technical and political complications associated with enabling the data stored in these systems to be shared with other institutions.

Despite my somewhat dim view of any immediate progress toward a universal solution in this area, it should be realized that the closest thing to a longitudinal electronic patient record currently existing is, in many cases, the anatomic pathology information systems. A patient is likely to have many physicians, and their record will be scattered about these physicians' offices. However, since anatomic pathology LIS's contain not only hospital cases, but also referral cases and a growing number of outreach cases from physicians in the community (as pathology practices grow their outreach programs), the pathology information system becomes the most complete longitudinal record of the patient's medical history. This certainly increases the value of that information, for patients, for the pathologists, and for clinical and basic research. Many of these opportunities are discussed further below.

Disease-Based Integrative Reports

The need for data integration is already here. With the increasing number of specialized tests which can be performed on tissue specimens (not simply immunohistochemistry and electron microscopy but also chromosomal analyses, polymerase chain reactions, drug susceptibility studies, molecular marker assessments, gene rearrangement studies, etc.), a single specimen often results in multiple reports. Since the turnaround time for these procedures varies significantly, the data resulting from these multiple studies is being fragmented within the medical record. Not only is the clinician often the one forced to make sense of the segmented data provided as a result of their request for our consultation, but we occasionally hinder this process.

Pathology laboratories have scored a number of significant failures in this area. Because of the separation of histology and clinical laboratory services at many institutions, a bone marrow biopsy and aspirate obtained from the patient at the same time are often reported separately, and may even be conflicting. Because electron microscopy interpretation is often performed by a different pathologist than the one doing the light microscopic examination of the tissue, I have seen examples of electron microscopy "addendums" reaching a different conclusion about the origin of a particular neoplasm than the histology-based portion of the report. Not only is conflicting information present in the same resulting report, but there is often no attempt by either party to reconcile or explain the discrepancy. Clinicians are left to flip back and forth through the report trying to figure out what it all means.

However, we have had some important successes as well. Many pathology laboratories have developed specialized workflow for hematologic specimens, integrating biopsy and cytology and immunohistochemistry and flow cytometry data into one, coherent report with one final diagnosis. Pathologists will integrate the results of liver function tests into their assessment of a medical liver biopsy, and no wise bone pathologist will place a definitive diagnosis on a bone mass without knowing the radiological assessment of its aggressiveness. (I know I just said this a few pages ago, but it seemed worth repeating.) These are examples of reports which integrate the histologic examination with the data derived from other disciplines to produce far more clinically useful reports than any of the elements by themselves.

The goal of the whole being greater than the sum of the parts has ushered in the new concept of a "disease-based pathology report". In much the same way that a clinician who requests a cardiology consultation would expect to receive a report which summarizes all of the relevant data from physical examination, laboratory tests, electrocardiography, and echocardiography into one bottom-line assessment and treatment recommendation, the thought is that specimens submitted to the laboratory would similarly result in a multidisciplinary summary, assessment, and plan. Thus, rather than the clinician receiving, separately, a bone marrow smear report and a bone marrow biopsy report and a flow cytometry report and peripheral blood cell counts and a cytogenetic report, they would be able to receive a "hematologic neoplasm assessment report". Similarly, by extension, clinicians could receive a "diabetes status" report, integrating data from blood tests, kidney biopsy, ophthalmologic exam, and urinalysis. Other examples would include transfusion reaction assessments, coagulopathy workups, and several endocrine workups. Opponents to the disease-based reports argue that this is simply regurgitation of data already in the medical record, increasing the volume of the record and introducing opportunities for errors. Proponents offer that a consolidated report enables the more efficient practice of medicine and provides pathologists an opportunity to emphasize our roles as consultants, adding value to the data we generate. As mentioned, this is already being done to some extent, often informally, but that sets the stage for expansion of this activity into new areas.

Of course, a number of issues will need to be examined and addressed. If I include the results of a radiological evaluation in my composite report, and that radiological evaluation is later rethought and amended, how will I be notified of that so that I can address it and potentially amend my composite report? This is not a new issue. Whether done formally as an integrated report or not, anatomic pathology assessments and diagnoses are almost always tempered by our understanding of the clinical situation, and when our knowledge of the clinical status changes, that often requires us to rethink our interpretation. Additionally, if the disease-based report is to integrate data generated by multiple medical disciplines, is the pathologist always the best person to do this integration? Is this an independently billable activity? Certainly there is a professional component to the task, but some may argue that that professional component is already incorporated into the individual tests. Finally, from what information system will these disease-based reports be generated? Should it be the anatomic pathology information system, or the laboratory medicine information system, or the central electronic medical record system which is the composite repository for all of the primary data elements? Does the answer have to be the same for all disease-based reports? The possible use of institutional electronic medical record systems to generate these reports is another argument in favor of the pathologist being involved in the design and deployment of these systems.

An important step toward achieving control of the data integration process will be to maintain custodianship of the tissue we receive for evaluation. As new molecular tests become available which can be performed on patient tissue, laboratories to perform these tests are popping up all over the institution. Pathologists must be careful that our role in this process is not reduced to that of dividing up the tissue into appropriate sized chunks and sending it off to other laboratories. Whenever possible, this advanced testing should be done within the pathology department. When not possible, the reports from these tests should come back to the pathology department and the pathologist should integrate all of the individual data elements into a single, composite report. Since most hospitals already require that all tissue removed from a patient go through the pathology laboratory, we are in a position to make this happen, but if we fail to seize this opportunity, we may lose it forever.

New Information Systems Structured for Outcomes Research

Pathology is the study of disease. Every pathologist has uttered this phrase dozens of times, often in response to queries from friends or relatives asking "now, tell me again, what is it that you do?" However, it would serve us well to pay attention to our response more carefully. Pathology is the study of disease... not just the histology of disease, or the morphology of disease, or the molecular biology of disease, but the whole disease. An important part of the study of disease is finding out what happens to patients after we make our diagnoses. It has always puzzled me somewhat that pathologists seem to be quite willing to forego learning about the subsequent clinical course of these patients, and that no practical mechanism has been developed to provide us with routine feedback on the outcomes of our patients.

If combined with patient outcome data, the potential of the data stored in pathology information systems to improve and advance our understanding of human disease, to better stratify patients for treatment, and to improve patient outcome and quality of life, is unparalleled by any literature resource or technology in existence today. One can easily imagine roles for pathology information systems in public health monitoring, cohort analysis for data-based treatment decisions and up-to-date evidence-based prognoses.

Current Pathology LISs are Not Ideally Suited for Research

Despite the fact that anatomic pathology information systems contain a tremendous amount of highly valuable data for potential use in clinical research, that data is not structured in a way that allows optimum use of the information.

Anatomic pathology information systems traditionally do not store raw data, but rather interpretations of that data, and they store those interpretations in the worst possible way for data retrieval: free-text. If, given a particular patient with a particular tumor, one wants to look at outcomes of similar patients with similar tumors, the computer system can identify similar patients (age, gender), but how will it identify similar tumors? The first step is identifying patients with the same diagnsosi. A variety of coding and keyword-based searching techniques can be used for this, and these are discussed in more detail in Chapter 11. However, not all patients with the same diagnosis have similar lesions. Very few pathology information systems can be searched to identify patients with, for example, node-negative breast cancer between 2 and 3 cm in greatest dimension. This is because tumor size and lymph node status generally do not exist as independently searchable fields. Certainly, the information is there, perhaps in the final diagnosis, perhaps in the gross description. But developing a search algorithm to consistently and accurately extract this data from free text, taking into account the varying styles of individual pathologists and the fact that units are not always consistent (cm, mm, inches), is essentially impossible. To facilitate this type of searching in the future, new ways of storing the data upon which the diagnoses are made will need to be developed. Structured or checklist-based reporting (see Chapter 7 for a detailed discussion) provides a potential solution, because it is possible not only to more easily extract data from the report if certain elements are always stored in the same place, but also the actual components themselves can be stored as individually searchable criteria. Structured reporting will also assure completeness of reporting and satisfy new, soon to be imposed regulations. It should be noted that even such "specific" information as TNM staging data is not sufficient "detail", since these staging criteria are not immutable, and what is today a T2 lesion may, next year, be reclassified as a T1 or a T3 lesion. Recognizing this variation in staging criteria over time, the American College of Surgeons' Commission on Cancer has adopted a new staging model for tumor registries known as "collaborative staging", in which up to fifteen individual data elements are stored for each tumor diagnosed, and then algorithms can be used to calculate the stage for various staging systems. As the staging criteria change, the algorithms can be updated and even applied to historical data, allowing better comparisons within longitudinal data sets spanning years of diagnostic criteria.

Another shortcoming in the way data is stored in anatomic pathology information systems is that it is stored in a specimen-based rather than a patient-based structure. This has evolved around the transactional focus of current information systems, which to date have been concerned predominantly with practice management issues. However, it is often necessary to assimilate clinical and diagnostic data from several specimens to appropriately classify a patient's disease status. Take for example the instance in which a patient has a PAP smear, interpreted as a high grade squamous lesion. A colposcopy is performed, and a biopsy is diagnosed as invasive squamous cell carcinoma. A hysterectomy is performed and evaluated as a Stage I lesion, but within 2 months a biopsy of a clinically palpable inguinal node shows locally metastatic disease, and the patient is appropriately upstaged. Six months later, a pulmonary metastasis is identified. Five specimens have been received, yet, this patient does not have five cancers of various stages, but rather one tumor. There needs to be a way to handle this data as a single tumor, and to base treatment and outcomes information on that classification.

Pathologists must have access to information systems which are structured to allow for disease based clinical outcomes research. Many options exist for how to achieve this, but the first decision should be whether to integrate this capability into existing transactional systems or to set up a separate data repository into which the pathology information is exported. Both have advantages and disadvantages. For a number of reasons, a second data-repository dynamically linked to the transactional system is likely to be the best solution, but also carries with it the greatest risk of conveying the impression that it is then "some one else's problem" to make this work. Pathology departments, and pathologists in particular, must remain vested in this effort and in fact should be the architects of these systems, since full access to this data during signout will be crucial to integrating this information into patient care decisions.

Institutional Tumor Registries

Most institutions already have an information system which meets many of the structural and informational requirements of a system designed for clinical research. This rich source for outcomes data at most hospitals is their internal tumor registry. Although the information will be limited to patients diagnosed with malignant neoplasms, this is an excellent place to start, and one could argue that these are the patients for whom the outcome data is of greatest value to the surgical pathologist. Diagnosis and treatment of malignancies currently receives a lot of attention from clinicians and the public in general, and there are a number of government and private funding sources to address improvements in this area.

Current tumor registry systems tend to be remarkably underutilized locally. Although they provide valuable data to state and national organizations which, presumably, make good use of the information, in many cases little use is made of it at the institution collecting the data, beyond providing numbers for administrative reports. In part, this is due to the fact that many commercially available tumor registry systems have been stripped down to the bare bones needed to meet externally mandated reporting requirements, making them poorly suited to customized searching and data analysis. Additionally, hospitals managing the staff responsible for data entry into these systems have streamlined their operations so much that there is little in the way of available resources to coordinate data searching, case identification, or analysis requests.

Pathology departments should be running tumor registries (with financial support from the hospitals, of course, since they bear the regulatory requirements which tumor registries exist to meet). Granted, running a tumor registry caries with it a number of requirements and responsibilities for reporting to state and federal organizations, but the value of this data far outweighs these administrative headaches.

The data stored in tumor registry systems is perhaps the cleanest data in any clinical information system, because regulations require it to be complete, because it includes data compiled from multiple sources, and most importantly because it is manually curated. This last fact is crucial: data pooled electronically is nice as a starting point, but nowhere near approaches the value of data manually abstracted, reviewed, and encoded by trained individuals. The data is also already structured in the appropriate fashion for the outcomes research information to which pathologists need to have access as part of their role as data integrators. The data in these systems is stored by tumor diagnosis rather than by specimen or visit, and a significant amount of relevant diagnostic, treatment, and follow-up data is included.

Arguments in favor of pathology departments managing tumor registries are easy to make. Since very few treatments for malignancies are made without at least one tissue based diagnosis having been reviewed locally, essentially every patient in the tumor registry system will have had at least one pathology specimen reviewed or processed by the pathology department, and in fact the pathology information system is the source of much of the data in the tumor registry system. At many institutions, this data is already transferred in some electronic fashion.

A close marriage of tumor registry and pathology information systems will create opportunities for more accurate and more complete abstracting of data. Currently, pathologists analyze each cancer case in detail, often integrating information obtained from the clinicians and from other diagnostic procedures as well as from the gross and microscopic examination of the specimen(s), and then communicate their findings and interpretations in the form of a written report. Months later, an abstractor in the tumor registry will read over this written report, and try to extract the exact same information which, months earlier, the pathologist had readily available. Having both information systems under the same management, and having pathologists who understand the importance of recording and documenting this information in a granular form creates new opportunities for more accurate and timely "transfer" of the data into tumor registries. In addition, pathologists often have access to data not otherwise available to tumor registrars. Many pathology laboratories serve a much larger geographical area than the patient catchment area for the institution. The pathology department will potentially have access to prior biopsies done in an outpatient setting, or have reviewed material processed and evaluated elsewhere in preparation for the patient receiving treatment locally. In contrast, tumor registry systems have traditionally been much better at recording other potentially relevant stratifying information about the patients which may not be routinely available to pathologists. This would include such information as family, social, and occupational history. Most importantly, tumor registries have well established mechanisms for collecting and integrating patient treatment and outcome data, information which pathology information systems were not designed to accommodate. Creating an environment in which the pathologists have full, real-time access to the information in the tumor registry systems (among others), and the registrars have full, real-time access to the information in pathology information systems (among others), especially if that environment encourages collaboration between these two groups, will promote better patient care, more accurate diagnosis and treatment decisions, and truly invaluable opportunities for on-going clinical research.

It may take a long time for any one institution to accumulate enough data about any particular disease process to provide effective statistically relevant outcomes and profiling data. This would be greatly accelerated by creation of multi-institutional databases. This is not likely to be in the form of a real, central repository of data, but rather as a virtual multi-institutional data federation (see Chapter 6 for more details), seamlessly interconnected by some common interface.

As pathology departments and their information systems more and more become a storehouse of longitudinal patient data, pathology departments will become increasingly involved in assuring patient safety through dissemination of information to appropriate treating physicians.

Pathology Informatics and Biomedical Research

The data stored in pathology information systems is incredibly valuable for clinical research, especially as some of the changes discussed in the previous sections become a reality. However, pathology departments also have in their possession the single most valuable commodity for basic biomedical research – archived human tissues linked to that clinical data.

Research use of tissues carries with it a number of politically and socially charged issues. The past few years have seen a rapidly evolving sense of "ownership" of pathology tissue and the associated data, and this must be taken into account in designing any system for identifying tissue for research. Not too long ago, there would have been few who would have argued with the fact that this tissue "belonged to pathology". However, it is now more commonly felt that the tissue, if linkable to the patient of origin, still belongs to the patient, and if unlinked from the patient, belongs to the scientific and medical community as a whole. Federal legislation and other external regulations (see Chapter 12) are also weighing in heavily on this issue.

As the custodians of patient tissue, pathologists must also consider their on-going obligations to their patients. Definitions such as "excess tissue" are being rethought: as new molecular tests become available which can further stratify patients into different diagnostic and prognostic groups, the desire to perform those tests on archived tissue and potentially alter current treatments accordingly require that some of that archived tissue still be available and not have been exhausted for research. Clearly, ways of making this valuable resource more readily available without compromising patient confidentiality and the possible future care of the patient need to be worked out, but this is beyond the scope of the current discussion. However, these solutions will require careful oversight, difficult decision making, and a strong information management infrastructure.

One of the unfortunate realities about the past and current use of tissue for research is that, to date, it has been largely a unidirectional process. Tissue is identified, extracted from pathology archives, and then disappears into researcher's laboratories. There has been very little work invested into building reference databases into which the results from the research can be stored and used to feed back into decision support. To a certain extent, this has been because the output of modern research studies is becoming almost unmanageable. Traditionally, a particular gene or protein was linked to a particular outcome risk. If sufficient reliability and reproducibility was established, that test became clinically available – a test could be ordered, and the result reported and stored. But this model will not work for some of the new tests being developed, tests which produce not simply a single number, but rather a huge array of data. This data will not integrate into existing transactional information systems, and argue instead for building data warehouses specifically designed and optimized for data mining and research. Chapter 6 discusses this topic in more detail.

The increasing battery of diagnostic tests which evaluate both single as well as thousands of molecular events allow objective stratification of patients and patient tissue into groups which may have diagnostic and/or prognostic significance. Correlation studies with outcomes information are needed to assess and validate that possible significance. Many argue that as more and more of these tests become available, the morphologic examination of the tissue under the microscope will no longer be necessary. (Parenthetically, what is it that everyone who does not routinely use a microscope have against microscopes? I find the recurrent desire that non-anatomic pathologists seem to have for getting rid of the microscope as a diagnostic instrument quite intriguing. People are willing to view with fascination the multi-pseudo-colored outputs of gene array experiments or the myriad of overlapping mass spectroscopy peaks which represent the protein expression profile of tissue, and to accept the potential future role these large data sets might eventually have in telling us about the molecular characteristics of the lesion. Yet, they fail to realize that the morphologic appearance of the tissue is simply another intricate, highly detailed read-out of the aggregate and interacting gene and protein expression levels of the cells making up that tissue, a read-out which the trained anatomic pathologist has become incredibly adept at processing and interpreting. Personally, I think that what makes people uncomfortable with the pathologist's interpretation of the morphological phenotype is that it is a subjective process, and not every pathologist will process the data in the same way. Apparently, there are some who would rather have a more "objective", computer driven interpretation which will be more consistent, even if less correct. But I digress....) Pathologists must not view these new tests as "competition", but rather a new battery of tools at our disposal to provide better patient care. Pathologists should be closely involved in the development and assessment of these tools, and do so enthusiastically and objectively, contributing our years of experience to that assessment. And we must be the first to adopt those tests which prove valuable for patient care, integrating that information, and all available information (including the morphologic interpretation) into our overall evaluation of the specimen.

"Basic" Informatics Research

The majority of this text has focused on what I defined in the first chapter to be "translational informatics research", namely the application of existing information technologies and algorithms to the day to day practice of pathology. That is where my particular interests lie. However, there is clearly the need for the development of some new algorithms and new technologies to fully leverage the amount of information potentially valuable for the practice of medicine.

Information Extraction from Text

Chapter 11 introduced retrieval of anatomic pathology reports by diagnosis, and the capabilities and limitations of keyword searching in contrast to pre-coded reports. So much of the medical data that exists today exists only in the form of free-text, and the increasing documentation requirements being imposed on physicians is only increasing the amount of that text. This includes not only pathology reports, but also admission notes, operative reports, discharge summaries, and outpatient progress notes. As many organizations are beginning to move toward electronic patient records, these documents are being stored electronically. In many cases, they are even generated electronically. For those instances in which "free-text" reports are generated in an automated fashion from the entry of a limited number of key data elements, there should be a way to store those key data elements as individually identifiable and searchable data elements from the beginning, so that they do not need to be re-extracted at some later time. For those documents which are generated as free dictations, new information-extraction tools based on natural language processing algorithms need to be developed to at least semi-automate this process. Retrospectively, such tools could be used to further unlock the tremendous value of tissue archived in pathology departments by making the diagnostic reports on those tissues more searchable and retrievable. These information extraction tools will need to have the appropriate level of sophistication to deal with negation logic, changing terminologies, and reports of different formats. If subsequently linked to particular controlled vocabularies, these information extraction tools would enable the development of auto-coding software, vastly increasing the available resource of consistently encoded medical documents.

An environment already exists in which such tools could be developed and tested. Tumor registrars spend most of their day manually scanning through a variety of free text reports, extracting information and re-entering it for reporting purposes. In this setting, newly developed information extraction software could be run against these same reports, and the results compared to data manually extracted. This would provide quality and accuracy assessment of the software. To the extent to which the software is successful, it will be readily received by tumor registrars, facilitating their daily activities, and therefore they are likely to be quite amenable to such trials.

Information Extraction from Images

This past decade has seen the appearance of "electronic cytotech-nologists", instruments which are effective at, and have even been "approved" for, the screening of exfoliative cervical cytologic specimens.

Under the proper circumstances and with a sufficient number of samples, these machines can designate a portion of the slides examined as needing no further evaluation – meaning they are never screened by a human. This new paradigm has opened the door for electronic image-based diagnoses, and created a need for new algorithms for information extraction from digitized images.

Traditional image analysis has focused on quantitative measurements of density and color, and the variation of these parameters spatially across the image. Electronics are very good at absolute density assessments, far better, in fact, than are humans. The human eye and brain are too easily distracted by surrounding structures (Figure 13-4). This explains, in part, the superior performance of instruments which quantitatively assess intensity of immunohistochemical stains. Subtle differences in intensity can be used to automatically segment an image into component parts, and perform differential analyses on those parts. An example of this would be software which takes an image, identifies where the nuclei are, measures the area of each nucleus, sums that data, and divides by the area of the cytoplasm, calculating a nuclear:cytoplasmic ratio. Additional density and chromatic analysis tech-

Figure 13-4: Absolute density determination. The human eye is not well suited for determining the absolute density of image information separated by intervening and different backgrounds. The two small squares shown here are actually the exact same shade of gray, but do not appear to be because of the different background.

niques can measure nuclear contours, or even extract subtle textural differences between different chromatin patterns, extracting potentially important differences which the human eye cannot appreciate.

In contrast, the human eye, especially a trained one, is particularly good at recognizing patterns, and even subtle differences in patterns, differences which cannot be adequately described in words or by any mathematical representation, can be readily distinguished. This has been largely responsible for the success of surgical pathology as a discipline. The automated image analysis techniques used for cytologic specimens do not have to take into account cell-cell relationships, and as such address a relatively simpler problem. New image analysis algorithms will be needed to analyze histologic sections. Some of these are starting to appear, drawing on techniques developed for the automated processing of aerial satellite photographs. There are some diagnoses in surgical pathology today which are made based on a single microscopic field. Evaluation of prostatic core biopsies for the presence or absence of adenocarcinoma is one of those. One is often faced with an "atypical" focus, which one has to determine as representing a benign proliferation, adenocarcinoma, or falling into that indeterminate category "atypical small acinar proliferation".   It may eventually be possible to take a digital photograph of that focus and upload it to a web site which will then return a probability assessment as to the likelihood that the focus represents a malignant process.

A far more compelling role for whole slide imaging may emerge as automated image analysis routines are tuned to discriminate histologic images. This whole-slide approach significantly increases the amount of "noise" in which to find the diagnostic signal, and far more sophisticated techniques will be needed. Even the "simple" problem of identifying artifacts in histologic sections is not trivial from an electronic perspective.

The potential use of computerized image analysis techniques has caused some early adopters of digital imaging to steer away from lossy compression algorithms like JPEG. I think that concern is unnecessary. Automated analysis of histologic images is years off, and there is no way to predict what level of image detail will be needed for any such analysis to work. Additionally, even if appropriate archival images were available, it is unlikely that there would be a great need to go back and re-analyze them. Should that be necessary for some research project, the original glass slides, or the tissue blocks, will still be available, so this contingency can be addressed when the need arises.

New Knowledge Management and Data Presentation Tools
Tremendous amounts of data are becoming available via the internet. By this, I do not mean simply the billions of text-based web pages, but more specifically both medical literature and curated databases of genes, protein expression patterns, and diseases. It is not always very easy to draw upon this body of knowledge in a way which fits into the workflow of a practicing pathologist.   As the field of medicine evolves toward "personalized medicine" in which treatment decisions are based on the individual genetic makeup of the patient or their tumor, knowledge management tools to tap into these publicly available databases will be essential.

The explosion of data which needs to be managed is not limited to reference material. Many of the new diagnostic modalities being developed yield large data sets as their result. New approaches are needed to display the data generated by these tests. People in general, including pathologists, are not particularly good and assimilating large series of numeric data. Graphical data, however, can be much more readily interpreted. The large data sets generated by many of these new diagnostic tests (immunohistochemical panels, gene-arrays, tumor specific protein expression profiles, etc.) has created the need for tools to display the vast amount of "data" in such a way that it can be converted into usable "information". The informatics sub-field of data display and human-computer interfaces will need greater attention over the coming years.

Decision Support Systems

A number of "expert systems" have come and gone over the past decades. These systems were essentially large databases which were touted to be able to make diagnoses based on the user's response to a handful of context-selected questions. The poor success of these has induced a somewhat reflexive withdrawal among physicians when the topic is broached. However, there is quite a difference between "computer-made-diagnoses" and "computer-assisted-diagnosis", the former being the claim of these early expert systems and the latter referring to the use of computer-based tools during the diagnostic process. Many of the areas discussed above constitute the beginning of decision support systems. In the automated PAP-smear screening field, a step toward automated diagnosis is to have the instrument screen a slide, and then via a robotic microscope stage, direct the cytotechnologist or the cytopathologist to the handful of fields determined to be the "least normal", allowing them to then make the final call. One could equally imagine other computer-based tools which take large data sets as input, filter through them, and then present as output the most relevant data for the pathologist to integrate into his/her final evaluation. Decision support systems will need to draw upon vast amounts of data and present suggestions to the pathologist in a highly interactive fashion. Such decision support systems represent the culmination of all of the ongoing basic and translational informatics research in pathology.

Modeling of Biological Systems

One of the roles of the pathologist has always been to predict the future, initially predicting the behavior of a particular tumor and now, more commonly, predicting the responsiveness of a disease to a particular therapy. The process by which this has been done has largely been correlation between starting points and ending points, with little in the way of substance in between. Increasing knowledge about genes, proteins, and biochemical pathways has begun to unlock some of the mechanisms which connect a particular diagnosis with a particular outcome. Computerized modeling of whole biological systems looks like it may some day become a reality. With the appropriate inputs, underlying knowledge of component interactions, an awful lot of statistics, and sufficient computing power, computerized modeling may be able to assist physicians in selecting the appropriate level of aggressiveness for treatment of a particular patient.

Summary and Conclusions

This book has attempted to provide the reader with a broad overview of a number of topics related to pathology informatics, while providing sufficient detail to also serve as a reference. Walking that line in attempting to appeal to readers with a wider range of backgrounds and interests is not easy, and I hope I have been at least partially successful.

Pathologists as well as other non-physician members of the discipline must become and remain proficient in the use of informatics tools. I have little doubt that when immunohistochemistry first made its appearance in the diagnostic laboratories, there were probably a number of groups which thought this "new technology" was something that others would worry about but which they could largely ignore. Those groups have either recognized their error and reversed their decision, or are no longer practicing pathology. Information management is a similar wave passing over our discipline. Those who do not acquire the skills to deal with it will be similarly swept away.

The early chapters of this book introduced a number of core topics in general informatics, building the foundation necessary to better understand and discuss issues more pertinent to pathology informatics in particular. Subsequent chapters focused on using informatics in the current day-to-day as well as the future practice of anatomic pathology. A number of practical issues, problems, and solutions have been discussed to facilitate pathologist involvement in the growing informatics infrastructure in their practices. These tools can and should be used today, but will also guide us through the changing face of medicine in the years to come.

If the future of the pathologist as a diagnostic specialist is to be obtained, pathology departments, led by strong informatics groups, must move aggressively to develop the skills and the informatics infrastructure necessary to leverage the information explosion. We must eagerly adopt new diagnostic and prognostic modalities as they become available, must rethink how and why we store data electronically, and be willing to progressively look to the future value of this information even in the absence of short term benefits. Recognizing, accepting, and supporting the role that pathology informatics will have in shaping that future is crucial, and we must avoid the impression that this is merely a "technical" activity best relegated to others. Finally, we must leverage our existing and growing informatics infrastructure to explore new options for data storage, analysis, interpretation, and presentation.

As has been said in many different settings, the best way to predict the future is to be part of the force making the future. The future of the pathologist as the diagnostic specialist is both desirable and attainable, but that future is not being reserved for us. Its realization will require aggressive incorporation of new technologies into our practices and training programs, and the development of a new generation of pathology informatics capabilities to support this integration. If we do not act now to secure our future, someone else's vision of the future will be forced upon us.

INDEX

Active Server Pages, 115
Address book database
  entity-relationship diagram for, 136
  modeled as index cards, 123
  modeled as table, 124
Administrative safeguards, 337–338
Advanced Research Projects Agency, 103
Amending reports, 299
American College of Surgeons, 346–348
American Standard Code for Information
    Interchange, 72–73
Anatomic pathology information systems,
    207–232, 369–370
  automated reporting, 214
  bar code technology, 223–225
  checklist-based/itemized/synoptic
      reporting, 218–221
  computer assisted report distribution, 213
  customizability, 227
  data conversion, 228-232
  diagnosis, case identification by, 214
  digital image acquisition, 216–217
  digital images in reports, 217
  electronic interfaces, 215–216
  electronic signout, 214–215
  high technology features, 215–227
  identification of previous specimens, 213
  informatics activities, 227–228
    evaluation, in anatomic pathology,
        211–228
  information technology impact, categories
      of, 211–212
  legacy information systems, data recovery
      from, 228–232
  literature databases, online, access to,
      227–228
  management reporting tools, 215
  multi-site/lab support, 223
  outreach support, 222
  pathology web sites, 228
  size of display field, 194
  specimen tracking, 212
  speech recognition technology, 225–227
  traditional features, 212–215
  workflow, 207–209
API. See Application Programming Interface
Application access to databases, 141–144
Application Programming Interface,
    168–169
Application software, 55–65
  backward compatibility, 56
  bytecode compiler, 60
  compiler, 57
  computer programming, 56–62
    interpreter, 59
    object code, 57–60
    source code, 57–60
  converting source to executable object
      code, process of, 58–60
  cross-compilers, 58–59
  executable object code, 57–60
  Integrated Development Environment,
      58–59
  interaction with operating system, 55–56
ARPA, 103
ARPANet, 104
ASCII. See American Standard Code for
    Information Interchange
ASP. See Active Server Pages
Attachment of documents, Multipurpose
    Internet Mail Extensions protocol,
    116–117
  MIME, 116–117
Attributes
  definition, 123
  entity-attribute-value data model, 139-140
  redundant, 126
  repeating, 125

Auto-coding, medical documents, 323–324
Automated reporting, 214
Autopsy environment, digital imaging in, 256–257

Babbling, 87
Back end, client-server model, 143
Backup tapes, 157
Backward compatibility, 56
Bandwidth, 89–91
Bar codes, 223–225
  one dimensional, *vs.* two dimensional, 224
Batch files, interfaces, 288–289
Best-of-breed approach, 202
Big-endian, 22
Billing, 216
  batch interface, 296–297
Binary digit, 21
Binary Large Objects, 148
Bioinformatics, 3
  clinical informatics, separation between, 4
Biological systems, modeling, 378–379
Biomedical informatics, 3
Biomedical research, pathology informatics, 372–374
Bit, 21
BLOBs. *See* Binary Large Objects
Bluetooth, 40
Boolean query, 317
Bridges, 99–100
Broadcast networks, 86, 93–97
Bus architecture, 20–21
Bus network, 86–87
Bytecode compiler, 60
Bytes, 23

Cable modems, 47–48
Cables and connectors
  coaxial, 91
  Ethernet, 45
  firewire, 39
  monitor, 34
  small computer system interface, 37
  universal serial bus, 38
  video, 269-271
Cache, 29–30
Cameras, 255
  digital, 256
  one chip, 267
  three chip color, 267
  video, 266–268
Cardinality, 123
Carrier-sense/multiple access, 96

Case identification by diagnosis, 303–324
  coding, evolution of, 304–305
  coding systems, in anatomic pathology, 310–316
  controlled vocabulary, elements of, 307–310
  Current Procedural Terminology, 310–311
  information retrieval, 316–324
    evolution of, 304–305
  International Classification of Diseases, 311–314
  keyword-based information retrieval, 317–319
  natural language processing, 316–324
    in clinical domain, 320–321
    information retrieval, 323–324
      auto-coding, medical documents, 323–324
      keyword queries, expansion of, 323
  Systematized Nomenclature of Medicine, 314–315
  term identification in biomedicine, 321–323
    term classification, 322
    term mapping, 322–323
    term recognition, 321–322
  terminology, 305–310
  Unified Medical Language System, 316
Cathode ray tubes, 31
CCD. *See* Charge Coupled Device
CD. *See* Compact Disc
Central Processing Unit, 27
  speed of, 27–28
CERN. *See* European Laboratory for Particle Physics
Charge Coupled Device, 266
Checklist-based/itemized/synoptic reporting, 218–221
Checklist questions, College of American Pathologists, 343 346
Checksum, 105
Client-server model
  back end, 143
  front end, 143
Client-side-processing, world wide web, 114–115
  JavaApplets, 114
  JavaScript, 114
Client web browser, viewing web page on, 112
Clinical and Laboratory Standards Institute, 350–353
Clinical data repository, 190

Clinical informatics, 3–4
  bioinformatics, separation between, 4
Clinical Laboratory Improvement
  Amendments of 1988, 348–350
CLSI. *See* Clinical and Laboratory
  Standards Institute
Clustered Index, 150
CMOS. *See* Complementary Metal Oxide
  Semiconductor
Coding systems, in anatomic pathology,
  310–316
  Current Procedural Terminology, 310–311
  evolution of, 304-305
  International Classification of Diseases,
    311–314
  Systematized Nomenclature of Medicine,
    314–315
  Unified Medical Language System, 316
College of American Pathologists, checklist,
  342–346
  questions, 343–346
Collision detection, 96–97
Color depth, 238–241
Color video cameras, 266–267
Color lookup table, 241
Color mixing, 239
Commission on Cancer, 347
  Cancer Program Standards, 347
Common Gateway Interface, 115
Communication handler, 288–289
Compact disc, 42–43
  drives, 36, 43
Compilers, 57
Complementary Metal Oxide
  Semiconductor, 268
Component video, 270–271
Composite video, 271
Computer assisted report distribution, 213
Computer languages, spectrum of, 61
Computer processing speed, 28
Computer programming, 56–62
  interpreter, 59
  object code, 57–60
  source code, 57–60
Computer programs execution, 60
Computerized patient record, 190, 364–368
Concept negation, 320–321
Concept orientation, 308–309
Concept permanence, 309
Conference room
  setup, 275
  video microscopy for, 273–276
Consumerism, 357–358

Contention protocol, 95–96
Context representation, 309
Continuous-tone graphics, 80
Controlled vocabulary, 30
  elements of, 307–310
Converting source to executable object code,
  process of, 58–60
CPR. *See* Computerized patient record
CPT. *See* Current Procedural Terminology
CPU. *See* Central Processing Unit
Cross-compilers, 58–59
CRTs. *See* Cathode ray tubes
Current pathology legacy information
  system, research, 368–370
Current Procedural Terminology, 310–311,
  331
Custodianship of tissue, 368
Custom conversion programming, 231
Customizability, 227

Data backup, recovery, 155–157
Data communication rates, bits-per-second,
  35
Data concurrency, 154–155
Data conversion, 229
Data entry constraints, 210
Data exchange, 287–302
  admission/discharge/transfer interface,
    293–296
  billing batch interface, 296–297
  communication handler, 288–289
  interface architecture, 287–292
  interface languages, 289–292
    health level 7, 292
    message formats, 290–291
  interface (translation) processor, 289
  for pathology information systems,
    293–301
  results interface, 297–301
Data federation, 197
Data locking, 157–160
Data persistent model, synoptic reporting,
  219
Data provider, pathologist as, 359
Data repositories, 195–196
  centralized, 196-199
  federations, 196
Data storage in computer, 21–23
Data storage devices, 41–44
  compact disc, 42–43
  Digital Video/Versatile Disc, 43–44
  flash memory drive, 44
  floppy disks, 42

hard disk, 42
magnetic storage devices, disks, 41–42
memory stick, 44
Syquest, 44
zip drive, 44
Data types, 145–149
Database abstraction, 144
Database management system, 140–161
  capabilities of, 145–161
  data backup and recovery, 155–157
  data concurrency, 154–155
  data locking, 157–160
  data types, 145–149
  index maintenance, 149–150
  query optimization, 150–152
  referential integrity, 152–154
  transaction deadlocks, 160–161
Database normalization, 136–138
Database server, communication with, 179, 181
Databases, 121–172
  application access to databases, 141–144
  architecture, 124–140
  database abstraction, 144
  database management system, *See* Database Management System
  entity-attribute-value data models, 139–140
  multi-table databases, 127–131
    hierarchical databases, 128–129
    network databases, 129–130
    object oriented databases, 130–131
    shortcomings of non-relational database architectures, 131
  relational databases, 131–138
    database normalization, 136–138
    entity-relationship diagrams, 135–136
    primary and foreign keys, 132–135
  single table databases, 124–126
    redundant fields, 126
    repeating fields, 125–126
  SQL, 166–172
    application plan, generation of, 166
    database language, 161–172
    embedded, 166–167
    execution of application plan, 166
    module, 167–168
    optimization, 166
    parsing, 165
    processing statements, 165–166
    SELECT statement, 163–165
    validation, 166
  terminology, 122–124

world-wide-web-based access to databases, 169–172
Datagrams, 105
Date storage, 71
Deceased individuals, 336
Decimal numbers, 146–147
Decision support systems, 378
Declarative referential integrity, 153
Degree of entity, 123
Desktop computers, 1–82
  bus architecture, 20–21
  cable modems, 47–48
  cache, 29–30
  Central Processing Unit, 27
    speed of, 27–28
  components, 26–49
  connecting to internet, 47
  data representation, 66–76. *See also* Digital data representation
  data storage in computer, 21–23
    binary digit, 21
    byte, collection of bits, 22
    bytes, large quantities of, terms used to describe, 23
  data storage devices, 41–44. *See also* Data storage devices
  dial-up modem, Internet service Provider, 46
  Digital Subscriber Line modem, 48
  executable software, *See* Software
  flat-text ASCII file, 78
  input/output devices, 34-40. *See also* Input/output devices and controllers
  integrated design, vs modular design, 20–21
  Integrated Services Digital Network, 47
  Local Area Network, 46
  local networking, Network Interface Card, 45–46
  memory, 24-26, 30–31. *See also* Memory
  modem, 46
  mother board, 20
  network connection, 45–49
  non-executable software, 65–82. *See also* Software
  parallel computing, 28–29
  Point-to-Point Protocol, dial-up modem, 46
  processor, 26–30
    architecture, 28
  Serial Line Internet Protocol, dial-up modem, 46

video display controller, 31–34. *See also*
    Video displays
wireless, 48
DHCP. *See* Dynamic Host Configuration
    Protocol
Diagnosis
    case identification by, 214, 303–324. *See
        also* Case identification
    index by, 285–286
Diagnostic radiology, analogy to, 282–283
Diagnostic specialist, pathologist as, 360
Dial-up modem
    Internet Service Provider, 46
    Point-to-Point Protocol, 46
Digital communication, 89
Digital data, binary representation, 21
Digital data representation, 66–76, 166
    binary format, 66–69
    dates, times, storage, 71
    floating point data, 68–71
        double precision, 68
        exponent, 68–70
        number storage, 70
        sign bit, 68
        significand, 69–70
        single precision, 68
    graphical data, 73–76
        bitmapped graphics, 74
            pixels, 74
        vector images, 74–75
    integers, 66–68
    operating systems, variability between,
        70–71
    textual data, 72–73
        American Standard Code for
            Information Interchange, or
            ASCII, 72–73
        character, 76–78
        Unicode Character Set, 73
Digital data transmission on wire, 89
Digital display resolutions, 32
Digital image acquisition, 216–217
Digital imaging, 233–264
    acquisition, 246, 254–257
    autopsy environment, 256–257
    camera, digital, 256
    color depth, 238–241
    compression, 243–245
    for digital projection, 249–250
    elements, 245–248
    integrated imaging, 258–260
    Joint Photographic Experts Group, 243
    modular imaging, 261–264

photomicroscopy, 257
pixel, 236–237
pixel density, 237–238
practical aspects, 248–258
    for printing, 250–254
resolution, 237
size, 242
specifications, 236–242
storage, 242–247, 257–258
surgical pathology gross room, 257
utilization, 247–254
vs. traditional photography, 234
Yale imaging process, 261–264
Digital Subscriber Line, 48
Digital video, 271–273
Digital video projector, 247–248
Digital video signals, 273
    analog video signals, conversion to, 272
Digital Video/Versatile Disc, 43–44
DIMMs. *See* Dual Inline Memory Modules
Direct Memory Access, 36
Direct program access to databases, 141
Disclosures of health information, 330, 334
Disease-based integrative reports, 366–368
Disks, data stored on, 42
Distributed processing, 179–181
DMA. *See* Direct Memory Access
Document retrieval, 315
Domain knowledge, 132
Domain name system, 108–109
DSL. *See* Digital Subscriber Line
Dual Inline Memory Modules, 26
Dumb terminal, 177
Dynamic database driven web page, process
    of delivering, 171–172
Dynamic Host Configuration Protocol, 107
Dynamic non-robotic telemicroscopy
    system, 278
Dynamic random access memory, 24, 30
Dynamic robotic telemicroscopy, 278
Dynamic Structured Query Language, 167
Dynamic telemicroscopy, 277

E-mail. *See* Electronic mail
EEPROM. *See* Electrically Erasable and
    Programmable Read Only Memory
Electrically Erasable and Programmable
    Read Only Memory, 25
Electronic interfaces. *See* Interfaces
Electronic mail, 115–120
    on internet, 120
    Internet Message Access Protocol,
        117–118

Post Office Protocol, 117
  Internet Message Access Protocol,
      contrasted, 118–120
  security, 120
  simple mail transfer protocol, 116–117
  viruses, 120
Electronic medical record systems, 189–206
  anatomic pathology outreach services,
      205–206
  centralized data storage, access, 195–199
  data centralization, 192–195
  obstacles to adoption of, 199–205
      economics, 200–201
      universal patient identifier, 202–205
      vendor choice, 201–202
  patient safety, 191
  professional society recommendations,
      191–192
  resurgence of interest, 190–192
  wireless technology, 191
Electronic signout, 214–215
Embedded Structured English Query
      Language, 166–167
Encapsulated Postscript, 82
Endian, 22
Engineering
  defined, 8
  informatics as, 8–9
Entity, 122
Entity-attribute-value data models, 139–140
Entity-relationship diagram, 135–136
EPROM. *See* Erasable and Programmable
      Read Only Memory
Erasable and Programmable Read Only
      Memory, 24
Ethernet, 97–98
  data frame, structure, 105
  icon, connector, 45
  standard, 98
European Laboratory for Particle Physics,
      HyperText Transfer Protocol, 104
Excess tissue, 373
Executable object code, 57–60
Executable software, 51–65. *See also*
      Software
eXtensible Markup Language, 291
External peripheral devices, 34–35
Extranet, defined, 174

FDDI. *See* Fiber Distributed Data Interface
      protocol
Federated databases, 197-199
Fiber Distributed Data Interface protocol, 93

Fiber optic cabling, 91
Fields, 122–123
File Transfer Protocol, 103–104
Files, storing images in, 242–245
Firewall, 174
First normal form, 137
Flash memory drive, 44
Flash ROM, 25
Flat-text files, 78–79
Floating point data, 68–71
  double precision, 68
  exponent, 68–70
  number storage, 70
  sign bit, 68
  significand, 69–70
  single precision, 68
Floppy disks, 42
Floppy drives, 44
Forces reshaping medicine, 356–358
Foreign key, 134–135
Formal definitions, 309
Free speech, 226
FROM clause, 163–165
Front end, client-server model, 143
FTP. *See* File Transfer Protocol
Fully instantiated, defined, 306
Future developments, 355–361

Gateway, 101
Generic single precision floating point
      number, 69
Government, future role of, 202
Graphical data storage, 73–76
  bitmapped graphics, 74
      pixels, 74
  vector images, 74–75
      bitmapped images, distinction between,
          76
Graphical interchange format, 80–81

Hard disks, 42
Hardware, desktop computers. *See* Desktop
      computers
Headless session, 181
Health Insurance Portability and
      Accountability Act, 325–342
  administrative safeguards, 337–338
  adoption of standards, 328
  business associate, 331
  covered entity, 330
  disclosure, 330
  electronic transactions, code sets, 331
  general provisions, 330–331

history of, 328–330
individually identifiable health
    information, 330–331
national identifiers, 340–342
physical safeguards, 339
principles of, 327
privacy regulations, 332–337
protected health information, 330
research use, anatomic pathology
    information systems, 334–337
security regulations, 337–340
security standards
    availability of data, 337
    integrity of data, 337
    unauthorized access, 337
technical safeguards, 340
universal patient identifier, 202-203
Hierarchical databases, 128–129
HIPPA. *See* Health Insurance Portability and
    Accountability Act
History of internet, 103–105
HTML. *See* Hypertext markup language
Hubs, 98–99
Human subject, defined, 335
Hybrid entity, 332
Hypertext markup language, 112–114
HyperText Transfer Protocol, 104

ICANN. *See* Internet Corporation for
    Assigned Names and Numbers
ICD. *See* International Classification of
    Diseases
IDE. *See* Integrated Drive Electronics
IDF*TF. *See* Inverse Document Frequency
    times Term Frequency
IEEE. *See* Institute of Electrical and
    Electronic Engineers
Image acquisition, 246, 254–257
Image compression, 243–245
Image file formats, 80-82
    continuous-tone graphics, 80
    Encapsulated Postscript, 82
    graphical interchange format, 80–81
    Joint Photographic Experts Group, 81–82
    object-based image file format, 82
    pixel-based image file format, 81
    Portable Network Graphics, 81
    Tagged Image/Interchange File Format, 81
    Windows Meta File, 82
Image quality, 283–284
Image quality category, 255
Image resolution, 237–238
Image sizes, 242

Image storage, 246–247, 257–258
Image utilization, 247–254
Images for digital projection, 249–250
Images for printing, 250–254
IMAP. *See* Internet Message Access Protocol
Index by diagnosis, 285–286
Index maintenance, 149–150
Indirect treatment relationship, 332–333
Individually identifiable health information,
    330–331
Informatics, defined, 1
Informatics activities, evaluation, in
    anatomic pathology, 211–228
Informatics perspective, issues to consider,
    335–336
Informatics process, 2
    life cycle of, 10
Information retrieval, 316–324
    evolution of, 304–305
Information system management
    enterprise vs specialty solution, 185–186
    institutional management, vs departmental
        management, 188–189
    off-the-shelf software, vs custom-built
        software, 187–188
    philosophical spectra of, 183–189
Information technology impact, categories
    of, 211–212
Information Technology Services, 6–7
Information technology support domination,
    184
Input/output devices and controllers
    bluetooth, 40
    compact disc drives, 36, 42-43
    data communication rates,
        bits-per-second, 35, 41
    Direct Memory Access, 36
    hot swappable, 38
    Institute of Electrical and Electronic
        Engineers, 39
    Integrated Drive Electronics, 36
    magnetic disk drives, 36
    parallel devices, 35–37
    peripherals, 34-35
    printer port, 35–36
    serial connectors, 38
    serial devices, 37–40
    Small Computer Systems Interface, 36–37
    Universal Serial Bus, 38–39
    wireless communications, 39–40
Institute of Electrical and Electronic
    Engineers, 39
Institution email, 120

Institutional electronic medical record
    systems, 364–365
Institutional management, vs departmental
    management, 188–189
Institutional medical record number, 204
Institutional tumor registries, 370–372
Integer data storage, 66–68, 146
Integrated, single circuit board, 20
Integrated Development Environment, 58–59
Integrated Drive Electronics, 36
Integrated imaging, 258–260
Integrated Services Digital Network, 47
Interface cards, 98
Interfaces, 215–216, 287–302
    admission/discharge/transfer interface,
        293–296
    architecture, 287-292
    billing batch interface, 296–297
    communication handler, 288–289
    elements of, 288
    languages, 289–292
        health level 7, 292
        message formats, 290–291
    outreach material, 299–301
    results interface, 297–301
    results interfaces, 299–301
    translation processor, 289
Internal peripheral devices, 34–35
International Classification of Diseases,
    311–314, 331
    Health Insurance Portability and
        Accountability Act designated code
        set, 312
    for Oncology, 313–314
International Standard Organization, 88
Internet, 102–120
    domain name system, 108–109
    history of, 103–105
    internet protocol, 106–108
    port numbers, 110
    protocol header, 106–107
    top-level domains, 109
    transmission control protocol, 105–111
        ports, sockets, 110–111
Internet Corporation for Assigned Names
    and Numbers, 109
Internet Message Access Protocol, 117–118
    Post Office Protocol, contrasted, 118–120
Internet Service Provider, dial-up modem, 46
InterNIC, central agency assigning
    addresses, 107
Inverse Document Frequency times Term
    Frequency, 319

ISDN. *See* Integrated Services Digital
    Network
ISO. *See* International Standard Organization
ISP. *See* Internet service Provider
ITS. *See* Information Technology Services

Java Server Pages, 115
JavaApplets, 114
JavaScript, 114
Joint Photographic Experts Group, 81–82,
    243, 250
    compression, 243–245, 250–252
JPEG. *See* Joint Photographic Experts Group
JSP. *See* Java Server Pages

Keys, primary, foreign, 134
Keyword-based information retrieval,
    317–319
Keyword queries, expansion of, 323

LAN. *See* Local Area Network
Legacy information systems, 207–232
    data recovery from, 228–232
Licensing issues, 280
    software, 62-65. *See also* Software
Literature databases, online, access to,
    227–228
Little-endian, 22
Local Area Network, 46, 83–84
Longitudinal electronic patient records,
    365–366

Magnetic disk drives, 36
Magnetic disks, formatting, 42
Magnetic storage devices, disks, 41–42
Mainframe systems, 176–179
    early, 177
Management reporting tools, 215
Mantissa, 69–70
Many-to-many relationships, 130
Markup-tags, 113
Media access control, 97
Medical informatics, 10
Medical intranets, 173–176
Memory
    main computer memory, 30-31
        memory location, address, 30–31
    Dual Inline Memory Modules, 26
    dynamic random access memory, 24, 30
    Electrically Erasable and Programmable
        Read Only Memory, 25
    Erasable and Programmable Read Only
        Memory, 24

Flash ROM, 25
non-volatile random access memory, 25
Programmable Read Only Memory, 24
Read Only Memory, 24
Single Inline Memory Module, 25–26
Message collision, 93
Microarray analysis, 4
pathology informatics, 4
Microscope-mounted camera, 274
MIME. *See* Multipurpose Internet Mail
Extensions
Mirroring, 33
Modeling, biological systems, 378–379
Modems, 46
Modular design, *vs.* integrated design,
desktop computers, 20–21
Modular imaging, 261–264
Mother board, 20
Multi-site access, 285
Multi-site/lab support, 223
Multi-table databases, 127–131
hierarchical databases, 128–129
network databases, 129–130
object oriented databases, 130–131
shortcomings of non-relational database
architectures, 131
Multi-user database, prevention of
modifying data in memory, 159
Multiple hierarchies, 309
multi-axial, versions of, 315
Multipurpose Internet Mail Extensions
protocol, 116–117

National Health-Plan (payer) identifier, 341
National identifiers, 340–342
National Provider Identifier, 341
National Television System Committee,
formatted signal, 268
Natural language processing, 316–324
in clinical domain, 320–321
information retrieval, 323–324
auto-coding, medical documents,
323–324
keyword queries, expansion of, 323
NEC. *See* Not elsewhere classified
Negative integers, 67
Network bridges, 99
Network communication logic, 91–98
Network connection, 45–49
Network databases, 129–130
Network interconnectivity devices, 98–102
bridges, 99–100
gateway, 101

network interface cards, 98
repeaters and hubs, 98–99
routers, 101–102
switches, 100–101
Network Interface Card, 45–46
Networking
broadcast networks, 93–97
communication, 87–102
bandwidth, 89–91
network communication logic, 91–98
network protocols, 88–89
Ethernet, 97–98
standard, 98
token passing logic, 92
Networking topologies, 84–87
bus network, 86–87
ring network, 85–86
star network, 84–85
New data streams, 358
Nomenclature, 305–306
Non-executable software, 65–82 (*See also*
Software)
Non-procedural language, 161–162
Non-relational database architectures,
shortcomings of, 131
Non-robotic telemicroscopy system, 278
Non-volatile random access memory, 25
Nonsemantic concept identifiers, 309
Normal forms, 138
Nosology, 307
Not elsewhere classified, designation as, 310
NPI. *See* National Provider Identifier
NTSC. *See* National Television System
Committee
NULL, 148–149

Object based graphics, 74–75
Object-based image file format, 82
Object code, source code, relationship
between, 58
Object oriented databases, 130–131
ODBC. *See* Open DataBase Connectivity
Off-the-shelf software, vs custom-built
software, 187–188
One chip cameras, 267
One dimensional bar codes, 223–224
One-to-many relationships, 128
Online protocol, 117
Ontology, 306
Open database connectivity, 169
Open Systems Interconnect model, 88-89
Operating system add-ons, 53–55
device drivers, 53–55

services, 55
Operating systems, 52–53
Ordering concepts, classification system, 306
OSI. *See* Open Systems Interconnect
Outcomes research, new information
        systems structured for, 368–372
Outreach material, 222, 299–301
Ownership, pathology tissue, 373

PAL. *See* Phase Alteration Line
Parallel computing, 28–29
Parallel devices, 35–37
Passive star network, 84
Pathologist
        as data provider, 358–359
        as diagnostic specialist, 359–361
Pathology conference rooms, video
        microscopy for, 273–276
Pathology departments managing tumor
        registries, arguments for, 371–372
Pathology informatics
        as academic activity, 9–13
        as applied discipline, 7
        basic informatics, 6
        defined, 1–5
        developmental informatics unit, 8
        future of discipline, 13–15
        Information Technology Services, 6–7
        skill set in, 13
        spectra of, 6–13
        as subspecialty, 13–16
        technical support, line between, 4
        translational informatics, 6
Pathology informatics programs, 362–363
        leadership for, 363
        scope of, 363
Pathology tissue, ownership, 373
Pathology training program, 15–16
Pathology web sites, 228
Patient identifier, 202–205
Patient reports, embedding images in, 253
Peripheral data storage devices, 41–44. *See
        also* Data storage devices
Peripherals
        external peripheral devices, 34–35
        internal peripheral devices, 34–35
Phase Alteration Line, 268–269
Photomicroscopy, 257
Pixel, 31, 236–237, 250
        density, 237–238
                effect on image quality, 251
        number of, 249
        resolution, density, 238

Pixel-based image file format, 81
Point-to-Point Protocol, dial-up modem, 46
Polled communication protocol, 94
Polled logic, 94–95
POP. *See* Post Office Protocol
Portable Network Graphics, 81
Ports, 110–111
Post Office Protocol, 117
        Internet Message Access Protocol,
                contrasted, 118–120
Primary key, 132–134
Printer port, 35–36
Prior material, access to, 285
Privacy regulations, 332–337
Procedural referential integrity, trigger,
        153–154
Processors, 26–30
Programmable Read Only Memory, 24
Propagation delay, 86
Proportional time sharing, 94
Protected health information, 330
        amendment of, 334
Protocol, internet, 106–108
Publication quality photographs, 253–254

Quality of image, 234, 274–275
Query optimization, 150–152

RAM. *See* Random Access Memory
Random Access Memory, 23–24
Raster graphics, 74
Read Only Memory, 24
Real time communication mode, 288
Record, 122
Redundancy, recognition of, 310
Redundant fields, 126
Referential integrity, 152–154
Regulations, 325–354
        American College of Surgeons, 346–348
        Clinical and Laboratory Standards
                Institute, 350–353
        Clinical Laboratory Improvement
                Amendments of 1988, 348–350
        College of American Pathologists,
                checklist, 342–346
        Health Insurance Portability and
                Accountability Act, 325–342. *See
                also* Health Insurance Portability and
                Accountability Act
Relational databases, 131–138
        database normalization, 136–138
        entity-relationship diagrams, 135–136
        primary and foreign keys, 132–135

Removable long term storage media, 44–45
    floppy drives, 44
    Syquest, 44
    zip drive, 44
Repeaters, 98–99
Repeating fields, 125–126
Reports, 351
    incorporating digital images into, 217
Research informatics, 374–379
    anatomic pathology information systems,
        334–337
    data presentation tools, 377–378
    decision support systems, 378
    images, information extraction from,
        375–377
    modeling, biological systems, 378–379
    text, information extraction from, 375
Resident training, 285
Results interfaces, 297–301
Ring network, 85–86
ROM. *See* Read Only Memory
Routers, 101–102
Routing, 107

S-video, 271
Science
    defined, 8
    informatics as, 8–9
Scope, pathology informatics, 1–18
Screen resolution, 31
SCSI. *See* Small Computer System
        Interface; Small Computer Systems
        Interface
Second normal form, 137–138
Security
    of electronic mail, 120
    regulations for, 337–340
SELECT statements, 163–165
Serial devices, 37–40
Serial Line Internet Protocol, dial-up
        modem, 46
Server-side-processing, 114–115, 170
    Active Server Pages, 115
    Common Gateway Interface, 115
    Java Server Pages, 115
    language, to generate dynamic web page,
        171
Signed integers, 66
SIMM. *See* Single Inline Memory Module
Simple mail transfer protocol, 116–117
Simultaneous data modification, without
        record locking, 158
Single Inline Memory Module, 25–26

Single table databases, 124–126
    redundant fields, 126
    repeating fields, 125–126
Sixteen-bit color, 240–241
SLIP. *See* Serial Line Internet Protocol
Small Computer Systems Interface, 36–37
SMTP. *See* Simple mail transfer protocol
Sniffer programs, 120
SNOMED. *See* Systematized Nomenclature
        of Medicine
Social security, proposal to use as national
        identifier, 204–205
Sockets, 110–111
Software, 51–82
    digital data representation, 66–76, 166.
        See also Digital data representation
    executable software, 51–65
        application software, 55–65
            backward compatibility, 56
            bytecode compiler, 60
            compiler, 57
            computer programming, 56–62
                interpreter, 59
                languages, high level and low
                    level, 61-62
                object code, 57–60
                source code, 57–60
            converting source to executable
                object code, process of, 58–60
            cross-compilers, 58–59
            Integrated Development
                Environment, 58–59
            interaction with operating system,
                55–56
            syntax, 57
            text files, 56–58
        operating system add-ons, 53–55
            device drivers, 53–55
            services, 55
        operating systems, 52–53
            operating system, 52
            run on specific processors, 53
        system software, 51–55
    licensing, 62–65
        freeware, 63
        internet, way of distributing software,
            63
        medical environments, open source
            software in, 65
        open source, 63–64
        shareware, 63
    non-executable, 65–82
        backward compatibility, 77

extension, 76
flat-text files, 78–79
image file formats, 80–82. *See also*
Image file formats
portable document format, 79–80
proprietary format, 77
Source code, object code, relationship
between, 58
Source databases, data in, inconsistencies
between, 198–199
Specimen tracking, 212
Specimens, identification of, 213
Spectra of informatics disciplines, 3
Speech recognition technology, 225–227
SQL. *See* Structured Query Language
Stain ordering/tracking, 213
Star network, 84–85
Static telemicroscopy, 276
Storage of data, 369–370
Streaming, 87
Structured Query Language, 161
access to database from computer
programs, 166–172
application plan
execution of, 166
generation of, 166
database language, 161–172
dynamic, 167
embedded, 166–167
module, 167–168
optimization, 166
parsing, 165
processing statements, 165–166
static, 167
validation, 166
Surgical pathology gross room, digital
imaging in, 257
Switches, 100–101
Synchronization signals, 269
Synoptic reporting, 4, 218-221
Syquest, 44
System software, 51–55
Systematized Nomenclature of Medicine,
314–315
Systeme Electronique Couleur Avec
Memoire, 269

Table scan, 149
Tagged Image/Interchange File Format, 81
Taxonomy, classification is fully
instantiated, 306
TCP/IP. *See* Transmission Control
Protocol/Internet Protocol

Technical support, pathology informatics,
line between, 4
Tele-education, 281
Teleconsultation, 280–281
Telemicroscopy systems, 276–281
technologies, 277
tele-education, 281
teleconferencing, 281
teleconsultation, 280–281
telemicroscopy technology, 276–279
telepathology, 279–280
uses for, 279–281
Telepathology, 279–280
defined, 279
Term identification in biomedicine, 321–323
term classification, 322
term mapping, 322–323
term recognition, 321–322
Terminal emulation software, 178
Terminology, 305–310
Text files, 56–58
Textual data storage, 72–73
American Standard Code for Information
Interchange, 72–73
character, 76–78
strings, 73
Thin-client technology, 181–183
Third normal form, 138
Three chip color cameras, 267
Time sharing protocol, 93
Times, storage of, 71
American formats, 71
custom schemes, 71
electronic interfaces, 71
European formats, 71
Tissue
custodianship of, 368
excess, 373
ownership, 373
Token passing logic, 92
Tools of infomatics, use of by practicing
pathologist, 14–15
Top-level domains, 109
Training program, pathology, 15–16
Transaction deadlocks, 160–161
Transaction log, 156
data recovery, 157
Transactions, 155
Translation processor, 289
Translational informatics, 6
Transmission control protocol, 105–111
ports, sockets, 110–111

Transmission Control Protocol/Internet
    Protocol, 104
Tumor registries, 370–372
Tuples, 123
Twenty-four bit color, 240
Twisted-pair copper cabling, 90–91
Two dimensional bar codes, 224–225
Two-step dual storage imaging solution, 262
.txt files. *See* Flat-text files

UMLS. *See* Unified Medical Language
    System
Unauthorized access, protection health care
    information from, 193
Unified Medical Language System, 316
Unique Health Identifier for Individuals,
    341–342
Universal patient identifier, 202–205
Universal Serial Bus, 38–39
Unshielded twisted-pair copper cabling,
    90–91
Unsigned integers, 66
USB. *See* Universal Serial Bus
UTP. *See* Unshielded twisted-pair

Vector *vs.* bitmapped images, 75
Video camera, 266–268
Video connectors, standard, 270
Video display connections, icon, connector
    diagrams for, 34
Video displays, 31–34
    cathode ray tubes, 31
    connector types, 33–34
    display resolutions, 32
    full color, 33
    mirroring, 33
    multiple video controllers, 33
    pixels, 31
    wide versions, 32–33
Video microscopy, 266–276
    cables, 269–271
    component video, 270–271
    composite video, 271

connectors, 269–271
digital video, 271–273
    signals, 273
for pathology conference rooms, 273–276
S-video, 271
    video camera, 266–268
    video signals, 268–269
Video projector, 274
Video signals, 268–269
Virtual microscopy, 278–279
Viruses, electronic mail and, 120

WAN. *See* Wide Area Networks
Web, 111–115
Web-based interface, to image repository,
    screen shots, 263
Web browser, 110
Web server, 111–112
WHERE clause, 163–165
Whole-slide imaging, 362
Wide Area Networks, 84
Wide-field digital microscopy, 281–286
Windows Meta File, 82
Wireless communications, 39–40
Wireless Fidelity, 48
Wireless networking, 49
Word-by-word search, 317
Word indices, 317
Workflow issues, 210, 260
World wide web, 111–115
    access to databases, 169–172
    client-side and server-side processing,
        114–115
    hypertext markup language, 112–114

XML. *See* eXtensible Markup Language

Yale Pathology Informatics Program, 7,
    261–264

Zip drives, 44